CHRONIC FATIGUE SYNDROME

CHRONIC FATIGUE SYNDROME

An Integrative Approach to Evaluation and Treatment

Edited by
MARK A. DEMITRACK, M.D.
SUSAN E. ABBEY, M.D.

Foreword by Stephen E. Straus, M.D.

THE GUILFORD PRESS
New York   London

Last digit is print number: 9 8 7 6 5 4 3 2

Library of Congress Cataloging-in-Publication Data

Chronic fatigue syndrome: an integrative approach to evaluation and treatment / edited by Mark A. Demitrack, Susan E. Abbey; foreword by Stephen E. Straus.
       p.   cm.
    Includes bibliographic references and index.
    ISBN 1-57230-038-8
    1. Chronic fatigue syndrome—Psychological aspects.
    2. Psychotherapy.   I. Demitrack, Mark A.   II. Abbey, Susan E.
    [DNLM: 1. Fatigue Syndrome, Chronic—psychology.   2. Fatigue Syndrome, Chronic—therapy.   3. Fatigue Syndrome, Chronic—etiology.
WB 146 P974 1996]
RB150.F37C474   1996
616'.047—dc20
DNLM/DLC
for Library of Congress   95-26739
                                                                    CIP

To Lucy and Molly; I have no greater gift than the love
and support you have provided.

MAD

To Jamie, Alanna, Charlie, and Henry—
for play postponed.

SEA

Contributors

SUSAN E. ABBEY, M.D., Program in Medical Psychiatry, The Toronto Hospital, University of Toronto, Toronto, Ontario, Canada

MARK A. DEMITRACK, M.D., Department of Psychiatry, University of Michigan Medical Center, Ann Arbor, Michigan

N. CARY ENGLEBERG, M.D., Division of Infectious Diseases, University of Michigan Medical Center, Ann Arbor, Michigan

LAURA FAGIOLI, Ed.M., Harvard Medical School, Brigham and Women's Hospital, Division of General Medicine and Primary Care, Boston, Massachusetts

JORDAN GRAFMAN, Ph.D., Cognitive Neuroscience Section, National Institutes of Health, National Institute for Neurological Disorders and Stroke, MNB, Bethesda, Maryland

ANTHONY L. KOMAROFF, M.D., Harvard Medical School, Brigham and Women's Hospital, Division of General Medicine and Primary Care, Boston, Massachusetts

THOMAS J. LANE, M.D., New Britain General Hospital, New Britain, Connecticut

PETER MANU, M.D., Hillside Hospital, Long Island Jewish Medical Center, Glen Oaks, New York

DALE A. MATTHEWS, M.D., Georgetown University Medical Center, Washington, D.C.

MICHAEL C. SHARPE, M.A., M.R.C.P., M.R.C.Psych., University of Oxford, Department of Psychiatry, Warneford Hospital, Oxford, United Kingdom

STEPHEN E. STRAUS, M.D., Laboratory of Clinical Investigation, National Institute of Allergy and Infectious Diseases, NIH, Bethesda, Maryland

SIMON C. WESSELY, M.D., King's College Hospital and the Institute of Psychiatry, Denmark Hill, London, United Kingdom

Foreword

C hronic fatigue syndrome is evolving—not in character, but in concept—and it is doing so at such a rapid rate that it is difficult to project what textbooks will say of the disorder a decade from now.

My own interests in the syndrome became rooted, about 15 years ago, in an assessment of a few patients who remained ill after recovering otherwise fully from the defining features of infectious mononucleosis: fever, pharyngitis, and lymphocytosis. These patients were left with a residue of debilitating fatigue and malaise, and laboratory findings suggested that their infections might not have resolved fully. A description of these patients—and others like them elsewhere—helped crystallize a model based on a persisting Epstein–Barr virus infection (Dubois et al., 1984; Jones et al., 1991; Straus et al., 1985). In those early days of the AIDS epidemic, the notion that additional chronic diseases are attributable to viruses could not help but achieve some resonance in the community, and the various written and electronic media had become so pervasive as to place a hypothesis of this type at every doorstep.

Epstein–Barr virus was subsequently shown by several careful studies to plan no specific role in chronic fatigue syndrome, but the possibility that other viruses—new lymphotropic herpesviruses, enteroviruses, and retroviruses of real or imagined type—cause the syndrome continues to be pursued at the periphery of the main research stream (Bowles et al., 1986; Buchwald et al., 1992; DeFreitas et al., 1991; Flugel et al., 1992; Gow et al., 1991; Hellinger et al., 1988; Horowitz et al., 1985; Josephs et al.,

1991; Khan et al., 1993; Marshall et al., 1991; Sumaya, 1991; Yousef et al., 1988). It will prove difficult to totally dispense with this model because negative studies are never viewed as conclusive, because periodically we discover new candidate microbes, and because technology affords ever more sensitive means of detecting and studying them, but the concept will languish for lack of rigorous support, as have so many other earlier models of chronic fatigue.

The gradual displacement of the virologic model appeared inevitable by 1987, when the Centers for Disease Control promulgated a case definition for chronic fatigue syndrome that acknowledged the futility of requiring any markers of infections for diagnosis. The model's adumbration was hastened and permitted most by formulation of alternative hypotheses of disease pathogenesis (Holmes et al., 1988; Straus, 1994).

The recognition that chronic fatigue syndrome may not represent a chronic infection gradually drew into the field an enlarging repertoire of expertise encompassing epidemiology, immunology, neurology, endocrinology, psychology, psychiatry, and rheumatology, among others. Each of these disciplines contributed fresh perspectives to the field, but they remain largely disparate visions that have yet to be woven into a tapestry depicting fully what chronic fatigue syndrome is, how it relates to other, better appreciated disorders, and how it is best managed.

For example, it is apparent that physical deconditioning is an element of chronic fatigue syndrome (Riley et al., 1990). Exercise physiologists inform us that deconditioning could play a role in disease—certainly in perpetuating or exacerbating it, if not contributing to its origins. Moreover, many chronic fatigue syndrome patients sleep abnormally, and the protracted failure to attain adequate restorative sleep is also seen as contributing to both the roots of chronic fatigue syndrome and its continuation (Moldofsky, 1993; Morriss et al., 1993).

Despite these and several other fragmentary images of chronic fatigue syndrome, two dominant alternative models are evolving: one is based on a putative immune dysregulation, and one attempts to explain the syndrome's neuropsychological and mood features. These models are not mutually exclusive, and attempts are being made to draw a unifying hypothesis incorporating elements of each of them. Unfortunately, the scientific foundations for an overarching explanation of chronic fatigue syndrome of this type remain tenuous.

Evidence of immune dysregulation in chronic fatigue syndrome has accumulated, and it is even possible that infection could trigger such changes (Strober, 1994). Numerous studies reveal that chronic fatigue syndrome patients and normal controls differ in terms of immunoglobulin responses, lymphocyte phenotype, and *in vitro* cytokine release (Chao et al., 1991; Gupta & Vayuvegula, 1991; Klimas et al., 1990; Landay et al., 1991; Lloyd et al., 1992; Straus et al., 1993; Tirelli et al., 1993). Regrettably, the existing data do not show these immunologic findings to be consistent, nor are they reflective of illness severity. Moreover, it is unclear whether any such immune dysregulation bears an etiologic importance in the syndrome or is merely secondary to other aspects of the disease phenotype.

Competent evaluation of patients could not long disregard the remarkable prevalence of neuropsychological and affective problems in chronic fatigue syndrome (DeLuca et al., 1993; Katon et al., 1991; Kruesi et al., 1989; Manu et al., 1988; Sheffers et al., 1992; Taerk et al., 1987; Wessely & Powell, 1989). Here, too, there are inconsistent results, and causality is uncertain; nonetheless, a variety of interesting lines of investigation are being pursued. Demitrack himself first developed the concept that aberrant release of corticotropin-releasing hormone contributes to the neuroendocrine and behavioral stigmata of chronic fatigue syndrome (Demitrack, 1994; Demitrack et al., 1991). Recent epidemiologic studies in England showed that the persistence of fatigue after an acute viral illness is strongly dependent on preexisting and comorbid psychiatric factors (Bruce-Jones et al., 1994; Cope et al., 1994).

However these and the many other seemingly disparate research findings are reconciled, we now appreciate that neuropsychologic and psychiatric problems in chronic fatigue syndrome can assume such import and magnitude as to make the mental health professional an essential element of the team approach to the chronic fatigue syndrome. In the earlier days of chronic fatigue syndrome research, the value of mental health evaluation or psychopharmacologic intervention was not only neglected but actively resisted, and the physician was often disinclined to argue with the decision.

As chronic fatigue syndrome evolved conceptually from an infectious or postinfectious disorder to one acknowledged to impinge on multiple aspects of health and performance, it moved in concert beyond the capacity of the general practitioner and internist to encompass the total needs of the patient (Hirata-Dulas et al., 1994). There is a place for pain management, for sleep hygiene, for rehabilitation, and for occupational therapy. For many patients, there is also the need for expert assessment and treatment of mood and of behaviors that thwart recovery (Butler et al., 1991; Goodnick & Sandoval, 1993; Gracious & Wisner, 1991; Lloyd et al, 1993; Sharpe, 1993). There is a need for the mental health professional to help study chronic fatigue syndrome if we are to comprehend its dimension and essence. Demitrack, Abbey, and their able coauthors provide a practical and contemporary overview for those willing to face these challenges.

STEPHEN E. STRAUS, M.D.

REFERENCES

Bowles, NE, Richardson, PJ, Olsen, EGJ, Archard, LC. Detection of Coxsackie-B-virus-specific RNA sequences in myocardial biopsy samples from patients with myocarditis and dilated cardiomyopathy. *Lancet* 1986; 1:1120–1123.

Bruce-Jones, WDA, White, PD, Thomas, JM, Clare, AW. The effect of social adversity on the fatigue syndrome, psychiatric disorders and physical recovery, following glandular fever. *Psychol Med* 1994; 24:651–659.

Buchwald, D, Cheney, PR, Peterson, DL, Henry, B, Wormsley, SB, Geiger, A, Ablashi, DVM, Salahuddin, SZ, Saxinger, C, Biddle, R, Kikinis, R, Jolesz, FA, Folks, T, Balanchandran, N, Peter, JB, Gallo, RC, Komaroff, AL. A chronic illness characterized by fatigue, neurologic and immunologic disorders, and active human herpes virus type 6 infection. *Ann Int Med* 1992; 116:103–113.

Butler, S, Chalder, T, Ron, M, Wessely, S. Cognitive behaviour therapy in chronic fatigue syndrome. *J Neurol Neurosurg Psychiatry* 1991; 54:153–158.

Chao, CC, Janoff, EN, Hu, S, Thomas, K, Gallagher, M, Tsang, M, Peterson, PK. Altered cytokine release in peripheral blood mononuclear cell cultures from patients with the chronic fatigue syndrome. *Cytokine* 1991; 3:292–298.

Cope, H, David, A, Pelosi, A, Mann, A. Predictors of chronic "postviral" fatigue. *Lancet* 1994; 344:864–868.

DeFreitas, E, Hilliard, B, Cheney, PR, Bell, DS, Kiggundn, E, Sankey, D, Wroblemska, Z, Palladino, M, Woodward, JP, Koprowski, H. Retroviral sequences related to human t-lymphotropic virus type II in patients with chronic fatigue immunodysfunction syndrome. *Proc Natl Acad Sci USA* 1991; 88:2922–2926.

DeLuca, J, Johnson, SK, Natelson, BH. Information processing efficiency in chronic fatigue syndrome and multiple sclerosis. *Arch Neurol* 1993; 50:301–304.

Demitrack, MA. Neuroendocrine aspects of chronic fatigue syndrome: Implications for diagnosis and research. In Straus, SE, ed., *Chronic fatigue syndrome.* New York: Marcel Dekker, 1994; 285–308.

Demitrack, MA, Dale, JK, Straus, SE, Lane, L, Listwak, SJ, Krüesi, MJP, Chrousos, GP, Gold, PW. Evidence for impaired activation of the hypothalamic–pituitary–adrenal axis in patients with chronic fatigue syndrome. *J Clin Endo Metab* 1991; 73(6):1224–1234.

DuBois, RE, Seeley, JK, Brus, I, Sakamoto, K, Ballow, M, Harada, S, Bechtold, TA, Pearson, G, Purtilo, DT. Chronic mononucleosis syndrome. *S Med J* 1984; 77(11):1376–1382.

Flugel, RM, Mahnke, C, Geiger, A, Komaroff, AL. Absence of antibody to human spumaretrovirus in patients with chronic fatigue syndrome. *Clin Infect Dis* 1992; 14:523–524.

Goodnick, PJ, Sandoval, R. Psychotropic drug treatment of chronic fatigue syndrome and related disorders. *J Clin Psychiatry* 1993; 54(1):13–20.

Gow, JW, Behan, WMH, Clements, GB, Woodall, C, Riding, M, Behan, PO. Enteroviral RNA sequences detected by polymerase chain reaction in muscles of patients with postviral fatigue syndrome. *Br Med J* 1991; 302:692–696.

Gracious, B, Wisner, KL. Nortriptyline in chronic fatigue syndrome: A double-blind, placebo-controlled single case study. *Biol Psychiatry* 1991; 30:405–408.

Gupta, S, Vayuvegula, B. A comprehensive immunological analysis in chronic fatigue syndrome. *Scand J Immunol* 1991; 33:319–327.

Hellinger, WC, Smith, TF, Van Scoy, RE, Spitzer, PG, Forgacs, P, Edson, RS. Chronic fatigue syndrome and the diagnostic utility of antibody to Epstein–Barr virus early antigen. *JAMA* 1988; 260(7):971–973.

Hirata-Dulas, CAI, Halstenson, CE, Peterson, PK. Medical therapy of chronic fatigue syndrome. In Straus, SE, ed., *Chronic fatigue syndrome*. New York: Marcel Dekker, 1994; 387–404.

Holmes, GP, Kaplan, JE, Gantz, NM, Komaroff, AL, Schonberger, LB, Straus, SE, Jones, JF, Dubois, RE, Cunningham-Rundlls, C, Pahwa, S, Tosato, G, Zegans, LS, Purtilo, DT, Brown, N, Schooley, RT, Brus, I. Chronic fatigue syndrome: A working case definition. *Ann Int Med* 1988; 108:387–389.

Horowitz, CA, Henle, W, Henle, G, Rudnick, H, Latts, E. Long-term serological follow-up of patients for Epstein–Barr virus after recovery from infectious mononucleosis. *J Inf Dis* 1985; 151(6):1150–1153.

Jones, JF, Streib, J, Baker, S, Hergerger, M. Chronic fatigue syndrome: 1. EBV immune response and molecular epidemiology. *J Med Virol* 1991; 33:151–158.

Josephs, SF, Henry, B, Balachandran, N, Strayer, D, Peterson, D, Komaroff, AL, Ablashi, DV. HHV-6 reactivation in chronic fatigue syndrome. *Lancet* 1991; 337:1346–1347.

Katon, WJ, Buchwald, DS, Simon, GE, Russo, JE, Mease, PJ. Psychiatric illness in patients with chronic fatigue and those with rheumatoid arthritis. *J Gen Int Med* 1991; 6:277–285.

Khan, AS, Heneine, WM, Chapman, LE, Gray, HE, Woods, TC, Folks, TM, Schomberger, LB. Assessment of a retrovirus sequence and other possible risk factors for the chronic fatigue syndrome in adults. *Ann Int Med* 1993; 118:241–245.

Klimas, NG, Salvato, FR, Morgan, R, Fletcher, MA. Immunological abnormalities in chronic fatigue syndrome. *J Clin Microbiol* 1990; 28:1403–1410.

Kruesi, MJP, Dale, JK, Straus, SE. Psychiatric diagnosis in patients who have chronic fatigue syndrome. *J Clin Psychiatry* 1989; 50:53–56.

Landay, AL, Jessop, C, Lennette, ET, Levy, JA. Chronic fatigue syndrome: Clinical condition associated with immune activation. *Lancet* 1991; 338(8769):707–712.

Lloyd, AR, Hickie, I, Brockman, A, Hickie, C, Wilson, A, Dwyer, J, Wakefield, D. Immunologic and psychologic therapy for patients with chronic fatigue syndrome: A double-blind, placebo-controlled trial. *Am J Med* 1993; 94(2):197–203.

Lloyd, AR, Hickie, I, Hickie, C, Dwyer, J, Wakefield, D. Cell-mediated immunity in patients with chronic fatigue syndrome, healthy control subjects and patients with major depression. *Clin Exp Immunol* 1992; 87(1):76–79.

Manu, P, Lane, TJ, Matthews, DA. The frequency of the chronic fatigue syndrome in patients with symptoms of persistent fatigue. *Ann Int Med* 1988; 109:554–556.

Marshall, GS, Gesser, RM, Yamanishi, K, Starr, SE. Chronic fatigue in children: Clinical features, Epstein–Barr virus and human herpesvirus 6 serology and long term follow-up. *Pediatr Infect Dis J* 1991; 10:287–290.

Moldofsky, H. Fibromyalgia, sleep disorder and chronic fatigue syndrome. In Bock, GR, Whelan, J, eds., *Chronic fatigue syndrome,* Ciba Foundation Symposium 173. New York: John Wiley & Sons, 1993; 262–279.

Morriss, R, Sharpe, M, Sharpley, AL, Cowen, PJ, Hawton, K, Morris, J. Abnormalities of sleep in patients with the chronic fatigue syndrome. *BMJ* 1993; 306(6886):1161–1164.

Riley, MS, O'Brien, CJ, McCluskey, DR, Bell, NP, Nicholls, DP. Aerobic work capacity in patients with chronic fatigue syndrome. *BMJ* 1990; 301:953–956.

Scheffers, MR, Johnson, RJ, Grafman, J, Dale, JK, Starus, SE. Attention and short-term memory in chronic fatigue syndrome patients: An event-related potential analysis. *Neurology* 1992; 42:1667–1675.

Sharpe, MC. Non-pharmaceutical approaches to treatment. In *Chronic fatigue syndrome,* Ciba Foundation Symposium 173. New York: John Wiley & Sons, 1993; 298–317.

Straus, SE, ed. *Chronic fatigue syndrome.* New York: Marcel Dekker, 1994.

Straus, SE, Fritz, S, Dale, J, Gould, B, Strober, W. Lymphocyte phenotype analysis suggests chronic immune stimulation in patients with chronic fatigue syndrome. *J Clin Immunol* 1993; 13(1):30–40.

Straus, SE, Tosato, G, Armstrong, G, Lawley, T, Preble, OT, Henle, W, Davey, R, Pearson, G, Epstein, J, Brus, I. Persisting illness and fatigue in adults with evidence of Epstein–Barr virus infection. *Ann Int Med* 1985; 102(1)7–16.

Strober, W. Immunological function in chronic fatigue syndrome. In Straus, SE, ed., *Chronic fatigue syndrome,* 207–237. New York: Marcel Dekker, 1994.

Sumaya, CV. Serologic and virologic epidemiology of Epstein–Barr virus: Relevance to chronic fatigue syndrome. *Rev Inf Dis* 1991; 13(suppl 1):S19–S25.

Taerk, GS, Toner, BB, Salit, IE, Garfinkel, PE, Ozersky, S. Depression in patients with neuromyasthenia (benign myalgic encephalomyelitis). *Int J Psychiatry Med* 1987; 17(1):49–56.

Tirelli, U, Pinto, A, Marotta, G, Crovato, M, Quaia, M, dePaoli, P, Galligioni, E, Santini, G. Clinical and immunological study of patients with chronic fatigue syndrome: A case study from Italy. *Arch Int Med* 1993; 153:116–117.

Wessely, S, Powell, R. Fatigue syndromes: A comparison of chronic "postviral" fatigue with neuromuscular and affective disorders. *J Neurol Neurosurg Psychiatry* 1989; 52:940–948.

Yousef, GE, Bell, EJ, Mann, GF, Murugesan, V, Smith, DG, McCarney, RA, Mowbray, JF. Chronic enterovirus infection in patients with postviral fatigue syndrome. *Lancet* 1988; 1:146–150.

Preface

Our interests in chronic fatigue syndrome began early in our professional careers. Over time, clinical care of patients with this condition, and research activities in understanding its causes and consequences came to occupy a considerable portion of our work. It became apparent to us that a full appreciation of the importance of a biopsychosocial perspective of chronic fatigue syndrome was lacking in the standard of care for this condition. As a clinical reality, chronic fatigue syndrome (and its historical ancestors) has shown an amazing resilience, by resisting a convincing compartmentalization into any existing medical or psychiatric nosology. This resilience has been fueled by its ability to evoke passionately held beliefs about underlying etiologic mechanisms, frequently based on little to no objective evidence. It is unfortunate, most of all for the patients, that these passions often collide, and result in an obfuscation of rational discourse on this issue.

It was because of our beliefs that chronic fatigue syndrome exists, and that the greater medical and psychiatric community were ill-informed about the controversies surrounding it, that we began to think seriously about educational activities which might at least assist in demarcating the terrain involved. Portions of our efforts have been represented in a continuing medical education course on chronic fatigue syndrome which has been presented on more than one occasion at the annual meeting of the American Psychiatric Association. Many of the contributors to this volume have taught in versions of that course. Late one night, during our participation in the first Ciba Foundation Symposium on chronic fatigue syndrome, we formalized our thoughts about publishing a volume which would review our clinical and theoretical approach to this syndrome.

This book is the culmination of those ideas, and encompasses what we feel is our best understanding of an integrative approach to chronic fatigue syndrome. We hope that clinicians, researchers and patients who take the time to read this text will find our thoughts to be useful. We would also hope that over time, approximations such as the one we offer here become part of an iterative process, with ever-increasing levels of scientific rigor and useful clinical application. However, in reviewing the historical background which leads to chronic fatigue syndrome, it is sometimes hard not to feel that the process is more a circular one. Time will certainly be the judge.

We would like to acknowledge the hard work of our collaborators, who have endured endless phone calls and faxes. Thanks are also extended to Dr. Paul Garfinkel for his wisdom and patience, the Canadian Psychiatric Research Foundation and the Ontario Ministry of Health for research training funding, Drs. Laurie Gillies, Anne Hennessy, Mary Moskowitz, and Maggie Wilson for their unstinting support, Adrianne Hlavenka for her diligence in pursuing references and Christine MacKinnon for skillful preparation of the manuscript. Particular accolades are also to be directed to Mr. Seymour Weingarten and the staff of Guilford Press, and to Ms. Nancy Marcus Land for her good humor.

Finally, this book would certainly not have come about without the thoughtful teaching provided by the patients we have seen, who, through their distress, have expanded our understanding of the nature of chronic fatigue syndrome.

MARK A. DEMITRACK, M.D.
SUSAN E. ABBEY, M.D.

Contents

SECTION III: TREATMENT

I
BACKGROUND

1

Historical Overview and Evolution of Contemporary Definitions of Chronic Fatigue States

Mark A. Demitrack, M.D.
Susan E. Abbey, M.D.

. . . antiquarian research attains oftentimes the wisdom of
philosophy and the perfection of art; since it is demonstrated again
and again that what we call modern science is really ancient; that
the latest truths are but survivals of the oldest. . . .
—GEORGE M. BEARD (1880)

The recent resurgence of interest in fatigue as a discrete clinical syndrome has been accompanied by vigorous assertions that the contemporary appearance of such chronic fatigue states represents a novel clinical entity. On the other hand, it is clear that clinical syndromes characterized by profound fatigue and associated constitutional debility are not new in medical literature. In this chapter, we propose that the remarkable technical advances in biomedical research technique, particularly in the domains of infectious diseases, immunology, and the neurosciences, have, in fact, provided a more refined reinterpretation of clinical realities that were similarly perceived, albeit with more coarse resolution, by earlier investigators.

The chapter provides a selective historical review of several important clinical syndromes that, we believe, serve as templates for an understanding of the development of the contemporary definitions of chronic fatigue syndrome. The most important observations to emerge from this review are the recurring theme of central nervous system dysfunction, and the preeminent role of stress and behavioral symptoms in the development and clinical expression of the illness. It is not surprising, therefore, that many of the more successful therapeutic options have often involved psychopharmacologically and psychotherapeutically active maneuvers. These general insights have prompted the preparation of this text, and they suggest to us that psychiatry has been, and will remain, an integral part of the multidisciplinary approach to the treatment of this clinical syndrome.

EXHAUSTION, NERVOUSNESS, AND NEURASTHENIA

In one of the earliest descriptions, Sir Richard Manningham wrote, in 1750, of the "febricula" or "little fever." This illness presented with a profound sense of lassitude, accompanied by a bewildering variety of constitutional complaints, but few objective clinical findings: "[T]he symptoms of the febricula, or little, low, continued fever, are these . . . transient chilliness . . . a mist before the eyes . . . listlessness, with great lassitude and weariness all over the body . . . little flying pains . . . and sometimes the patient is a little delirious and forgetful. . . ."

Manningham noted the association of this condition with stressful circumstances, and observed its preponderant incidence in females, particularly of the upper social classes. One of the more lasting clinical terms for this set of symptoms was neurasthenia, a name coined by George Miller Beard, a 19th-century American neurologist. He chose this title, combining the Greek words for "nerve" (νευρον) and "strength" (σθενοσ), to refer to the principal source of the debility: a lack of strength in the nervous substance of the individual. In his initial clinical descriptions of this illness (Beard, 1869, 1880), he emphasized that neurasthenia may arise from an acute or chronic disease, or itself may be acute or chronic in its course, and may give rise to an array of clinical sequelae, including "dyspepsia, headaches, paralysis, insomnia, anaesthesia, neuralgia, rheumatic gout, spermatorrhea in the male, and menstrual irregularities in the female. . . ." Like Manningham, Beard reported the prevalence of the illness to be greatest in the upper socioeconomic class, hence his consideration that this clinical syndrome represented a disease unique to civilized society, an "American nervousness" that arose from the demands of "brain work" inherent in the habits and occupational risks of industrialized society: "Among the special exciting causes of neurasthenia may be mentioned the pressure of bereavement, business and family cares, parturition and abortion, sexual excesses, the abuse of stimulants and narcotics, and civilized starvation, such as is sometimes observed even among the wealthy order of society, and sudden retirement from business. . . ."

These views have led to some speculation that neurasthenia represented a socioculturally defined illness that subsumed within its framework a range of functional somatic syndromes—a culturally sanctioned form of illness behavior (Abbey & Garfinkel, 1991). Indeed, as an extension of this view, it has been suggested that the ultimate realization of the role of psychiatric illness and psychological factors as principal determinants of the development of neurasthenia is precisely what has led to its repeated decline in popularity and subsequent reemergence with a new organic pathophysiological mantle as each generation of medical researchers attempts to hold the entity in its grasp.

Despite the controversy that surrounded Beard and his public presentation of this syndrome in his day, his contributions to the organization of a definitional structure and a diagnostic approach to neurasthenia were considerable. Noting the difficulty in accurately diagnosing the condition, he pointed out the importance of specifically discerning the presence of comorbid illnesses, which may have a tremendous influence on the outcome of the illness: ". . . the diagnosis . . . of neurasthenia is obtained partly by the positive symptoms and partly by exclusion . . . [it] may be associated with anemia and with almost every conceivable form of organic disease. . . . In such cases it is sometimes very difficult to ascertain whether it is the cause or the effect. The history of the symptoms will help us to decide this question. . . ."

In the same generation, a separate clinical entity emerged in the medical literature. J. M. DaCosta, an American physician, described a clinical syndrome he had observed in a group of over three hundred soldiers he treated during and in the aftermath of the Civil War (DaCosta, 1871). He termed this entity the "irritable heart" of the soldier. This syndrome is of particular interest to the present discussion for several reasons: (1) there exists a close symptom similarity of this condition with Beard's description of neurasthenia; (2) the preeminent role of stress in the development of this syndrome echoes the claim, as in neurasthenia, for central nervous system involvement in the pathophysiology of the illness; and (3) the historical fate of this entity followed the same path as that for neurasthenia—namely, an increasing realization of the important role for psychological distress in the risk for, and in the course of, the syndrome, and a subsequent rejection of these clinical entities by the general medical community as unworthy of further study.

DaCosta reported the usual clinical presentation to be heralded by gastrointestinal symptoms, usually diarrhea, occurring in an apparently previously healthy soldier who was in the midst of a significant degree of combat-related stress. Shortly following the gastrointestinal disturbance, the functional debility worsened to include persistent dizziness and exertional fatigue, especially aggravated by a return to battle. Finally, spontaneous palpitations developed, accompanied by episodic tachyarrhythmias, which appear notably similar to contemporary descriptions of panic attacks. The treatment of the condition invariably involved removal of the soldier from the stressful military context, and the administration of a variety of tonics and cardiac medicinals, which produced varying degrees of amelioration of symptoms. In enumerating the symptoms of the affliction, DaCosta noted that the sudden palpitations were the pathognomonic feature, present in all cases. These episodes could occur "at all times of the day or night . . . most readily excited by exertion, . . . but attacks also occurred when the patient was lying quietly in bed, disturbing his rest or waking him up . . . ." These palpitations were usually accompanied by "headache, dimness of vision, and giddiness," and by pain in the chest, radiating to all parts of the body. Shortness of breath or the sensation of choking was also common, often in association with hyperventilation. Of the remaining observed symptoms, nervous disorders and digestive disturbances were frequently seen. The former were characterized largely by headache, giddiness, vertigo, and disturbances of sleep. The digestive complaints were protean, although diarrhea was reported as the most common presenting complaint. Notably absent were any physical signs other than the rapid heartbeat. Pathological changes in the heart itself were not observed in one case that went to autopsy due to death from unrelated causes.

Regarding the inciting or premorbid causes of this condition, DaCosta was at a loss to elucidate a specific factor; however, the uniform occurrence of hard field service immediately preceding the symptoms was emphasized. There is also indication that preexisting factors were important in many individuals, as suggested by a history of rheumatic pain and previous episodes of shortness of breath and palpitations prior to their military service. The course of symptoms was one of almost uniform improvement upon removal from the stressful wartime experience. The majority of cases described progressed to full or nearly full recovery upon follow-up. Although DaCosta entertained, and then dismissed, the role of malingering as a causative factor in this illness, an investigation of psychological factors was absent in his initial manuscript. Nevertheless, viewed from a contemporary light, the parallels with panic and other anxiety disorders is striking.

The initial enthusiasm of these and other terms for this syndrome was enormous. Indeed, the use of a model that emphasized an organic pathology of the nerve cell permitted a socially acceptable diagnosis. Furthermore, the construct lent itself to easy self-diagnosis and self-treatment. The ready availability (and lack of government regulatory controls) of a wide range of patent medications facilitated this process. However, by the turn of the century, it was becoming increasingly apparent to most clinicians that the psychological dimensions of the illness were an undeniable reality. In 1906, Lane noted that "the prolonged influence of depressing emotions is the common exciting cause [of neurasthenia] . . . it is well recognized that a pathological fatigue is rarely caused by simple hard work, mental or physical, unless some depressing emotional element is also present . . . ." Dicks (1933) articulated the frustration of many physicians when he stated:

> Neurasthenia, as a clinical entity, is elusive. Everywhere we meet with the statements that it is rare . . . yet no name is more often upon the lips of our profession . . . . The word serves its most useful purpose perhaps as a vague generic term for almost any psychological disorder other than frank insanity; it appeases the layman's thirst for a label without shocking a false self-esteem. . . . Matters become more serious when, with its implication of a definite pathology, it satisfies the physician that he has arrived at a full diagnosis. . . . I submit that the concept has outlived its usefulness; that the symptoms described under the heading of neurasthenia can for the most part be related to other disorders; and that what remains . . . should be called by some name that does not commit us to an obsolete theory . . . .

In his three Goulstonian lectures of 1941, the eminent British cardiologist Paul Wood delivered an even more forceful and definitive rejection of the purported pathophysiologic constructs underlying the illness, which by that time was referred to by an ever-enlarging nomenclature that varied with the specialty expertise of the investigator. He wrote, "I urge the rejection of all these terms . . . nor do I feel morally bound to suggest a substitute, for I believe that the recognition of this syndrome, as such, will die . . . ." The reason for his assertion of its early demise was again the increasing realization of the profound influence of premorbid and concurrent psychological factors in the generation of the symptoms of the syndrome. Wood based his conclusions on the observations of over 300 patients evaluated at the Effort Syndrome Unit of the National Hospital for Diseases of the Heart. He chastised the medical profession and implicated iatrogenic factors as common contributors to the development of this syndrome: "[T]he failure to diagnose rheumatic carditis may be a bad mistake, but its diagnosis where none exists is worse . . . no greater blame can be attached to a psychiatrist who fails to make a physical examination than to a physician who fails to probe the mind. . . ." In his view, a careful review of DaCosta's original material and of the patients he himself evaluated revealed that constitutional susceptibility, family history, infection, neurosis, and physical and mental stress were substantial factors responsible for producing the full syndrome. In other words, Wood proposed that the effort syndromes emerged from a complex interplay of psychological and biological risk factors. Moreover, he noted that the attitude of the physician could be enormously influential in exacerbating the patient's abnormally active fear and nervousness. Indeed, he stated, "Patients should be informed of their illness, and treated as psychoneurotics; their distaste for this label may prove quite helpful. . . . The patient must be induced to believe that he is suffering from the effects of emotional disturbance, and not from any disease or alteration of visceral function . . . ."

By this time, it was clear that a major conceptual shift had occurred. The profoundly confident view of a specific "deficiency of nervous strength," advanced by Beard, was ultimately regarded, in the advancing knowledge base of contemporary medicine, to be a caricature of any potential disturbance in neural substrate. This view evolved in conjunction with more detailed observations of the behavioral antecedents and sequelae of the syndrome. The result of these two developments was the rejection of neurasthenia and its related representations in the literature. It was felt that once a more detailed reflection on the morbid medical conditions associated with the neurasthenic condition was definitively addressed and a more thoughtful appraisal of the psychological state of the individual was performed, nothing would remain in Beard's previously established category. The latter process was assisted, in large part, by the rise of psychiatry as an independent medical discipline, and by its desire to establish definite categories of illness with associated pathologic intrapsychic mechanisms. In retrospect, it is clear that this compromise position served only as an intermediate solution. It satisfied the desire of the medical community to dispense with concepts that were regarded as archaic and detrimental to patients and physicians alike. Furthermore, it attempted to erase the discomfort faced by the nascent modern medical community when confronted with clinical syndromes that defied easy interpretation, were multifactorial in nature, and demonstrated a complex development in time. These syndromes exist at the terribly gray zone where the observable and unobservable events that exchange between physician and patient come together.

PROLONGED RECOVERY FROM INFECTIOUS ILLNESS

No sooner had Paul Wood attempted to drive the final nail into the coffin of neurasthenia and its related syndromes, than an alternate model was emerging to account for these elusive illnesses. In this section, we review two separate but interrelated threads leading to this model—threads that have served in an important way to advance our appreciation of the uselessness of a strictly Cartesian approach to the problem of chronic fatigue.

Acute brucellosis is a bacterial illness caused by one of three types of bacteria: brucella meletensis, brucella abortus, or brucella suis. This illness, transmitted by cattle, was quite common prior to the routine pasteurization of milk. Beginning in 1934, Alice Evans, a bacteriologist working for the U.S. Public Health Service, began to describe a syndrome she referred to as chronic brucellosis (Evans, 1947). She observed that, in addition to its acute forms, there was clear evidence of the ability of the brucellar organism to persist in animals in the form of latent, localized infections, with no obvious signs of disease. She speculated that a similar state of chronic, occult disease may occur in humans, and proposed that such an illness may be the underlying diagnosis in many cases previously labeled as neurasthenic. At that time, it was known that the brucellar organism could localize and multiply within phagocytic cells of the reticuloendothelial system, where it could evade the bactericidal effect of administered antibiotics. In view of the previously observed propensity for neurasthenia to develop often in the aftermath of an infectious stress, the putative model of brucella as a chronic, difficult-to-detect infectious illness was attractive. However, because there was no reliable method to determine the presence of a chronic brucellar infection, this claim was difficult to prove or disprove. Its validity rested largely on clinical anecdote and generalization from animal forms of the disease.

In 1951, Wesley Spink published an extensive report on the nature of chronic brucellosis in which he carefully reviewed the experience of his clinical service at the University of Minnesota. In order to address the question of which factors were important in the symptomatic perpetuation of the illness, he studied the clinical outcome of 65 individuals who had developed documented acute brucellosis but had received no specific antibiotic therapy for their disease. Interestingly, because most of his cases were drawn from dairy farmers or workers in the local meat-packing industry, the majority of his sample of 65 patients were men (77%), a figure that is the reverse of most published gender ratios for chronic fatigue syndrome and that differed from the typical description of the population at risk for neurasthenia. Defining persistence of illness as not simply the absence of recovery of laboratory normality, but the actual cessation of symptomatic distress, Spink determined that 46% of the initial sample manifested persistent symptoms lasting more than one year, the definition of chronicity employed in his study. Of this group, only five were females. Seventeen subjects in this latter group eventually were shown to have clearly demonstrated evidence of relapsing illness or a localized infectious lesion. In thirteen patients (20% of the total sample), persistent symptoms were unaccompanied by any objective evidence of active disease. By use of formal psychiatric consultation, Spink determined that there was demonstrable evidence of formal psychiatric debility in over half of this sample, and, in two additional individuals, "the state of their health was intimately related to the outcome of claims for compensation . . . ." In only four individuals was there no evidence for any psychiatric disturbance. In an additional follow-up study of 61 patients with documented acute brucellosis, who had been treated with antibiotics for their disease, Spink observed a virtually identical percentage of patients (20%) who remained symptomatic after one year and had no organically demonstrable cause for their debility.

From these data, Spink proposed three possible explanations. First, this group of patients may indeed have a specific persistence of active brucella infection, a proposal that could not be defended or refuted with certitude. Second, the persistent symptoms are nonspecific and correspond to the previous categories of neurasthenia or psychoneurosis. Alternatively, he noted that these symptoms may be causally unrelated to the primary infectious process, or they may indicate an underlying central nervous system vulnerability directly aggravated by the activity of the acute brucella disease. On this point, he speculated that "patients bordering on a personality disorder or emotional disturbance may be tipped over into a functional state of chronic ill health by an attack of acute brucellosis . . . individuals with functional complaints or personality difficulties may have an exaggeration of these manifestations following acute brucellosis . . . ." The third possible mechanism he proposed was that the infectious process resulted in direct organic damage to the cerebral cortex that could be causally related to the behavior seen in the chronically ill patients.

In an important extension of Spink's work, a collaborative group of investigators from the Departments of Medicine and Psychiatry at the Johns Hopkins University attempted to explore these proposed mechanisms for the development of chronic brucellosis more directly. Over a series of years, these investigators completed a number of landmark studies that are as relevant today as then (Cluff et al., 1959; Imboden et al., 1959). Their initial reports focused on a group of individuals who worked in a laboratory setting where clinical samples of brucella organisms were processed. In two separate communications, they reported follow-up medical and psychological characteristics of a group of 60 individuals who had clearly documented infection with either brucella meletensis or brucella suis 4 to 8 years before.

Repeated clinical assessments and serologic studies were performed at approximately 6-month intervals on a group of 24 of the original 60 subjects who were available for contact. Eight patients had no clinical symptoms within a year after the acute illness; they were referred to as the acute recovered group. Sixteen of the 24 patients had persistent symptomatic complaints after 1 year of follow-up; this group was referred to as the chronic group. The symptoms reported by this group fluctuated in severity, but few patients were ever symptom-free. In order of frequency, the reported symptoms included: fatigue, headache, nervousness, depression, leg ache or back ache, generalized aching, and sexual impotence. Six patients in the chronic group, who eventually resolved their symptoms, were referred to as the chronic recovered group. The chronic symptomatic group was composed of ten patients whose symptoms were not resolved during the course of follow-up. All of the patients had been treated with appropriate antibiotic therapy for the initial acute infection. In addition, both of the chronically ill groups were given an additional course of antibiotics, without clinical effect.

There was no difference among the groups with regard to age (approximately 35 years), year of onset of the acute illness, symptoms present during

the acute infection (duration or maximum level of fever), pattern of serological response, or physical abnormalities. An extensive medical assessment was
performed on all patients. The electroencephalogram (EEG) was used for
specific assessment of central nervous system dysfunction. Nine subjects had
abnormal EEGs. Two of these individuals had a past history of head injury;
the remaining seven were equally distributed among the acute recovered and
chronic groups. There was no evidence that the chronically ill groups had
had more intimate contact with the brucella organism in the course of their
work than had the subjects in the acute group, nor was there any evidence of
increased hypersensitivity of the two chronically ill groups to intradermal
challenge with the brucella antigen. The investigators also inquired as to
whether the diagnosis of chronic brucellosis had been assigned largely by a
particular clinic physician, but no specific indication of an iatrogenic source
of the chronicity could be found. They concluded that two of the hypotheses
proposed by Spink to explain chronic brucellosis—the persistence of active
brucella infection, or the presence of direct central nervous system damage as
a result of the infection—were not supported by the evidence uncovered in
this study. In their next report, they focused their attention on the third possibility: that the development of chronic brucellosis was intimately linked to
psychological events present in and experienced by the individual.

They noted that psychological risk could have an impact on the resolution of the acute brucella infection in several ways. Chronic brucellosis may
reduce the capacity of individuals to adapt to their environment by inducing
a state of unwellness due to some persistent abnormal physiologic events. In
this model, psychological distress is an emergent event, a reactive psychological response to the primary pathophysiologic process producing the disease.
Alternately, the presence of psychological stress may have altered the resistance of the individual, hence producing constitutional inability to fight off
the chronic infectious process. They felt that both of these proposals were less
than likely in light of the results of the comprehensive medical assessment
noted above. A final hypothesis was that the illness termed chronic brucellosis was, in essence, a psychoneurosis, and hence was mislabeled.

A blindly scored psychological assessment was performed on all 24 subjects. Portions of the Wechsler Adult Intelligence Scale were included to assess general intellectual function. The Bender–Visual Motor–Gestalt test
was employed to assess motor coordination and perceptual confusion. Personality was assessed using the Minnesota Multiphasic Personality Inventory
(MMPI). The authors also devised for this study a "neurotic index" composed of the averages of the hypochondriasis, depression, and hysteria subscales. In addition, a separate "morale-loss" index was developed by one of
the authors and included in the analysis. The Self-Concept scale was employed, and, finally, a formal psychiatric interview was conducted, though
not in a blinded manner.

The results of the studies revealed that although there was a higher percentage of professional employees, and hence a higher general intelligence level, in the two recovered groups, when adjustments for intellectual ability were made, there was no evidence of impairment in intellectual function among all three groups. Similarly, the performance of the subjects on the Bender–Visual Motor–Gestalt test did not reveal any significant difference among the groups. In contrast to these findings, the assessment of personality variables demonstrated significant differences. In particular, the depression and psychasthenia scores, the morale-loss index, and the average neurotic index were all significantly higher in both of the chronically ill groups compared to the acute recovered group. The Self-Concept scale also revealed a higher number of positive self-concepts in the acute recovered group compared to the chronic groups. It was of particular interest that, between the two chronic groups, the chronic symptomatic group tended to view themselves as relatively normal with respect to emotional health, but poorly with respect to physical health, while in the chronic recovered group, the reverse self-percept was evident. Upon formal psychiatric interview, further differences were apparent. In the opinion of the interviewing psychiatrist, the chronic symptomatic patients were more resistant, in general, to the discussion of personal issues than were the two recovered groups. Interestingly, the chronic symptomatic patients also tended to consider the chronic brucellosis with which they were afflicted to be capable of producing virtually any type of subjective physical discomfort. In reviewing the specific biographical data reported by all the groups, the authors noted that there was gross evidence of psychologically traumatic events or circumstances in childhood in 11 of the 16 chronically ill patients compared to 2 of the 8 acute recovered individuals (Fisher's exact test, $p < .05$). At the time of the illness or during the year before or after the acute phase of the illness, it was also noted that 11 of the 16 chronically ill subjects were experiencing stresses of some sort compared to none of the 8 recovered patients. These stresses ranged in severity from death or serious illness in a close family member to failure at work.

The Johns Hopkins study investigators concluded from their work that there was little evidence to support the view that chronic brucellosis was the result of direct damage to the central nervous system, or that it reflected an ongoing infectious illness. They stated that, "taken together, the results presented in this and the preceding paper support the view that chronic brucellosis consists essentially of an emotional disorder . . . ." They emphasized that the historical evidence of emotional upset in the chronic patients, which preceded by many years the onset of the symptomatic acute infection, along with the evidence of increased levels of emotional disturbance in the two chronically ill groups, led to the notion that the emotional disturbance was the critical variable leading to persistence of symptoms. In their words, "in the wake of acute brucella infection there is almost always a period of lassitude or fatigability. In the depressed patient, these otherwise transient symptoms merge imperceptibly with depressive fatigue and lassitude and thus appear to be perpetuated . . . ." The degree of synchrony between the emotional disturbance and the attack of acute brucellosis dictated the relative risk of developing the chronic condition.

Intrigued by these results, these investigators reasoned that the specific psychological factors involved in delaying the symptomatic recovery from acute brucellosis might also be applicable to other acute infections. To address this issue, they embarked on one of the few well-designed prospective studies in this area (Imboden et al., 1961a, 1961b). Taking advantage of the impending influenza epidemic in 1957, they proposed obtaining a pre-illness psychological assessment in a large susceptible population, and then studying patterns of recovery in those individuals who later contracted the influenza virus. To accomplish this project, Imboden, Canter, and Cluff administered the MMPI, the Cornell Medical Inventory (CMI), and a brief social questionnaire to a group of 600 employees at Fort Detrick, an Army base in Maryland. This was a unique opportunity because all employees of the base were required to report to the central dispensary in the event of any symptoms of illness. All those reporting to the dispensary during the winter of 1957–1958 with apparent influenza were required to return for follow-up evaluation within 3 to 6 weeks of the onset of the illness. A review of symptoms and a physical examination were performed at each visit. Serological tests for influenza were performed with hemagglutination-inhibition testing, and, in a few subjects, viral isolation was attempted from pharyngeal washings.

Twenty-six persons arrived in the dispensary during that winter—an attack rate of 5%, which was similar to the incidence of influenza in the surrounding areas of Maryland during that year. When the subjects returned to the clinic 3 to 6 weeks later, 14 individuals had recovered and 12 reported the persistence of symptoms similar to those described by the chronic brucellosis patients. The most common symptoms was tiredness or weakness; other symptoms included cough, anorexia, insomnia, headache, and depression. All of the patients were male, with the exception of one woman in the symptomatic group. There was no difference in the pattern or character of symptoms associated with the acute illness between the groups, nor was there any difference in the physical signs, laboratory findings, or complications of the acute infection between the persistently symptomatic group and those subjects who recovered in less than 3 weeks. However, when the scores obtained from the psychological tests administered 3 to 6 months in advance of the infection were examined, interesting differences were observed. The total score on the CMI and the subscale scores on the depression and morale-loss indices of the MMPI were significantly higher in the symptomatic group. The authors noted that the differences between symptomatic and recovered groups on the MMPI subscale scores were virtually identical to the differences seen in their previous study of acute recovered and chronic symptomatic patients with brucellosis, despite the fact that these values were obtained well in advance of the clinical illness in the influenza study, and hence could not be attributed to the infectious process itself. In discussing these results, the authors speculated that, in the patients with an evident pre-illness propensity to depression, there was a greater tendency for some degree of depressive symptoms to arise during the acute infection. The clinical symptoms of depression (e.g., fatigue, lack of energy or interest, vague somatic concerns) tended to merge with the weakness and fatigability normally present during the acute infection: "[T]his intermingling of symptoms in the convalescent period obscures the endpoint of the physical illness from the views of both patient and physician . . . ."

The importance of these studies cannot be overemphasized. They represented a notable advance in the specification of psychological symptoms and their relation to recovery from acute infectious episodes. Although a historical continuity between the older concepts of neurasthenia and DaCosta's syndrome and the modern-day descriptions of chronic fatigue states cannot be determined with complete certainty, the similarity of symptom presentation among all these conditions is compelling. Hence, these studies serve as precursors for a more complete appreciation of the forces that have led to the formal definitions of chronic fatigue syndrome, to be delineated later in this chapter. Despite these considerations, it is clear that the researchers in the Johns Hopkins group still maintained a largely dichotomous view of the relation between the psychological state of the individual and their subsequent response to an infectious disease. Although a more thorough discussion of this topic is well beyond the scope of this chapter, it is instructive to mention briefly some additional prospective studies that demonstrate the need for a more synthetic view of the relation between the domains of physiological stress and psychological stress.

In July 1969, the entire freshman cadet class at the United States Military Academy at West Point was entered into a prospective study examining the seroepidemiology of infectious mononucleosis (Hallee et al., 1974). A total of 1,401 cadets were studied over a 4-year time span. Upon entry into the Academy, blood was obtained from each cadet, and a comprehensive series of questionnaires was administered, including detailed assessment of demographic characteristics, psychosocial status, and personality variables. The seroepidemiology of Epstein–Barr virus infection was assessed by obtaining interval blood samples from any cadet who sought treatment in the infirmary for an acute respiratory disease. When a case of infectious mononucleosis was identified, the roommates of the infected cadet were also bled and were followed for 2 months, through detailed symptom questionnaires and serial bleedings, to assess the spread of the infection to susceptible and exposed contacts. Upon entry into the study, 63.5% of the class had serologic evidence of prior exposure to the Epstein–Barr virus, but only 5.6% of these cadets gave a history compatible with clinical infectious mononucleosis. No evidence of clinical infectious mononucleosis was observed in these cadets throughout the remainder of their time at the Academy. Of the remaining seronegative subjects at entry to the Academy 54 (12.4%) seroconverted during their freshman year; over the 40 months of observation in this report, a total of 46% of the cadets seroconverted during their time at the Academy. Only 26.4% of this latter group of cadets manifested clinical evidence of infectious mononucleosis. A companion report described the psychosocial risk factors that were associated with the development of infectious mononucleosis in this population (Kasl et al., 1979). The pattern of findings suggested that a specific set of factors, interpreted to indicate greater academic pressure, was associated with the development and clinical expression of infectious mononucleosis among the cadets who seroconverted during the school years. These factors included having their fathers described as "overachievers," higher levels of motivation for success, and poorer academic performance. Even more striking was the observation that these same psychosocial risk factors predicted the development of Epstein–Barr virus seroconversion among those cadets with *no apparent clinical disease.*

Cohen, Tyrrell, and Smith (1991) extended these observations in a more focused prospective study. Using the unique facilities of the Medical Research Council's Common Cold Unit, in Salisbury, England, they examined the frequency of documented clinical colds in subjects who were purposefully exposed to a range of common respiratory viral pathogens. A group of 394 healthy individuals were selected for this study. All the subjects, after being admitted to the Common Cold Unit, underwent a comprehensive psychological stress assessment that inquired about (1) the actual number of stressful life events experienced by the subjects during the past year and judged by them to have had a negative impact on their lives, (2) the degree to which the subjects felt that their current life demands exceeded their ability to cope, and (3) a measure of current negative affect. From this assessment, a composite "stress index" was operationalized. After the initial assessment, the subjects were given nasal drops containing a low infectious dose of one of five common respiratory viruses, or of saline. They had been quarantined in the Common Cold Unit for two days before the viral challenge and were quarantined for six days after. Daily clinical examinations were performed to assess the presence of symptoms and signs of acute infection. Analysis of the study results revealed that psychological stress was associated with increased risk for the development of clinical illness. Moreover, this increased risk was due to a specific relation between greater psychological stress and higher rates of infection. In other words, the association between psychological stress and infection rates could not be attributed to differential patterns of exposure;

hence, whether the subject was rooming alone or with a roommate who was also ill, no effect on the relationship was noted. The authors asserted that the pattern of results indicated a specific association of psychological stress and the resistance of the host to the development of infection.

These two studies suggest that the psychological–physiological dichotomy implicit in the work of the Johns Hopkins group needs extension. In short, the interaction of psychological stress and physiological stress (e.g., an acute infectious illness) is not a simple one. This interaction may occur at multiple levels within the psychobiology of the individual or at different points of time in the life of the individual. Stressful life experiences may, therefore, work to mold the personality, altering the manner in which the individual is likely to communicate the need for help and to respond to such help. These personality variables may, in turn, affect the frequency with which the individual exposes himself or herself to physiologically stressful events. As reflected in the latter two studies, we are becoming increasingly aware that the body's response to stress activates a cascade of physiological signals that result in complex intercommunications among the central nervous system, the endocrine system, and the immune system. For example, as suggested in the study by Cohen and his colleagues (1991), psychological stress may have a direct effect on altering the host response to an infectious challenge, independent of health practices or subjective reports of symptoms after infection has occurred.

EPIDEMIC NEUROMYASTHENIA

Contemporaneous with these studies of chronic brucellosis and the role of psychological variables in the recuperation from infectious illness, an alternate historical path was evolving—a path that also has particular relevance for a more complete appreciation of the contemporary case definitions of chronic fatigue states. This path concerns the observations of epidemic forms of illnesses which, again, closely resemble the syndromes mentioned above.

In association with the poliomyelitis epidemics in the early portions of this century, a number of reports described an unusual illness that often occurred in an explosive fashion in the midst of a local poliomyelitis epidemic (Acheson, 1959; Henderson & Shelokov, 1959). One of the earliest and best known outbreaks, at the Los Angeles County General Hospital in the summer of 1934, was described in detail (Gilliam, 1938). Among the subsequent occurrences reported were those in Akureyri, Iceland (Sigurdsson et al., 1950), Adelaide, Australia (Pellew, 1951), and upper New York State (White & Burtch, 1954); those among the hospital staff of the Middlesex Hospital, London, England (Acheson, 1954), among the student nurses of the Chestnut Lodge psychiatric hospital, Rockville, Maryland (Shelokov et al., 1957), among the nursing staff of Addington Hospital, Durban, South Africa (Hill, 1955), and among residents of the Florida community of Punta Gorda (Poskanzer et al., 1957); and, possibly the most discussed and controversial outbreak, the epidemic at the Royal Free Hospital, London, England (Crowley et al., 1957; Medical Staff, 1957). What was most remarkable about these illnesses was the protean nature of the symptoms. Though often having a core resemblance to poliomyelitis, including a variety of neurological symptoms (muscle weakness, headaches, profound fatigue, paresthesias and dysesthesias, confusion), there were other features that argued against the poliomyelitis virus as the pathogenic agent. These features included the remarkable absence of laboratory findings (normal cerebrospinal fluid, with none of the typical pleocytosis expected in polio), no or low fever, virtually no paralytic cases, and no mortality. The presence of dramatic behavioral symptoms—episodes of depression, nervousness, and mood lability—was frequently noted, as were the preponderance of young females affected by the disease and the apparently unique susceptibility of health care providers. We will describe the epidemics at the Los Angeles County General Hospital and the Royal Free Hospital in detail, because they encapsulate some of the most puzzling aspects of the illness. The reader is urged to examine the primary reference material of the other epidemics for supporting discussions.

In 1934, between May and December, 198 employees of the Los Angeles County General Hospital were cared for either in the clinics or in the hospital wards of that institution. The diagnosis at that time was poliomyelitis. However, a U.S. Public Health Service report published four years later (Gilliam, 1938) stated:

> If this diagnosis may be accepted in any large proportion of the cases, the epidemic is unique in the history of poliomyelitis because of the altogether unusual symptomatology, and the extraordinarily high attack rate in an adult population. If the disease were not poliomyelitis, the epidemic is equally extraordinary in presenting a clinical and epidemiological picture, which, so far as is known, is without parallel . . . .

The alarming context in which this illness emerged—a local and statewide epidemic of true poliomyelitis—must be taken into account. Among the cases in the surrounding epidemic that came to autopsy, the characteristic neuropathologic changes associated with poliomyelitis were observed. Virus was isolated in some autopsy cases, and, in one clinical instance, from nasal washings. It is highly probable that true cases of poliomyelitis were represented in the specific outbreak at the County hospital; however, by the time this specific epidemic was under way, the resemblance of this discrete epidemic to acute poliomyelitis was diffused by the clinical characteristics of the apparently novel illness. From May 5 to June 9, 1934, the population of patients admitted to the communicable diseases ward of the County hospital had nearly quadrupled, and the staff necessary to manage these patients had more than doubled. At the height of the epidemic, a physician was posted at the ambulance entrance gatehouse to question all prospective patients. Any patient giving a history "at all suspicious" for poliomyelitis was sent directly to the communicable diseases ward. The clinical presentation of the patients, which is described in detail, ranges widely. Discrete physical signs were few, and they rested largely on the identification of muscle weakness or joint stiffness, and on low-grade fevers. Cerebrospinal fluid was examined in 59 of the cases; in only 3 cases was there evidence of modest pleocytosis. No other laboratory abnormalities were apparent. The most common presentation was abrupt in onset, accompanied by pain (often described as "rheumatoid or influenzal in character") and headache. Other symptoms, which occurred in at least half of the individuals during the entire period of observation, included, in order of frequency, muscle tenderness, localized muscular weakness, muscle twitching, nausea, irritability, stiff neck or back, vomiting, and vertigo. The waxing and waning character of the symptoms was repeatedly noted, as was the wandering nature of the muscular weakness. In cases where muscular atrophy was recorded, the atrophy was considered to be out of proportion to the demonstrated weakness. Many patients recovered fully, but in the acute stages of the illness, disability was marked. On average, each patient lost 13.6 weeks of work.

When reading the text of Gilliam's report, it is difficult not to appreciate the degree to which observer bias may have obscured the true heterogeneity of the phenomenon under observation. Because of the ominous context of the immediate polio epidemic, a presumption of infectious illness was made and held, despite a lack of compelling evidence to support this assumption. Indeed, the context and the pattern of spread of the illness served as the principal observations bolstering the view of the cause as a unique infectious agent, probably viral in origin. Nevertheless, it is important to realize that the data analysis was based on clinical records collected at the time of the patients' care in the hospital and clinics; hence, the clinicians recording the information on which Gilliam and his team rested their conclusions had also approached the illness with the presumption that this was indeed poliomyelitis itself. The problems inherent in the lack of objectivity associated with such data are obvious. Furthermore, despite the intense and systematic scrutiny of the muscular symptoms, and of the basic age, gender, and occupational distribution of the study population, other clinical characteristics of the patients under study are less well described. In the final paragraph of the monograph, Gilliam notes: "It should, however, be pointed out that certain observers were of the privately expressed opinion that hysteria played a large role in this outbreak. While it cannot be denied that hysteria was an important factor in some cases, it appears extremely unlikely that many of the cases were purely hysterical in nature."

Some of the concerns raised in regard to the Los Angeles County General Hospital epidemic were revisited, and dealt with in greater detail in the literature, in association with the outbreak of a similar clinical syndrome in 1955 at the Royal Free Hospital, in London, England. We will discuss some of the clinical aspects of this illness and its unresolved controversy. The dramatic quality and speed of onset of the Royal Free Hospital epidemic probably made it even more striking than the Los Angeles outbreak. On July 13, 1955, a resident physician and a ward sister of the hospital were admitted for a clinical illness with features that were remarkably similar to those noted in the Los Angeles epidemic. By July 25, over 70 of the staff were ill, "and it was plain that there was in the hospital an epidemic of a highly infectious character, producing amongst other things manifestations in the central nervous system . . . ." The magnitude of the epidemic was so alarming, and the concern over the health of the patients so high, that the hospital was closed at that point and remained closed for nearly two and a half months. By the end of the reporting period in November, 292 members of the hospital staff had been affected, and 255 of them had been admitted to the hospital for care. Remarkably, although the hospital was fully occupied at the onset of the epidemic, only 12 of the patients present at that time developed the disease. The symptoms of the disease were variable in their pattern and intensity. Early symptoms were commonly malaise and headache, usually associated with a disproportionate degree of emotional lability and depressive symptoms. Other symptoms reported frequently at onset included sore throat, lassitude, vertigo, pain in limbs, nausea, dizziness, stiff neck, and back pain. The initial report (Medical Staff, 1957) notes that "the intensity of the malaise, particularly when related to the slight pyrexia in this disorder, requires emphasis . . . ." Physical signs were few, and laboratory examinations, including blood counts, Paul–Bunnell tests (for infectious mononucleosis), electrocardiograms, and cerebrospinal fluid analysis (in 18 cases), were normal. Electromyographic studies were reported as showing a pattern of asynchronous bursts of motor unit potentials. The illness had a clear pattern of prevalence among the young, resident, female nursing staff of the hospital. The course of the disease was variable, with waxing and waning of symptoms. Over half of the reported cases required in-hospital treatment for up to 2 months. It is of interest that the authors of the original report noted: "The protracted illness, with a large element of doubt in the mind of the victim as to the ultimate prognosis, naturally engendered considerable anxiety and depression. Functional manifestations in a few cases overlaid the organic picture, particularly in those cases longest in hospital . . . ."

An editorial entitled "A New Clinical Entity?" published in *Lancet* in May 1956, proposed the name *benign myalgic encephalomyelitis* for this syndrome. The author drew parallels between the outbreak at the Royal Free Hospital and other outbreaks (mentioned at the beginning of this section), and again emphasized that interest in these epidemic outbreaks had arisen against a backdrop of intense interest in central nervous system infections. That interest began not only with the worldwide epidemics of poliomyelitis, but also with the perplexing and devastating encephalitis lethargica that had permeated the European continent in the early part of this century. The operational definition supplied in the *Lancet* editorial for benign myalgic encephalomyelitis included (1) symptoms and signs of damage to the central nervous system, (2) protracted periods of muscle pain, (3) emotional disturbances in the convalescent period, (4) normal cerebrospinal fluid analysis, (5) involvement of the reticuloendothelial system, (6) an extended clinical course marked by frequent exacerbations, and (7) an ultimately benign clinical outcome.

Testimony to the importance of these epidemics has been given by the persistence of the name "myalgic encephalomyelitis" in the British and Canadian literature on this topic, and by the continuing controversy in regard to the cause(s) of these outbreaks. The development of a modern, interdisciplinary assessment of the nature of these illnesses began with a series of two follow-up articles on the Royal Free Hospital disease (McEvedy & Beard, 1970, 1973). In these articles, McEvedy and Beard presented a compelling reanalysis of the original case data. They contended that their analysis clearly supported a diagnosis of mass hysteria for the majority of the illnesses seen. At the very least, these reports emphasized the importance of more detailed and even-handed behavioral characterization of the population under study. In their first report, they reviewed in detail the original case material from the epidemic. They pointed out several general characteristics that supported a hysterical etiology for this illness: the high attack rate in females, the disparity between the level of malaise when contrasted with the low level of pyrexia, a core symptom constellation that shared many of the clinical features of a previous study of hysterical overbreathing, and the nonphysiologic, glove-and-stocking distribution of the anesthesia in the majority of cases. One of the authors was also able to reproduce, using themselves as test subjects, the electromyographic finding of asynchronous bursts of motor unit potentials seen in the original report. In their second report, McEvedy and Beard (1973) performed, 23 years after the initial outbreak, a controlled follow-up of 102 individuals affected in the original Royal Free Hospital epidemic. A variety of demographic characteristics and health history events were obtained, as well as the Eysenck Personality Inventory. Results of this study provided modest support for the contention that the affected population had an increased burden of medical and psychiatric debility many years before and after the acute stages of the disease.

Unfortunately, the approach taken by McEvedy and Beard was decidedly dichotomous: either the patients with Royal Free Hospital disease were suffering from a hysterical affliction or they weren't. As noted in the preceding section, the inadequacy of such an artificial distinction is becoming increasingly apparent.

It is of interest that epidemic illnesses such as those described in this section have rarely been reported in the medical literature in recent decades. However, considered in the context of these older studies, the revival of interest in chronic fatigue states as sequelae of acute or reactivated Epstein–Barr virus infection, which was sparked by the apparent clinical outbreak in Lake Tahoe in the early 1980s, may be seen as the historical heir to these prior epidemics. We would suggest that these previous studies offer important lessons that should help inform a clinical and research approach to this patient population. Indeed, these lessons are important if we are to advance our understanding beyond merely a more technically sophisticated reiteration of the findings of previous investigators. Some of the more important of these lessons concern an awareness of the effect, on both the patient and clinician, of the impact of bias in illness attribution in shaping the clinical presentation and course of the condition. In so doing, there is also a need to refrain from premature conclusions about the putative meaning of psychological or physiological symptoms present in the patients under study. Finally, these lessons underscore the importance of a comprehensive, interdisciplinary approach to clinical assessment and management. In this setting, psychiatry clearly plays a crucial role.

WHY IS A CASE DEFINITION IMPORTANT FOR CLINICAL ASSESSMENT? THE CENTERS FOR DISEASE CONTROL AND PREVENTION CASE DEFINITION

As noted in the preceding section, there has been a recent resurgence of interest in chronic fatigue states, in particular following a series of reports that began appearing in the early 1980s (Jones et al., 1985; Straus et al., 1985; Tobi et al., 1982). In these reports, a syndrome of persistent, unexplained fatigue was described, in association with a variety of constitutional symptoms reminiscent of the entities described above. These studies reported a spectrum of subtle abnormalities in cell-mediated and humoral immunity in these patients, along with atypical profiles of antibody responses to the Epstein–Barr virus and other viral antigens. These immunologic disturbances, coupled with the clinical observation that many of these patients developed the syndrome following an episode of acute infectious mononucleosis, led to the specific hypothesis that the illness was a manifestation of chronic Epstein–Barr virus infection. A new term had entered the popular vocabulary. However, as will be elaborated in other chapters in this text, several subsequent observations have challenged this idea and have suggested that, although immune stimulation may be present in these patients, *persistent* Epstein–Barr virus infection is almost certainly not a tenable explanation for most cases of the syndrome. First, the magnitude or pattern of the antibody titers bears little or no relationship to the severity of the clinical presentation. Second, controlled studies of sero-epidemiology have shown that enhanced activity of the Epstein–Barr virus may persist for as long as 30 to 104 months after the acute infection in otherwise asymptomatic individuals (Buchwald et al., 1987; Holmes et al., 1987; Horwitz et al., 1985). Third, a controlled trial of intravenous and oral acyclovir, an agent with moderate efficacy in combating the actively replicating Epstein–Barr virus, was without effect in these patients (Straus et al., 1988).

Quite rapidly, a confusion of names and operational definitions emerged in the professional and lay literature to describe this entity. It was not at all clear, though, that any group of investigators was using similar definitions or even systematically applying them. Comparability of research findings was therefore virtually impossible, and conclusions about what clinical or laboratory features were characteristic of this illness were indeterminable. To address this situation, in April 1987, the Centers for Disease Control and Prevention (CDC) convened a working group with the express charge of establishing a consensus case definition (Holmes et al., 1988). Clinicians and researchers with varying scientific backgrounds and levels of clinical familiarity with the topic composed the consensus panel. The original case definition is summarized in Table 1.1. Unanimous agreement was obtained in naming the newly operationalized syndrome "chronic fatigue syndrome" to highlight what was felt to be the most consistent and significant manifestation of the illness and to avoid the use of etiologically biased modifiers that were not applicable to all cases. Nevertheless, alternative names persist in the popular literature. One of the most prominent alternate names has been "chronic fatigue immune dysfunction syndrome," or CFIDS, suggested to emphasize what is perceived as the hallmark pathophysiology of the illness. The controversy surrounding the precise pathophysiology of the illness would suggest that premature closure on the nature of the illness by use of such a specific terminology could lead to a distortion of appropriate diagnostic assessment and treatment recommendations.

A number of issues regarding this original definition deserve comment. First, a fundamental emphasis has been placed on the *careful and systematic exclusion* of known entities which, early in their course, could mimic the presentation of this syndrome, such as systemic lupus erythematosus, rheumatoid arthritis, multiple sclerosis, or certain malignancies. The syndrome label is, therefore, applied only after an extended period of observation and evaluation and where diagnostic certainty is optimized. Second, the *absence of discrete laboratory testing,* which could be used to bolster confidence in the diagnosis of chronic fatigue syndrome, was underscored. Third, it was a somewhat implicit assumption that this definition captured *a heterogeneous cluster of individuals* rather than a single pathophysiological entity; hence, a theoretically neutral term, highlighting the hallmark clinical symptom, was specifically chosen.

TABLE 1.1. Centers for Disease Control and Prevention (CDC) Case Criteria for Chronic Fatigue Syndrome

Major Criteria (patient must fulfill major criteria 1 and 2):

1. New onset of persistent or relapsing, debilitating fatigue, or easy fatigability in person who has no previous history of similar symptoms, that does not resolve with bedrest, and that is severe enough to reduce or impair average daily activity below 50% of the patient's premorbid activity level for a period of at least 6 months.
2. Other clinical conditions that may produce similar symptoms must be excluded by thorough evaluation, based on history, physical examination, and appropriate laboratory findings.

Minor Criteria (patient must show 6 or more of the symptom criteria and 2 or more of the physical criteria; *or* 8 or more of the symptom criteria):

- *Symptom criteria* (must have begun at or after the time of increased fatigability, and must have persisted or recurred over a period of at least 6 months):

   1. Mild fever or chills (oral temperature between 37.5°C and 38.6°C)
   2. Sore throat
   3. Painful anterior or posterior cervical or axillary lymph nodes
   4. Generalized muscle weakness
   5. Myalgias
   6. Prolonged (24 hours or greater) postexertional fatigue
   7. Headaches
   8. Migratory arthralgia
   9. Neuropsychological complaints (including, photophobia, transient scotomata, forgetfulness, irritability, confusion, depression, poor concentration)
   10. Sleep disturbance
   11. Main symptom complex having an abrupt onset, over a few hours to a few days

- *Physical criteria* (must be documented by a physician on at least two occasions, at least one month apart):

   1. Low-grade fever (oral temperature 37.6°C to 38.6°C or rectal temperature 37.8°C to 38.8°C)
   2. Nonexudative pharyngitis
   3. Palpable anterior or posterior cervical or axillary lymph nodes

Criticisms were raised about this definition shortly after its publication in 1988 (Matthews et al., 1988). One of the most problematic aspects of the original definition was the mechanism to be employed to establish a clear delineation of the nature of "confounding" psychiatric illnesses. As the historical antecedents discussed in the previous sections have emphasized, a descriptive algorithm for the differentiation of primary psychiatric illnesses from chronic fatigue states remains elusive. With regard to the current definition, most investigators would agree that formally diagnosable psychiatric illnesses are present in well over half of all cases. Indeed, Katon and Russo

(1992) have recently suggested that the specific requirement in the case definition for multiple somatic symptoms leads to this overrepresentation of psychiatric illness in studies of chronic fatigue syndrome. It is difficult and often impossible to determine whether a psychiatric disorder is fully explanatory of the clinical presentation, a secondary manifestation of a primary disease process, or a coincident disease that modulates the presentation and course of the fatigue state. In response to this criticism, a revision of the case definition was formalized as the result of a joint workshop held in 1991 by the National Institute of Mental Health (NIMH) and the National Institute for Allergy and Infectious Disease (NIAID) (Schluederberg et al., 1992). The stipulations of this revision are summarized in Table 1.2. In practice, this change underscores the futility in attempting, in many cases, to distinguish

TABLE 1.2. Principal Modifications Based on the 1991 Workshop on the Definition and Medical Outcome Assessment of Chronic Fatigue Syndrome

Major medical exclusions:

Malignancy
Autoimmune disease
Inflammatory disease
Endocrine disease
Neurological disease
Chronic organic disease

Major psychiatric exclusions:

Psychotic illness, including: psychotic depression, bipolar illness, and
 schizophrenia
Substance abuse

Allowable comorbid medical and psychiatric conditions:

Fibromyalgia
Infectious mononucleosis
Adequately treated infection not typically associated with chronicity, including:
 toxoplasmosis, brucellosis, Lyme borreliosis
Nonpsychotic depressive disorders
Somatoform disorders
Anxiety disorders

Recommended assessment:

- *Laboratory (standard):* Urinalysis, complete blood count with differential,
  serum electrolytes, blood urea nitrogen, glucose, creatinine, calcium, thyroid
  function tests, erythrocyte sedimentation rate, antinuclear antibody testing
- *Laboratory (optional or as clinically indicated):* Serum cortisol, rheumatoid factor,
  immunoglobulin levels, tuberculin skin test, Lyme serology, HIV serology
- *Clinical examination (standard):* Complete history and physical examination,
  tender point examination, self-report health questionnaire, psychiatric interview (structured interview preferred)

between primary psychiatric illness and chronic fatigue syndrome on phenomenological grounds alone. The methodological approach proposed requires the specific a priori characterization of psychopathology, hence allowing, a posteriori, an examination of the interaction of psychopathology with the definition of chronic fatigue syndrome itself.

Assessment of the adequacy of this case definition and its implications for research and clinical practice is an area of continual review. A recent consensus conference—again, convened by the CDC—specifically reviewed the usefulness of the requirement for multiple unexplained physical symptoms in the formal definition. At the present time, scant data support the usefulness of the requirement in distinguishing a unique group of fatigued individuals. The one detectable consequence, as pointed out by Katon and Russo (1992), actually appears to be the incorporation of increasing levels of comorbid psychiatric illness in the overall population, most likely obscuring, rather than assisting in delineating a more biochemically and clinically homogeneous group. As a result of these deliberations, a second revision of the case definition has recently been published (Fukuda et al., 1994). Several changes have been proposed. Most notable was the recommendation to eliminate all of the physical signs from the case definition. General consensus and review of large clinical cohorts have established that the physical criteria were not only routinely unreliably documented, but were rarely present. Other principal changes were to reduce the number of unexplained medical symptoms necessary for the diagnosis of chronic fatigue syndrome to four, and to establish a category of idiopathic chronic fatigue for those individuals who manifest chronic fatigue but do not experience the additional physical symptoms. This latter distinction remains one of the more controversial aspects of the definition, and will undoubtedly be revisited as more systematic data accumulate to define an appropriate clinical and research definition. These most recent criteria are detailed in Table 1.3.

THE GREEN COLLEGE CRITERIA

Between the publication of the original CDC case definition and its first modification, an interdisciplinary consensus meeting was held in the United Kingdom, at Green College, Oxford, to address a number of perceived problems with the American definition (Sharpe et al., 1991). Specific sources of difficulty were highlighted, including the absence of specific recommendations on sampling procedures, comparison groups for study, or the use of reliable and valid instruments for symptom assessment and outcome. The stated aim of the working group was to "seek agreement amongst researcher workers on recommendations for the conduct and reporting of future studies of

TABLE 1.3. Centers for Disease Control and Prevention Revision of the Chronic Fatigue Syndrome Definition, 1994

Chronic fatigue syndrome:

- Clinically evaluated, unexplained, persistent or relapsing chronic fatigue ($\geq$ 6 months duration) that is of new or definite onset (has not been lifelong); is not the result of ongoing exertion; is not substantially alleviated by rest; and results in substantial reduction in previous levels of occupational, educational, social, or personal activities
- Four or more of the following symptoms are concurrently present for $>$ 6 months:
    1. Impaired memory or concentration
    2. Sore throat
    3. Tender cervical or axillary lymph nodes
    4. Muscle pain
    5. Multijoint pain
    6. New headaches
    7. Unrefreshing sleep
    8. Postexertion malaise

Idiopathic chronic fatigue:

- Clinically evaluated, unexplained chronic fatigue ($\geq$ 6 months' duration) that fails to meet the definition for chronic fatigue syndrome

Recommended clinical evaluation:

- Medical history and physical examination
- Mental status examination
- Laboratory screening battery to include: complete blood count with leukocyte differential, erythrocyte sedimentation rate, serum levels of alanine aminotransferase, total protein, albumin, globulin, alkaline phosphatase, calcium, phosphorus, glucose, blood urea nitrogen, electrolytes and creatinine, thyroid stimulating hormone, urinalysis

Exclusionary clinical diagnoses:

- Any active medical condition that could explain the chronic fatigue
- Any previously diagnosed medical condition whose resolution has not been documented beyond reasonable clinical doubt and whose continued activity may explain the chronic fatiguing illness
- Psychotic major depression; bipolar affective disorder; schizophrenia; delusional disorders; dementias; anorexia nervosa; bulimia nervosa
- Alcohol or other substance abuse within 2 years prior to the onset of the chronic fatigue and at any time afterward

patients with chronic fatigue . . . specifically . . . which patients should be included, how such studies should be approached, and . . . the minimal data
that should be reported . . . ."

The summary proceedings of the meeting are outlined in Table 1.4. Important in this definition, and distinct from the original American proposal,
was the specification of two broad categories for study: chronic fatigue syndrome and postinfectious fatigue syndrome (historically contiguous with the
entity myalgic encephalomyelitis, and presumably intended to replace it).
The former entity is essentially identical to the original American definition
without the specifically itemized "minor criteria." The latter category was a

TABLE 1.4. The Green College, Oxford, Definitions and Recommendations

Broad clinical syndromes:

- Chronic fatigue syndrome (CFS)

  1. Principal symptom is fatigue with definite onset and not lifelong
  2. Fatigue is severe, disabling, and affects physical and mental functioning
  3. Fatigue for at least 6 months, during which it is present at least 50% of the time
  4. Other symptoms may be included, such as:
     Myalgia
     Mood disturbance
     Sleep irregularity
  5. Definite medical and psychiatric exclusions:
     Established medical conditions known to produce chronic fatigue
     Schizophrenia
     Manic depressive illness
     Substance abuse
     Eating disorder
     Organic brain disease

- Postinfectious fatigue syndrome (PIFS)

  1. A subtype of CFS which follows or is associated with and infectious illness
  2. Patients must fulfill criteria for CFS as specified above, and, in addition, have:
     a. Definite evidence, including laboratory corroboration, of infectious illness at onset
     b. Full syndrome is present for at least 6 months after onset of infection

Elements considered essential to specify in reporting these syndromes:

- State which syndrome is being reported
- Measure degree of disability
- Specify criteria for inclusion and exclusion
- Indicate extent of clinical examination and investigation
- Specify method of assessment for associated psychiatric disorder

useful addition that separated out for study the unique group of subjects in whom an identifiable infectious stressor was clearly associated with the onset or course of the syndrome.

THE AUSTRALIAN GROUP DEFINITION

In addition to the formal consensus group definitions of chronic fatigue syndrome outlined above, another formal definition was published in 1988 (Table 1.5). This definition was proposed by Andrew Lloyd and colleagues in Australia, after a review of their first 100 patients. They concurred with the use of the name "chronic fatigue syndrome" as articulated by the CDC. Furthermore, they agreed that the hallmark symptom of fatigue—persistent or relapsing, of inexplicable cause, for at least 6 months' duration—was imperative in making the diagnosis. Their group differed, however, in the nature of the secondary criteria necessary for the full diagnosis. Two alternate criteria were specified; the presence of only one was necessary, in conjunction with the criterion of persistent fatigue to establish the diagnosis of chronic fatigue

---

TABLE 1.5. The Australian Definition of Chronic Fatigue Syndrome

Essential criteria:

1. Generalized, chronic persisting or relapsing fatigue of at least 6 months' duration, exacerbated by minor exercise, and causing significant disruption of usual daily activities

    and

2. Neuropsychiatric dysfunction, including impairment of concentration, and/or onset of short-term memory impairment

    and/or

3. Abnormal cell-mediated immunity indicated by reduction in absolute count of T8 and/or T4 lymphocyte subsets, and/or cutaneous anergy

Supportive criteria (not essential for the diagnosis of chronic fatigue syndrome):

- Myalgia
- Arthralgia
- Headaches
- Depression
- Tinnitus
- Paresthesias
- Sleep disturbance
- Lymphadenopathy
- Localized muscle tenderness
- Pharyngitis

---

syndrome. These two alternate criteria were: neuropsychiatric impairment and/or abnormal cell-mediated immunity. The criterion of impaired cell-mediated immunity makes the Australian group's case definition the sole definition to incorporate a laboratory marker in the diagnosis of chronic fatigue syndrome, though it is possible to meet this case definition without necessarily having the laboratory evidence of impaired cell-mediated immunity. Lloyd's group noted that, in a 12-month follow-up study of an additional 100 patients defined by this set of clinical and laboratory criteria, alternative medical diagnoses were uncovered in only two cases.

As with the Green College criteria, the Australian group's definition improved basic issues of nomenclature and helped to bring coherence to this field of clinical study. However, their specific inclusion of laboratory criteria in the definition has been criticized as premature, particularly given the lack of replicability of the specific pattern of the putative immune impairment present in this patient population, or the exact functional significance, if any, of such immune abnormalities (see Chapters 4 and 7, this volume).

CHRONIC FATIGUE SYNDROME AS A SPECTRUM CONDITION: RELATION TO FIBROMYALGIA

In contemporary research on chronic fatigue, it shortly became apparent that the emerging case definitions for chronic fatigue syndrome shared homology not only with certain psychiatric illnesses (as noted above), but also with certain other chronic, idiopathic illnesses. Arguably, the most important clinical entity in this regard is fibromyalgia. Fibromyalgia (previously referred to as fibrositis or fibromyositis) is a debilitating clinical condition characterized by widespread musculoskeletal pain. This pain has been typified by the presence of the so-called "tender points": well-demarcated and anatomically defined areas of heightened musculoskeletal tenderness. Indeed, the specific locations and number of tender points serve as one of the defining criteria for the syndrome as established by the American College of Rheumatology (see Table 1.6; Wolfe et al., 1990).

Although the organizing symptoms of fibromyalgia are pain and the presence of the distinctive tender points, the clear delineation of the syndrome as independent from chronic fatigue syndrome becomes less clear as the associated clinical symptoms present in patients with fibromyalgia are noted. These symptoms include fatigue, sleep disturbance, headache, depression, anxiety, and paresthesias. Further complicating the clinical picture is the observation that fibromyalgia, like chronic fatigue syndrome, often develops in the aftermath of an acute stressor, either physical (e.g., accidents or infections) or emotional. Several investigators have attempted to formally assess the relation between these two entities. Buchwald and colleagues (1987)

TABLE 1.6. Fibromyalgia—The American College of Rheumatology
1990 Criteria

---

1. History of widespread pain, defined as pain present in all of the following
   sites: left and right sides of the body, above and below the waist. Additionally, axial pain must be present.

and

2. The presence of pain in 11 of the following 18 bilateral tender point sites,
   upon digital palpation (approximate force of 4 kg; must elicit the subjective
   sensation of pain from the subject):

   • Occiput, at the suboccipital muscle insertions
   • Low cervical, at the anterior aspects of the intertransverse spaces at C5–C7
   • Trapezius, at the midpoint of the upper border
   • Supraspinatus, at origins, above the scapula spine near the medial border
   • Second rib, at the second costochondral junctions, just lateral to the junc-
     tions on upper surfaces
   • Lateral epicondyle, 2 cm distal to the epicondyles
   • Gluteal, in upper outer quadrants of buttocks in anterior fold of muscle
   • Greater trochanter, posterior to the trochanteric prominence
   • Knee, at the medial fat pad proximal to the joint line

---

provided a detailed clinical and laboratory report on a series of 50 patients
(46 women, 4 men) with primary fibromyalgia. They were specifically interested in detailing in the fibromyalgia patients the presence of symptoms characteristic of what was then referred to as the "chronic active Epstein–Barr
virus infection syndrome" (the CDC criteria for chronic fatigue syndrome
were still one year away from publication). They noted the high prevalence of
symptoms not previously thought to be characteristic of fibromyalgia,
namely recurrent sore throat (54% of subjects), recurrent rashes (47%), a history of allergies (64%), chronic cough (40%), recurrent adenopathy (33%),
and recurrent low-grade fevers (28%). In 55% of their sample, the onset of
illness was abrupt, in the aftermath of what appeared to the patient to be an
acute viral syndrome. In a study performed after the publication of the CDC
case definition for chronic fatigue syndrome, Goldenberg and coworkers
(1990) described the history and physical examination (including tender
points) of a series of 27 patients with debilitating fatigue of greater than 6
months' duration. Seventy percent of the sample of chronically fatigued subjects described the presence of diffuse musculoskeletal pain. In this group of
chronic fatigue patients, the tender point score was indistinguishable from the
score in a concurrent group of patients with fibromyalgia. The researchers
went on to note that, in their experience, more than 90% of patients with
chronic fatigue report persistent musculoskeletal pain; hence, the chronic fatigue sample described in their report "may underrepresent the association of
fibromyalgia with CFS . . . ."

The importance of the association between these clinical entities has been highlighted by the recommendation of the 1991 joint NIMH/NIAID workshop (Schluederberg et al., 1992), which recommended a tender point examination as part of the overall clinical assessment of chronic fatigue syndrome. Nevertheless, the specific relation between fibromyalgia and chronic fatigue syndrome is not clear. Some investigators have suggested that the similarity in clinical presentation among these various idiopathic syndromes argues for the presence of a common physiological abnormality (Hudson et al., 1992; Sternberg, 1993), which may occur along a spectrum of severity. If this latter point is true, then the presence of a discrete fibromyalgia syndrome within the context of a larger clinical syndrome of chronic, idiopathic fatigue may be of particular clinical relevance because recent studies suggest that this more focal constellation of painful musculoskeletal symptoms bodes poorly for long-term clinical outcome (Ledingham et al., 1993).

SUMMARY

Throughout medical history, clinical syndromes characterized by the principal symptom of fatigue or easy fatigability have recurred with remarkable regularity. The clinical expression of these conditions, as outlined in this chapter, strongly suggests a direct historical continuity among them, extending even to the modern concept of chronic fatigue syndrome. Constant themes associated with the study of these illnesses have been the importance of the psychological state of the individual, and their development in the aftermath of a variety of infectious illnesses. Of equal importance is the observation that a clear delineation of a discrete clinical disease among these entities has, so far, defied repeated attempts at analysis. On this latter point, Aronowitz (1991) has noted that "chronic fatigue syndrome, like its historical precedents, is a boundary condition that defines a set of debates about chronic illness in general: . . . whether, where, and how we might draw a categorical boundary between 'disease,' the objective manifestations of biological processes, and 'illness,' the subjective correlate, in the care of particular patients. . . ."

Viewed in this light, the probable clinical heterogeneity of this patient population can be more clearly appreciated. In other words, the historical perspective given in this chapter would suggest that chronically fatigued patients, including those who meet the current operational case definitions, may be more usefully regarded as a heterogeneous group of individuals with a variety of infectious and noninfectious antecedents (see Figure 1.1). We feel it is, therefore, clinically unreasonable at this time to presume that patients with chronic fatigue syndrome represent a discrete disease with a singular cause. Instead, a more useful formulation would characterize this

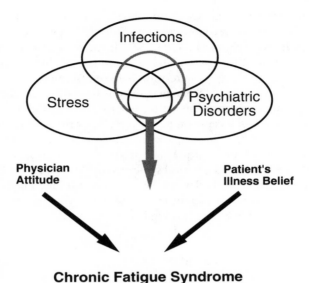

Chronic Fatigue Syndrome

FIGURE 1.1. The multidetermined nature of chronic fatigue syndrome: A risk factor model.

illness as a *clinical condition* rather than a diagnosis. In this sense, chronic fatigue syndrome is more analogous to a number of complex medical conditions, such as hypertension, where several direct and indirect factors (some of which may be psychological) lead to the development of the observable clinical syndrome. Such an approach rejects a unitary etiologic event to explain the condition, but nevertheless allows for the presence of shared pathophysiological processes, and emphasizes the interactive relation among many disparate factors.

With these considerations in mind, we hypothesize that, in chronic fatigue syndrome, specific pathophysiological antecedents (e.g., acute infection, stress, preexisting or concurrent psychiatric illness) may ultimately converge in a final common psychobiological pathway resulting in the clinical syndrome of chronic fatigue. We believe such a formulation provides a more congenial clinical and theoretical framework on which to integrate the varied biological and behavioral manifestations of the syndrome. The relative contribution of each of the antecedent factors toward increasing the morbid risk for the development of chronic fatigue syndrome in an individual patient may be difficult to specify with certitude. However, the current research case definitions are of direct relevance to clinical management: they serve as clinical algorithms, and they emphasize a risk factor model for the assessment of idiopathic fatigue states. In so doing, they may also foster an understanding of the potential influence of the physician's attitude and the illness belief of the patient on the clinical expression of the syndrome.

REFERENCES

Abbey, SE, Garfinkel, PE. Neurasthenia and chronic fatigue syndrome: The role of culture in the making of a diagnosis. *Am J Psychiatry* 1991; 148(12):1638–1646.

Acheson, ED. Encephalomyelitis associated with poliomyelitis virus: An outbreak in a nurses' home. *Lancet* 1954; 2:1044.

Acheson, ED. The clinical syndrome variously called benign myalgic encephalomyelitis, Iceland disease and epidemic neuromyasthenia. *Am J Med* 1959; April:569–595.

Anonymous (editorial). A new clinical entity? *Lancet* 1956; May 26:789–790.

Aronowitz, RA. The trouble with chronic fatigue. *J Gen Int Med* 1991; 6:378–379.

Beard, GM. Neurasthenia, or nervous exhaustion. *Boston Med Surg J* 1869; III(13): 217–221.

Beard, GM. A practical treatise on nervous exhaustion (Neurasthenia). Its symptoms, nature, sequences, treatment (2nd edition). New York: William Wood, 1880.

Buchwald, D, Sullivan, JL, Komaroff, AL. Frequency of "chronic active Epstein–Barr virus infection" in a general medical practice. *JAMA* 1987; 257(17):2303–2307.

Cluff, LE, Trever, RW, Imboden, JB, Canter, A. Brucellosis II. Medical aspects of delayed convalescence. *Arch Int Med* 1959; 103:70–77.

Cohen, S, Tyrrell, DAJ, Smith, AP. Psychological stress and susceptibility to the common cold. *New Engl J Med* 1991; 325:606–612.

Crowley, N, Nelson, M, Stovin, S. Epidemiological aspects of an outbreak of encephalomyelitis at the Royal Free Hospital, London, in the summer of 1955. *J Hygiene* 1957; 55:102–122.

DaCosta, JM. On irritable heart; A clinical study of a form of functional cardiac disorder and its consequences. *Am J Med Sci* 1871; 121:2–52.

Dicks, HV. Neurasthenia: Toxic and traumatic. *Lancet* 1933; Sept 23 (ii):683–686.

Evans, AC. Brucellosis in the United States. *Am J Pub Health* 1947; 37(2):139–151.

Fukuda, K, Straus, SE, Hickie, I, Sharpe, MC, Dobbins, JG, Komaroff, A, International Chronic Fatigue Syndrome Study Group. The chronic fatigue syndrome: A comprehensive approach to its definition and study. *Ann Int Med* 1994; 121(12):953–959.

Gilliam, AG. Epidemiologic study of an epidemic, diagnosed as poliomyelitis, occurring among the personnel of the Los Angeles County General Hospital during the summer of 1934. *Public Health Bull* 1938; 240:1–90.

Goldenberg, DL, Simms, RW, Geiger, A, Komaroff, AL. High frequency of fibromyalgia in patients with chronic fatigue seen in a primary care practice. *Arthritis Rheum* 1990; 33(3):381–387.

Hallee, TJ, Evans, AS, Niederman, JC, Brooks, CM, Voegtly, JH. Infectious mononucleosis at the United States Military Academy. A prospective study of a single class over four years. *Yale J Biol Med* 1974; 3:182–195.

Henderson, DA, Shelokov, A. Epidemic neuromyasthenia—clinical syndrome? *New Engl J Med* 1959; 260(15):757–764; 260(16):814–818.

Hill, RCJ. Memorandum on the outbreak amongst the nurses at Addington Hospital. *S A Med J* 1955; April 9:344–345.

Holmes, GP, Kaplan, JE, Stewart, JA, Hunt, B, Pinsky, PF, Schonberger, LB. A cluster of patients with a chronic mononucleosis-like syndrome: Is Epstein–Barr virus the cause? *JAMA* 1987; 257(17):2297–2302.

Holmes, GP, Kaplan, JE, Gantz, NM, Komaroff, AL, Schonberger, LB, Straus, SE, Jones, JF, Dubois, RE, Cunningham-Rundlls, C, Pahwa, S, Tosato, G, Zegans, LS, Purtilo, DT, Brown, N, Schooley, RT, Brus, I. Chronic fatigue syndrome: A working case definition. *Ann Int Med* 1988; 108:387–389.

Horwitz, CA, Henle, W, Henle, G, Rudnick, H, Latts, E. Long-term serological follow-up of patients for Epstein–Barr virus after recovery from infectious mononucleosis. *J Inf Dis* 1985; 151(6):1150–1153.

Hudson, JI, Goldenberg, DL, Pope, HG, Keck, PE, Schlesinger, L. Comorbidity of fibromyalgia with medical and psychiatric disorders. *Am J Med* 1992; 92:363–367.

Imboden, JB, Canter, A, Cluff, LE. Convalescence from influenza: A study of the psychological and clinical determinants. *Arch Int Med* 1961a; 108:115–121.

Imboden, JB, Canter, A, Cluff, LE. Symptomatic recovery from medical disorders. *JAMA* 1961b; 178(13):1182–1184.

Imboden, JB, Canter, A, Cluff, LE, Trever, RW. Brucellosis III. Psychological aspects of delayed convalescence. *Arch Int Med* 1959; 103:78–86.

Jones, JF, Ray, G, Minnich, LL, Hicks, MJ, Kibler, R, Lucas, DO. Evidence for active Epstein–Barr virus infection in patients with persistent, unexplained illnesses: Elevated anti-early antigen antibodies. *Ann Int Med* 1985; 102(1):1–7.

Kasl, SV, Evans, AS, Niederman, JC. Psychosocial risk factors in the development of infectious mononucleosis. *Psychsom Med* 1979; 41(6):445–466.

Katon, W, Russo, J. Chronic fatigue syndrome criteria. A critique of the requirement for multiple physical complaints. *Arch Int Med* 1992; 152:1604–1616.

Lane, C. The mental element in neurasthenia. *J Nerv Mental Dis* 1906; 33:463–466.

Ledingham, J, Doherty, S, Doherty, M. Primary fibromyalgia syndrome—An outcome study. *Br J Rheum* 1993; 32:139–142.

Lloyd, AR, Wakefield, D, Boughton, C, Dwyer, J. What is myalgic encephalomyelitis? *Lancet* 1988; 1:1286–1287.

Manningham, R. The symptoms, nature, causes, and cure of the febricula, or little fever. London: J Robinson, 1750.

Matthews, DA, Lane, TJ, Manu, P. Definition of the chronic fatigue syndrome [letter]. *Ann Int Med* 1988; 108:511–512.

McEvedy, CP, Beard, AW. Royal Free epidemic of 1955: A reconsideration. *Br Med J* 1970; 1:7–11.

McEvedy, CP, Beard, AW. A controlled follow-up of cases involved in an epidemic of "benign myalgic encephalomyelitis." *Br J Psychiatry* 1973; 122:141–150.

Medical Staff of the Royal Free Hospital. An outbreak of encephalomyelitis in the Royal Free Hospital Group, London, in 1955. *Br Med J* 1957; October 19:895–904.

Pellew, RAA. A clinical description of a disease resembling poliomyelitis, seen in Adelaide, 1949–1951. *Med J Australia* 1951; June 30:944–946.

Poskanzer, DC, Henderson, DA, Kunkle, EC, Kalter, SS, Clement, WB, Bond, JO. Epidemic neuromyasthenia. An outbreak in Punta Gorda, Florida. *New Engl J Med* 1957; 257(8):356–364.

Schluederberg, A, Straus, SE, Peterson, P, Blumenthal, S, Komaroff, AL, Spring, SB, Landay, A, Buchwald, D. Chronic fatigue syndrome research. Definition and medical outcome assessment. *Ann Int Med* 1992; 117(4):325–331.

Sharpe, MC, Archard, LC, Banatvala, JE, Borysiewicz, LK, Clare, AW, David, A, Edwards, RHT, Hawton, KEH, Lambert, HP, Lane, RJM, McDonald, EM, Mowbray, JF, Pearson, DJ, Peto, TEA, Preedy, VR, Smith, AP, Smith, DG, Taylor, DJ, Tyrell, DAJ, Wessely, S, White, P, Behan, PO, Rose, FC, Peters, TJ, Wallace, PG, Warrell, DA, Wright, DJM. A report—chronic fatigue syndrome: Guidelines for research. *J Roy Soc Med* 1991; 84:118–121.

Shelokov, A, Habel, K, Verder, E, Welsh, W. Epidemic neuromyasthenia. An outbreak of poliomyelitis-like illness in student nurses. *New Engl J Med* 1957; 257(8):345–355.

Sigurdsson, B, Sigurjonsson, J, Sigurdsson, JHJ, Thorkelsson, J, Gudmundsson, KR. A disease epidemic in Iceland simulating poliomyelitis. *Am J Hyg* 1950; 52:222–238.

Spink, WW. What is chronic brucellosis? *Ann Int Med* 1951; 35:358–374.

Sternberg, EM. Hypoimmune fatigue syndromes: Diseases of the stress response? *J Rheum* 1993; 20(3):418–421.

Straus, SE, Dale, JK, Tobi, M, Acyclovir treatment of the chronic fatigue syndrome: Lack of efficacy in a placebo-controlled trial. *N Engl J Med* 1988; 319(26): 1692–1698.

Straus, SE, Tosato, G, Armstrong, G, Lawley, T, Preble, OT, Henle, W, Davey, R, Pearson, G, Epstein, J, Brus, I, Blaese, RM. Persisting illness and fatigue in adults with evidence of Epstein-Barr virus infection. *Ann Int Med* 1985 Jan; 102(1):7–16.

Straus, SE, Dale, JK, Tobi, M, Lawley, T, Preble, O, Blaese, RM, Hallahan, C, Henle, W. Acyclovir treatment of the chronic fatigue syndrome. Lack of efficacy in a placebo-controlled trial. *N Engl J Med* 1988 Dec 29; 319(26):1692–1698.

Tobi, M, Morag, A, Ravid, Z, Chowers, I, Feldman-Weiss, V, Michaeli, Y, Ben-Chetrit, E, Shalit, M, Knobler, H. Prolonged atypical illness associated with serological evidence of persistent Epstein-Barr virus infection. *Lancet* 1982 Jan 9; 1(8263):61–64.

White, DN, Burtch, RB. Iceland disease: A new infection simulating acute anterior poliomyelitis. *Neurology* 1954; 4:506–516.

Wolfe, F, Smythe, HA, Yunus, MB, Bennett, RM, Bombardier, C, Goldenberg, DL, Tugwell, P, Campbell, SM, Abeles, M, Clark, P, Fam, AG, Farber, SJ, Fiechtner, JJ, Franklin, CM, Gatter, RA, Hamaty, D, Lessard, J, Lichtbroun, AS, Masi, AT, McCain, GA, Reynolds, WJ, Romano, TJ, Russell, IJ, Sheon, RP. The American College of Rheumatology 1990 criteria for the classification of fibromyalgia. *Arthritis Rheum* 1990; 33(2):160–172.

Wood, P. DaCosta's Syndrome (or effort syndrome). *Br Med J* 1941; May 24:767–772, May 31:805–811, June 7:845–851.

2

Idiopathic Chronic Fatigue: Depressive Symptoms and Functional Somatic Complaints

Peter Manu, M.D.
Thomas J. Lane, M.D.
Dale A. Matthews, M.D.

*I*diopathic chronic fatigue is common in primary care practice and is often assumed to be a symptom of a psychiatric disorder. In this chapter, we test this assumption by employing the database generated by the Connecticut Chronic Fatigue Study. We investigated the duration and severity of fatigue and the lifetime psychiatric symptoms of 200 consecutive patients with a chief complaint of chronic fatigue. All patients were given a standardized comprehensive medical evaluation and were administered a highly structured psychiatric interview. The patients with idiopathic chronic fatigue were compared with patients whose fatigue was attributable to a depressive disorder, a somatization disorder, a panic disorder, or chronic fatigue syndrome. The patients from the five diagnostic groups were similar with respect to age, female predominance, and duration and severity of fatigue. Compared with the appropriate control groups, the patients with idiopathic chronic fatigue had significantly fewer lifetime functional somatic complaints and affective and cognitive symptoms of mood disorders ($p < 0.005$). We conclude that idiopathic chronic fatigue does not resemble the psychiatric syndromes common among patients with chronic fatigue and deserves nosologic recognition and in-depth study.

Fatigue is one of the most common complaints in clinical practice and a symptom encountered in hundreds of diseases, being responsible for at least

10 million patient visits each year in the United States (National Center for Health Statistics, 1978). In the absence of physical illness, and after careful medical evaluation, most cases of chronic fatigue are given a psychiatric diagnosis such as major depression, panic disorder, somatization disorder, social phobia, or adjustment disorder (Allan, 1955; Katon et al., 1991; Kroenke et al., 1988; Manu et al., 1988; Morrison, 1980; Sugarman & Berg, 1984; Taerk et al., 1987; Wessely & Powell, 1989). However, recent prospective diagnostic studies of patients with chronic fatigue have shown that no physical or psychiatric diagnoses can be made in 10% to 30% of patients (Katon et al., 1991; Kroenke et al., 1988; Manu et al., 1988; Wessely & Powell, 1989). Some patients with unexplained chronic fatigue fulfill the diagnostic criteria for chronic fatigue syndrome (Holmes et al., 1988), a complex entity believed by some researchers to represent the clinical expression of a chronic, reactivated viral infection and/or an immune dysfunction (Bell et al., 1988; Buchwald et al., 1992; Klimas et al., 1990; Lloyd et al., 1989). The remaining patients with unexplained chronic fatigue have an idiopathic disorder that has not been explicitly studied, but has been interpreted to represent atypical manifestations of mood or somatization disorders (Greenberg, 1990; White, 1989).

This chapter presents the results of a study designed to test the assumption that the symptoms of patients with idiopathic chronic fatigue resemble the symptoms of depressive and somatization disorders, but fall short of fulfilling the standard criteria required for these diagnoses (American Psychiatric Association, 1987). To accomplish this goal, we compared idiopathic chronic fatigue patients to other groups of patients with a chief complaint of chronic fatigue. For a comprehensive analysis, in addition to control groups comprising patients with depressive and somatization disorders, we also used control groups of patients diagnosed to have panic disorder and chronic fatigue syndrome. The study utilized the database generated by 200 patients entered consecutively from November 1986 through October 1988 in the Connecticut Chronic Fatigue Study, a prospective clinical investigation of adult outpatients with a chief complaint of chronic fatigue. Previous publications of our group have used the database to describe, in detail, clinical characteristics of other groups of patients with chronic fatigue, but never those of idiopathic chronic fatigue patients (Kranzler et al., 1991; Lane et al., 1990; Manu et al., 1988, 1989a, 1989b, 1991; Matthews et al., 1991). The patients were examined by the authors, who are board-certified specialists in internal medicine, according to a protocol approved by the Institutional Review Board of the University of Connecticut and described in detail in Manu et al. (1988). Ninety-five percent of patients examined were white, and 91% were self-referred. Prior to being seen in the Chronic Fatigue Clinic of the University of Connecticut Health Center, the patients had been examined for their complaint of chronic fatigue by an average of 3.8 physicians.

EVALUATION PROTOCOL FOR CHRONIC FATIGUE

The 200 patients met the following entry criteria: (1) age 18 or older; (2) chief complaint of fatigue, tiredness, or lassitude, present at least one-half of waking hours during the month preceding the evaluation; and (3) no hospitalization during the 3 months prior to being examined in the Chronic Fatigue Clinic. All patients were asked to provide a narrative description of their illness, were queried in regard to the degree of their disability, and were asked to identify the provocative and palliative factors, and all of the symptoms associated with their fatigue. The patients also answered an extensive symptom checklist and were given a thorough physical examination. The following laboratory data were collected on all patients: complete blood count with differential white blood cell count; erythrocyte sedimentation rate; blood urea nitrogen; plasma levels of creatinine, sodium, potassium, chloride, bicarbonate, calcium, phosphorus, total protein, creatine phosphokinase, alanine aminotransferase, aspartate aminotransferase, alkaline phosphatase, lactate dehydrogenase, total and direct bilirubin, iron, total iron binding capacity, thyroid stimulating hormone, thyroxine, and triiodothyronine resin uptake; and urinalysis with microscopic examination of the sediment. Additional tests (e.g., antinuclear antibody, antibodies to the human immunodeficiency virus, Epstein–Barr virus, cytomegalovirus, heapatitis A and B viruses, toxoplasmosis, Borrelia Burgdorferi, as well as electroencephalograms, polysomonography, exercise testing, computerized axial tomography, and magnetic resonance imaging) were performed in individual patients if deemed necessary by the examining physician.

Psychiatric interviews of all patients were conducted by the authors using questions 16–100 and 210–213 of the third version of the Diagnostic Interview Schedule (DIS) of the National Institute for Mental Health, a highly structured method designed to elicit reliable and accurate psychiatric diagnoses conforming to standard criteria (Robins et al., 1981). These DIS questions elicit all the symptoms required for the diagnoses of somatization disorder, panic disorder, major depression, dysthymia, and mania. The DIS also assesses the severity, frequency, and distribution over time for all these symptoms.

PHYSICAL AND PSYCHIATRIC DIAGNOSES
OF CHRONIC FATIGUE PATIENTS

The diagnostic formulations were made according to *Cecil's Textbook of Medicine* (Wyngaarden & Smith, 1985) for physical disorders, the *Diagnostic and Statistical Manual of Mental Disorders,* third edition, revised (American Psychiatric Association, 1987) for psychiatric disorders, and Holmes and colleagues (1988) for chronic fatigue syndrome. These standards enabled the researchers

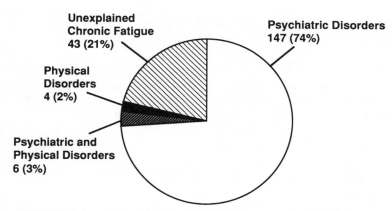

FIGURE 2.1. Etiologic diagnoses of 200 patients with chronic fatigue.

to classify the 200 patients into the following categories: (1) psychiatric disorders; (2) physical disorders; (3) physical and psychiatric disorders; and (4) unexplained chronic fatigue (Figure 2.1). Nine of the 43 patients with unexplained chronic fatigue fulfilled the working-case definition of chronic fatigue syndrome, leaving 34 patients with the diagnosis of idiopathic chronic fatigue.

Thirty-six of the 147 patients with psychiatric disorders had more than one diagnosis, and were excluded from further analysis. Of the remaining 111 patients, 86 were diagnosed to have only a depressive disorder (78 cases of major depression, 6 cases of dysthymia, and 2 cases of bipolar disorder), 15 patients met the criteria for somatization disorder, and 10 patients received a diagnosis of panic disorder (Figure 2.2).

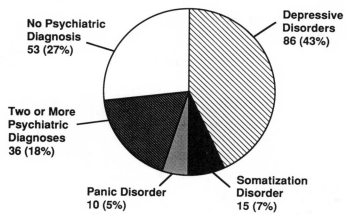

FIGURE 2.2. Psychiatric diagnoses of 200 patients with chronic fatigue.

Lifetime Psychiatric Symptoms in Idiopathic Chronic Fatigue

We compared the lifetime symptoms of depressive and somatization disorders recorded for the idiopathic chronic fatigue patients (group 1, $n = 34$) with those recorded for the group of patients given the diagnosis of depressive disorder (group 2, $n = 86$), somatization disorder (group 3, $n = 15$), panic disorder (group 4, $n = 10$), or chronic fatigue syndrome (group 5, $n = 9$) as the only identifiable disorders that could be etiologically linked to their chronic fatigue. Statistical significance was calculated by using the chi-square and two-tailed t testing, with the significance levels adjusted for the number of comparisons.

The 34 idiopathic chronic fatigue patients had an average age of 38 years and had been suffering from excessive tiredness for a mean of 11 years. Their female:male ratio was about 3:2. The patients with idiopathic chronic fatigue rated the severity of their fatigue at an average of 6.4 on a subjective scale going from 1 (negligible tiredness) to 10 (worst imaginable fatigue). The idiopathic chronic fatigue patients were similar to the patients from the four control groups in age, female predominance, duration of fatigue, and severity of fatigue. Excluding the symptoms of fatigue, fatigability, or lack of energy, patients with idiopathic chronic fatigue had an average of 2.5 depressive symptom clusters out of a maximum possible of 8 such clusters (dysphoria,

TABLE 2.1. Main Clinical Features of Patients with Chronic Fatigue

	Group 1: ICF ($n = 34$) Mean (SD)	Group 2: Depressive Disorder ($n = 86$) Mean (SD)	Group 3: Somatization Disorder ($n = 15$) Mean (SD)	Group 4: Panic Disorder ($n = 10$) Mean (SD)	Group 5: Chronic Fatigue Syndrome ($n = 9$) Mean (SD)
Age (years)	38.0 (11.9)	39.3 (11.5)	38.7 (10.2)	40.8 (10.1)	34.7 (6.5)
Female gender	58.8%	59.3%	86.7%	60.0%	55.6%
Duration of fatigue (years)	11.0 (11.5)	9.6 (11.7)	15.4 (14.7)	8.7 (7.2)	6.7 (6.4)
Severity of fatigue (1 = least, 10 = most)	6.4 (1.6)	6.6 (2.2)	7.1 (1.8)	6.9 (2.3)	7.2 (1.7)
Depressive symptoms score (min = 0, max = 8)	2.5 (2.1)	7.9 (3.0)[a]	3.5 (2.2)	3.7 (1.6)[c]	3.6 (1.9)
Functional somatic complaint score (min = 0, max = 35)	4.0 (2.6)	5.6 (3.3)[a]	13.5 (1.3)[b]	5.8 (2.6)[c]	5.0 (4.0)

[a] $p < .005$ for the difference between ICF and control.

[b] $p < .001$ for the difference between ICF and control.

[c] $p < .05$ for the difference between ICF and control.

anhedonia, change in weight or appetite, sleep disturbance, psychomotor agitation or retardation, worthlessness, difficulty with concentration and thinking, and morbid preoccupation). In contrast, patients diagnosed as having a depressive disorder reported an average of 7.9 symptom clusters. The average lifetime number of functional somatic complaints requiring medical evaluation was 4 among idiopathic chronic fatigue patients, substantially lower than the 13.5 such symptoms reported by patients with somatization disorder (Table 2.1).

The comparative analysis of the 16 individual depressive symptoms revealed statistically significant differences between idiopathic chronic fatigue patients and those given a diagnosis of depressive disorder. Patients with idiopathic chronic fatigue had a much lower frequency of all affective and cognitive symptoms of major depression. For example, only 28% of the patients reported a history of anhedonia, only 19% of the patients reported experiencing periods of worthlessness, and only 9% of the patients reported psychomotor retardation. The patients with idiopathic chronic fatigue also reported fewer vegetative symptoms associated with the clinical syndromes of mood disorders (Table 2.2).

TABLE 2.2. Frequency (%) of Lifetime Depressive Symptoms of Patients with Chronic Fatigue

	Group 1: ICF	Group 2: Depressive Disorder	Group 3: Somatization Disorder	Group 4: Panic Disorder	Group 5: Chronic Fatigue Syndrome
Mood symptoms					
Dysphoria	44.1	91.9[a]	66.7	90.0	44.4
Anhedonia	29.4	67.4[a]	6.7	40.0	22.2
Worthlessness	23.5	54.7[a]	13.3	10.0	0.0
Want to die	2.9	36.0[a]	13.3	20.0	0.0
Cognitive symptoms					
Suicidal ideation	14.7	48.8[a]	6.7	50.0	22.2
Morbid preoccupation	17.6	48.8[a]	33.3	40.0	22.2
Poor concentration	14.7	75.6[a]	33.3	20.0	66.7
Slowed thinking	14.7	53.5[a]	13.3	0.0	44.4
Vegetative symptoms					
Insomnia	29.4	67.4[a]	33.3	40.0	44.4
Hypersomnia	14.7	54.7[a]	20.0	10.0	55.5
Loss of appetite	11.8	33.7	20.0	0.0	22.2
Weight loss	2.9	30.2[a]	20.0	0.0	22.2
Weight gain	14.7	38.4	33.3	20.0	0.0
Retardation	8.8	57.0[a]	26.7	0.0	11.1
Agitation	2.9	22.1	6.7	10.0	0.0
Suicide attempts	2.9	8.1	6.7	20.0	0.0

[a] $p < .001$ for the difference between ICF and control.

The analysis of the lifetime prevalence of the 35 somatic symptoms of somatization disorder indicated that idiopathic chronic fatigue patients had significantly fewer complaints of abdominal pain, nausea, pain in the extremities (myalgias), dyspnea at rest, muscle weakness, and blurred vision than patients diagnosed as having somatization disorder. A major diagnostic feature of somatization disorder (i.e., feeling sickly most of one's life) was described in only 1 of the 34 patients with idiopathic chronic fatigue (Table 2.3).

NOSOLOGICAL AND METHODOLOGICAL IMPLICATIONS

In 1869, New York neurologist George M. Beard introduced the term neurasthenia, or "American nervousness," to define a condition characterized by chronic fatigue unexplainable by a known mechanism, but which he believed to be "developed, fostered and perpetuated with the advance of culture and refinement, and the corresponding preponderance of labor of the brain over that of the muscles" (Beard, 1869). Beard observed that women were more frequently affected by neurasthenia than men, especially "the sensitive white woman, with small inherited endowment of force; living indoors; torn and cursed by happy and unhappy love; waylaid at all hours by the cruelest of robbers, worry and ambition" (Beard, 1881). He also noted that "as would logically be expected, it [neurasthenia] is oftener met with in cities than in the country and it is more marked at the desk and in the counting room than in the shop or on the farm" (Beard, 1884).

Beard's description of chronic fatigue proved influential in 1894 when Freud extracted from it the symptom complex of anxiety neurosis (Freud, 1894), and again in 1903 when Janet used some of the patients' phobic and obsessive features to define psychasthenia (Janet, 1903). The 1968 edition of the *Diagnostic and Statistical Manual of Mental Disorders* of the American Psychiatric Association accepted neurasthenia as a condition "characterized by complaints of chronic weakness, easy fatigability, and sometimes exhaustion," different "from anxiety neurosis and psychophysiologic disorder in the nature of the predominant complaint, and from depressive disorder in the moderateness of the depression and the chronicity of its course" (American Psychiatric Association, 1968). The manual made note of the fact that "unlike hysterical neurosis, the patient's complaints are genuinely distressing to him and there is not evidence of secondary gain." However, the 1980 (American Psychiatric Association, 1980) and 1987 (American Psychiatric Association, 1987) editions of the *Manual* listed neurasthenia only in the subject index, and only to refer to the definition of dysthymia, a mood disorder. From 1982 through 1987, many cases of unexplained chronic fatigue were considered to represent chronic reactivated Epstein–Barr virus infection

TABLE 2.3. Frequency (%) of Functional Somatic Complaints of Patients with Chronic Fatigue

	Group 1: ICF	Group 2: Depressive Disorder	Group 3: Somatization Disorder	Group 4: Panic Disorder	Group 5: Chronic Fatigue Syndrome
Gastrointestinal symptoms					
Vomiting	5.9	11.6	20.0	10.0	22.2
Abdominal pain	20.6	30.2	93.3[a]	40.0	44.4
Nausea	11.8	23.3	53.3[a]	30.0	33.3
Bloating	17.6	26.7	60.0	20.0	22.2
Diarrhea	17.6	22.1	33.3	20.0	33.3
Food intolerance	14.9	11.6	26.7	0.0	33.3
Pain symptoms					
Painful extremities	20.6	25.6	86.7[a]	20.0	33.3
Back pain	32.4	19.8	80.0	30.0	11.1
Joint pain	17.6	24.4	73.3	20.0	33.3
Dysuria	0.0	4.7	6.7	0.0	0.0
Other pain	2.9	16.3	53.3[a]	0.0	11.1
Cardiopulmonary symptoms					
Dyspnea at rest	8.8	18.6	73.3[a]	20.0	0.0
Palpitations	17.6	26.7	40.0	60.0	11.1
Chest pain	14.7	30.2	60.0	30.0	33.3
Dizziness	29.4	25.6	53.3	60.0	44.4
Neurological symptoms					
Amnesia	0.0	3.5	6.7	0.0	11.1
Globus	23.5	25.6	26.7	10.0	11.1
Loss of voice	0.0	4.6	13.3	0.0	0.0
Deafness	2.9	3.5	6.7	0.0	0.0
Double vision	11.8	8.1	20.0	10.0	22.2
Blurred vision	11.8	24.4	53.3[a]	40.0	22.2
Blindness	8.8	2.3	20.0	0.0	0.0
Fainting	2.9	19.8	33.3	10.0	0.0
Seizure	2.9	1.2	0.0	0.0	0.0
Ataxia	8.8	17.4	26.7	20.0	0.0
Muscle weakness	11.8	34.8	80.0[a]	50.0	22.2
Sexual symptoms					
Burning in sex organs	0.0	3.5	20.0	0.0	0.0
Sexual indifference	23.5	12.8	46.7	20.0	11.1
Dyspareunia	0.0	7.0	20.0	0.0	0.0
Impotence	0.0	12.8	20.0	0.0	0.0
Female reproductive symptoms					
Dysmenorrhea	40.0	25.5	30.8	16.7	0.0
Irregular periods	40.0	27.4	46.2	0.0	60.0
Excessive menorrhagia	10.0	13.7	30.8	33.3	0.0
Vomiting during pregnancy	0.0	7.8	23.1	16.7	0.0
Sickly most of life	2.9	17.4	40.0[a]	10.0	0.0

[a] $p < .001$ for the difference between ICF and control.

(Jones et al., 1985; Straus et al., 1985; Tobi et al., 1982), a hypothesis later rejected (Buchwald et al., 1987; Hellinger et al., 1988; Holmes et al., 1987; see also Chapter 1, this volume).

Because neurasthenia was no longer available as a diagnostic label when we started our prospective study of patients with a chief complaint of chronic fatigue, we used idiopathic chronic fatigue as the name for the illness experienced by those of our patients who did not show evidence of a diagnosable physical or psychiatric disorder after comprehensive evaluations. This description corresponds most closely with the definition currently used in the United Kingdom, as developed by the Green College group (Sharpe et al., 1991). Although the symptom of chronic fatigue was apparently just as severe and persistent in patients with idiopathic chronic fatigue as it was in patients diagnosed as having a depressive disorder, the great disparity between the frequencies of depressive features recorded for these two groups suggests that idiopathic chronic fatigue does not resemble any of the standard clinical syndromes of major and minor depression. Strong evidence also indicated that patients with idiopathic chronic fatigue are remarkably different from chronic fatigue patients diagnosed as having somatization disorder. The magnitude of these differences suggests that idiopathic chronic fatigue is not the consequence of a classification bias, (i.e., a clinical syndrome falling short of one or two symptoms required for the diagnosis of a depressive or somatization disorder), but of a qualitatively different disorder.

Patients with idiopathic chronic fatigue appear to be most similar to those who fulfill the working case definition of chronic fatigue syndrome, a research construct proposed in 1988 to replace the diagnosis of chronic Epstein–Barr virus infection given certain patients with debilitating chronic fatigue (Holmes et al., 1988; see Chapter 1, this volume). In fact, it appears reasonable to propose the use of the two major diagnostic criteria for chronic fatigue syndrome to define idiopathic chronic fatigue as a condition characterized by disabling fatigue, persistent or recurrent for at least 6 months in the absence of any other medical or psychiatric diagnosis known to be associated with chronic fatigue, much as the current Green College criteria suggest (Sharpe et al., 1991). From this standpoint, chronic fatigue syndrome could be interpreted as a multisymptomatic and more severe subset of idiopathic chronic fatigue.

Idiopathic chronic fatigue undoubtedly affects millions of individuals and produces significant suffering, loss of productivity, and high emotional, social, and financial cost. We are ignorant of its biological underpinnings and uncertain of its natural history. We submit that idiopathic chronic fatigue deserves nosologic identity and a great deal of in-depth work in order to better characterize its clinical variants (including chronic fatigue syndrome), clarify its etiologies, and validate safe and effective treatments.

ACKNOWLEDGMENTS

Dr. Matthews was the 1989–1992 George Morris Piersol Teaching and Research Fellow of the American College of Physicians.

A version of this chapter was presented at the National Institute of Allergy and Infectious Diseases/National Institute of Mental Health *Workshop on the Definition and Medical Outcome Assessment of Chronic Fatigue Syndrome in Research,* Bethesda, Maryland, March 1991.

REFERENCES

Allan, F. The differential diagnosis of weakness and fatigue. *N Engl J Med* 1955; 231:414–418.

American Psychiatric Association. *Diagnostic and statistical manual of mental disorders, second edition* (DSM-II). Washington, DC: American Psychiatric Association, 1968.

American Psychiatric Association, Committee on Nomenclature and Statistics. *Diagnostic and statistical manual of mental disorders,* third edition (DSM-III). Washington, DC: American Psychiatric Association, 1980.

American Psychiatric Association, Committee on Nomenclature and Statistics. *Diagnostic and statistical manual of mental disorders,* third edition, revised (DSM-III-R). Washington, DC: American Psychiatric Association, 1987.

Beard, GM. Neurasthenia or nervous exhaustion. *Boston Med Surg J* 1869; 3:217–220.

Beard, GM. *American nervousness, its causes and consequences.* New York: G. P. Putnam's Sons, 1881.

Beard, GM. *Sexual neurasthenia, its hygiene, causes, symptoms, and treatment, with a chapter on diet for the nervous.* New York: E. B. Treat & Co., 1884.

Bell, EJ, McCartney, RA, Riding, MH. Coxsackie B viruses in myalgic encephalomyelitis. *J Roy Soc Med* 1988; 81:329–333.

Buchwald, D, Cheney, PR, Peterson, DL, Henry, B, Wormsley, SB, Geiger, A, Ablashi, DV, Salahuddin, SZ, Saxinger, C, Biddle, R, Kikiuis, R, Jolesz, FA, Folks, T, Balachandrau, N, Peter, JB, Gallo, RC, Komaroff, AL. A chronic illness characterized by fatigue, neurologic and immunologic disorders, and active human herpesvirus type 6 infection. *Ann Int Med* 1992; 116:103–113.

Buchwald, D, Sullivan, JL, Komaroff, AL. Frequency of "chronic active Epstein–Barr virus infection" in a general medical practice. *JAMA* 1987; 257: 2303–2307.

Freud, S. The justification for detaching from neurasthenia a particular syndrome: The anxiety neurosis (1894). In Freud, S, *Collected Papers, volume 1.* New York: Basic Books, 1959.

Greenberg, DB. Neurasthenia in the 1980s: Chronic mononucleosis, chronic fatigue syndrome, and anxiety and depressive disorders. *Psychosomatics* 1990; 31:129–137.

Hellinger, WC, Smith, TF, Van Scoy, RE, Spitzer, PG, Forgacs, P, Edson, RS. Chronic fatigue syndrome and the diagnostic utility of antibody to Epstein–Barr virus early antigen. *JAMA* 1988; 260:971–973.

Holmes, GP, Kaplan, JE, Gantz, NM, Komaroff, AL, Schonberger, LB, Straus, SE, Jones, JF, Dubois, RE, Cunningham-Rundles, C, Pahwa, S, Tosato, G, Zegans, LS, Purtio, DT, Brown, N, Schooley, RT, Brus, I. Chronic fatigue syndrome: A working-case definition. *Ann Int Med* 1988; 108:387–389.

Holmes, GP, Kaplan, JE, Stewart, JA, Hunt, B, Pimsky, PF, Schonberger, LB. A cluster of patients with mononucleosis-like syndrome: Is Epstein–Barr virus the cause? *JAMA* 1987; 257:2297–2302.

Janet, P. *Les obsessions et la psychasthénie.* Paris: Félix Alcan, 1903.

Jones, JF, Ray, CG, Minnich, LL, Hicks, MJ, Kibler, R, Lucas, DO. Evidence for active Epstein–Barr virus infection in patients with persistent, unexplained illnesses: Elevated anti-early antigen antibodies. *Ann Int Med* 1985; 102:7–16.

Katon, WJ, Buchwald, DS, Simon, GE, Russo, JE, Mease, PJ. Psychiatric illness in patients with chronic fatigue and those with rheumatoid arthritis. *J Gen Int Med* 1991; 6:277–285.

Klimas, NG, Salvato, FR, Morgan, R, Fletcher, MD. Immunologic abnormalities in chronic fatigue syndrome. *J Clin Microbiol* 1990; 28:1403–1410.

Kranzler, H, Manu, P, Hesselbrock, V, Lane, TJ, Matthews, DA. Substance use disorders in patients with chronic fatigue. *Hosp Comm Psychiatry* 1991; 42:924–928.

Kroenke, K, Wood, DR, Mangelsdorff, AD, Meier, NJ, Powel, JB. Chronic fatigue in primary care: Prevalence, patients characteristics, and outcome. *JAMA* 1988; 260:929–934.

Lane, TJ, Matthews, DA, Manu, P. Low yield of physical examinations and laboratory investigations in patients with chronic fatigue. *Am J Med Sci* 1990; 299:313–318.

Lloyd, AR, Wakefield, D, Boughton, CR, Dwyer, JM. Immunological abnormalities in the chronic fatigue syndrome. *Med J Aust* 1989; 151:122–124.

Manu, P, Lane, TJ, Matthews, DA. Somatization disorder in patients with a chief complaint of chronic fatigue. *Psychosomatics* 1989b; 30:388–395.

Manu, P, Mathews, DA, Lane, TJ. The mental health of patients with chronic fatigue: A prospective evaluation and follow-up. *Arch Int Med* 1988; 148:22130–2217.

Manu, P, Matthews, DA, Lane, TJ. Panic disorder among patients with chronic fatigue. *South Med J* 1991; 84:451–456.

Manu, P, Matthews, DA, Lane, TJ, Tennen, H, Hesselbrock, V, Mendola, R, Affleck, G. Depression among patients with a chief complaint of chronic fatigue. *J Affect Dis* 1989a; 17:165–172.

Matthews, DA, Lane, TJ, Manu, P. Antibodies to Epstein–Barr virus in patients with chronic fatigue. *South Med J* 1991; 84:832–840.

Morrison, JD. Fatigue as a presenting complaint in family practice. *J Fam Pract* 1980; 10:795–801.

National Center for Health Statistics. *Office visits to internists: The National Ambulatory Medical Care Survey, United States, 1975.* DHEW Publication No. 79-1787. Washington, DC: Public Health Service, 1978.

Robins, LN, Helzer, JE, Croughan, J, Ratcliff, KS. National Institute of Mental Health Diagnostic Interview Schedule: Its history, characteristics, and validity. *Arch Gen Psychiatry* 1981; 38:381–389.

Sharpe, MC, Archard, LC, Banatvala, JE, Borysiewicz, LK, Clare, AW, David, A, Edwards, RHT, Hawton, KEH, Lambert, HP, Lane, RJM, McDonald, EM, Mowbray, JF, Pearson, DJ, Peto, TEA, Preedy, VR, Smith, AP, Smith, DG, Taylor, DJ, Tyrell, DAJ, Wessely, S, White, P, Behan, PO, Rose, FC, Peteres, TJ, Wallace, PG, Warrell, DA, Wright, DJM. A report—Chronic fatigue syndrome: Guidelines for research. *J Roy Soc Med* 1991; 84:118–121.

Straus, SE, Tosato, G, Armstrong, G, Lawley, T, Prefle, OT, Henle, W, Davey, R, Pearson, G, Epstein, J, Brus, I, Blease, RM. Persisting illness and fatigue in adults with evidence of Epstein–Barr virus infection. *Ann Int Med* 1985; 102:7–16.

Sugarman, JR, Berg, AO. Evaluation of fatigue in a family practice. *J Fam Pract* 1984; 19:643–647.

Taerk, GS, Toner, BB, Salit, IE, Garfinkel, PE, Ozersky, S. Depression in patients with neuromyasthenia (benign myalgic encephalomyelitis). *Int J Psychiatry Med* 1987; 17:49–55.

Tobi, M, Morag, A, Ravid, Z, Chowers, I, Feldman-Weiss, V, Michaeli, Y, Ben-Chetrit, E, Shalit, M, Knobler, H. Prolonged atypical illness associated with serological evidence of persistent Epstein–Barr virus infection. *Lancet* 1982; 1:61–64.

Wessely, S, Powell, R. Fatigue syndromes: A comparison of chronic "postviral" fatigue with neuromuscular and affective disorders. *J Neurol Neurosurg Psychiatry* 1989; 52:940–948.

White, P. Fatigue syndrome: Neurasthenia revived. *Br Med J* 1989; 289:1199–1200.

Wyngaarden, JB, Smith, LH, eds. *Cecil's textbook of medicine,* 19th edition. Philadelphia: W. B. Saunders & Co., 1985.

3

Psychiatric Diagnostic Overlap in Chronic Fatigue Syndrome

Susan E. Abbey, M.D.

P sychiatric symptoms are common in the general population and occur in at least one-third of patients with a medical illness (Katon, 1987). They often occur transiently. However, they may cluster together and be of a severity to merit a psychiatric diagnosis as outlined in the *Diagnostic and Statistical Manual of Mental Disorders,* fourth edition, of the American Psychiatric Association (1994). When psychiatric symptoms are found in patients with a comorbid medical disease, these symptoms may represent (1) a coincidental finding unrelated to the medical disorder; (2) a symptom of the medical disorder or its treatment; or (3) a secondary reaction to the experience of illness and related disabilities (Rodin & Voshart, 1986). Psychiatric symptomatology is recognized to be part of a wide range of medical disorders (Derogatis & Wise, 1989; Lipkin, 1985; Stoudemire & Fogel, 1993). Although any given psychiatric symptom has a medical differential diagnosis in addition to a psychiatric differential diagnosis, there are some associations between psychiatric symptoms and medical disorders that are more common. Examples of these include depression with pancreatic cancer or following cerebrovascular accidents (Cohen-Cole et al., 1993) or anxiety in the context of pheochromocytoma or hyperthyroidism (Goldberg & Posner, 1993). Psychiatric symptomatology and, in particular, depressive symptomatology have been associated with increased morbidity and mortality in some medical disorders (Frasure-Smith et al., 1993; Silverstone, 1990). Unfortunately, the presence of prominent psychiatric symptomatology in conditions with a less clearly defined pathophysiology (e.g., chronic fatigue syndrome [CFS], irritable bowel syndrome, fibromyalgia, and temporomandibular joint dysfunction) may raise questions

48

as to the legitimacy of these conditions within the medical system. The presence of a high prevalence of psychiatric symptomatology and current or lifetime psychiatric diagnoses in patients with CFS has led to concerns that these findings will result in the delegitimation of the diagnosis. In juxtaposition to this is the clinical reality; there is treatment for psychiatric symptomatology associated with CFS and that treatment frequently improves the patient's quality of life. This chapter will review relevant issues related to psychiatric diagnosis in medical illness and will examine the psychiatric diagnostic categories where there is a potential overlap in phenomenology between the psychiatric diagnosis and CFS.

WHAT IS A PSYCHIATRIC DIAGNOSIS?

Much of the current controversy over diagnosis can be traced to fundamental questions about the meaning of the words "disease" and "diagnosis" (Guze, 1992), and whether chronic fatigue, CFS, and psychiatric disorders are diseases. Although tackling these fundamental questions is beyond the scope of this chapter, it is helpful to keep these questions in mind when considering CFS and its relationship to psychiatry. Therefore, the essential elements of this controversy will be summarized here. Medical anthropology and medical sociology distinguish between (1) a "disease," which is the physician's construction of a patient's experience in professional terms and typically requires a documentable "lesion" in terms of an abnormality in laboratory investigations or imaging studies, or a pathophysiology that can be inferred; and (2) an "illness," which refers to the subjective experience of the patient and his or her family (Kleinman, 1980). Others would argue that disease refers to a wide variety of conditions that are "regarded by the medical profession and the public as properly the responsibility of the medical profession" (Guze, 1970). However, both of these definitions emphasize the wide variety of factors (e.g., social, economic, and biological) that may be involved in deciding whether a given condition constitutes a disease from the perspective of physicians. The concept of diagnosis, which follows from a medical model, posits that different conditions are associated with different etiological factors, pathophysiological mechanisms, epidemiological characteristics, clinical features, and response to treatment interventions (Guze, 1992). It is clear that, as medical knowledge has grown, there has been a commensurate change in diagnostic classification systems and nomenclature. From a strictly medical perspective, diagnoses are useful for the purposes of clarity in communication between health care providers, and direction regarding the most helpful treatment interventions. However, diagnoses also carry social connotations and values that reflect wider social processes and impact on a variety of important socially and politically determined programs such as government and private disability and health care insurance programs.

Psychiatric diagnoses have been plagued by questions of reliability and validity. It has been proposed that the characteristics of a valid psychiatric diagnosis include predictions regarding etiology, pathogenesis, course, response to treatment, and associated familial psychopathology (Guze, 1992; Robins & Guze, 1970). A psychiatric diagnosis is validated through a five-phase process of clinical description, laboratory studies, separation and delineation from other disorders, follow-up studies of natural course and response to treatment, and family studies (Robins & Guze, 1970). Until recently, no technology existed to allow such validation for most psychiatric diagnoses. Thus, psychiatric diagnosis has relied on "the careful description and analysis of the patient's history and mental status" (Guze, 1992). With advances in technology and a number of the basic sciences, it is hoped that more refined and delineated psychiatric diagnoses will become possible.

The relationship among brain dysfunction, medical and psychiatric diagnoses, and disease is further complicated by the observation that "each body part has only a restricted repertoire of . . . manifestations. In general, the same restricted repertoire will be manifested in most illnesses affecting a certain part of the body, independent of etiology, though there may be variation in the manifestations as a function of the severity and type of disturbance" (Guze, 1992). Although our knowledge of central nervous system functioning remains primitive, it is increasingly clear that symptoms such as fatigue, depression, and psychosis are not the result of single abnormalities in nervous system functioning but may come about through a variety of final common pathways. These symptoms, which may be associated with specific brain neurochemical systems, can be affected by an assortment of different types of input occurring at a variety of levels of the central nervous system and associated with many different disease processes (Guze, 1992).

Comorbidity, or the presence of more than one clinical condition in a single patient, is a concept that is of increasing interest to psychiatry. The question of whether CFS and depression are comorbid conditions or different aspects of a single condition is difficult to answer. The concept of comorbidity is much easier to examine in nonpsychiatric contexts where there is greater clarity and diagnostic validity (Guze, 1992).

MECHANISMS UNDERLYING THE PRODUCTION OF PSYCHIATRIC SYMPTOMATOLOGY

A variety of mechanisms may underlie the occurrence of psychiatric symptomatology in patients with medical illnesses. These mechanisms include many primary biological mechanisms associated with disease processes as well as

TABLE 3.1. Postulated Mechanisms for Depression Associated with Medical Illness

---

When depression precedes medical illness

- Immunological or physiological changes due to depression
- Depression as an early symptom of illness
- Self-neglect or self-harm leading to illness
- Coincidental co-occurrence

When medical illness precedes depression

- *Biological mechanisms*
    Depression-inducing drugs used in treatment of illness
    Effects of underlying illness on neurochemical pathways mediating mood
    Immunological or endocrine effects
- *Psychological mechanisms*
    Damaged self-esteem, self-efficacy, self-worth
    Alterations in body image, sense of identity
- *Social mechanisms*
    Loss of social roles, activities
    Isolation, stigma, alienation
    Financial
    Other negative life events secondary to illness

Note: Adapted from Rodin et al. (1991, p. 131). Copyright 1991 by Brunner/Mazel, Inc., New York. Adapted by permission.

secondary neurobiological events occurring in response to psychologically or socially meaningful stressors. The postulated mechanisms for depression associated with medical illness have been described at length by Rodin et al. (1991) and are summarized in Table 3.1.

ASSESSING PSYCHIATRIC SYMPTOMATOLOGY IN MEDICAL DISORDERS

The problem of assessing psychiatric symptomatology in patients with medical disorders continues to bedevil both clinicians and researchers. The measurement or assessment of depression in the medically ill has received the most study (Rodin et al., 1991; Rodin & Voshart, 1986; Silverstone, 1991). It has been demonstrated that depressive symptoms are common, occurring in up to one-third of medically ill inpatients, and major depression is diagnosed in 6% to 10% of outpatient clinic samples (Katon, 1987). The problem of assessing the significance of somatic symptoms in making a diagnosis of major depressive episode in the medically ill has been particularly salient (Endicott, 1984; Kennedy et al., 1994; Rodin et al., 1991; Rodin & Voshart, 1986; Silverstone, 1991). Less attention has been paid to the question of cognitive and affective symptoms and the impact of medical illness on these groups of symptoms. It could again be argued that these symptoms are quite common in the medically ill, independent of the presence of a major depressive episode. The question of whether depressive symptoms are the result of physiological effects of the illness or occur independently is often difficult to answer. The DSM-III-R (American Psychiatric Association, 1987) and DSM-IV (American Psychiatric Association, 1994) instruct the clinician not to count symptoms that are due to the direct physiological effects of a substance or a medical condition. Nonetheless, it is often difficult to disentangle these issues in the clinical setting. This difficulty has led to a variety of proposals for how to deal with somatic symptoms: (1) an inclusive model in which they "count" toward the psychiatric diagnosis; (2) an exclusive model in which they are excluded from "counting" toward the psychiatric diagnosis; (3) a substitutive model in which alternative criteria substitute for the somatic symptoms (Cohen-Cole et al., 1993). A number of studies have emphasized the importance of assessing symptoms in the context of the nature of the medical diagnosis, the integrity of brain structure, the level of cognitive functioning, the degree of pain and physical disability, and the duration of illness (Fava & Molnar, 1987; Popkin et al., 1987; Silverstone, 1991). Recent research evidence suggests the need to assess the reliability of somatic symptoms in differentiating between depressed and nondepressed patients within specific disease categories. For example, a study of major depression in patients with end-stage renal disease found that depressed mood or loss of interest, feelings of worthlessness or excessive guilt, anorexia, weight loss, and slowed or mixed-up thoughts differentiated between depressed and nondepressed patients, but loss of energy, insomnia, and decreased sexual interest did not (Craven et al., 1987). Although research into these questions continues, current practice supports a comparison of the results obtained using inclusive and exclusive approaches (i.e. rates of psychiatric diagnoses are calculated including and excluding somatic symptoms that could be attributed to the medical diagnosis). This approach was first used in the study of psychiatric symptomatology in diabetic patients (Lustman et al., 1986) and has subsequently been used in some studies of chronic fatigue syndrome (Kruesi et al., 1989; Wessely & Powell, 1989; Wood et al., 1991).

FATIGUE AND PSYCHOPATHOLOGY

Fatigue has been associated with a variety of forms of psychopathology in addition to a range of medical disorders. The 19th century witnessed an explosion of interest in fatigue, and there were attempts to move beyond the objective description of fatigue to the study of the subjective experience of fatigue in a wide variety of settings (Berrios, 1990; Rabinbach, 1990). A number of investigators felt that the subjective experience of fatigue was beyond measurement, and their views precluded further study of the phenomenology of the feeling of fatigue. Alienists (asylum physicians) became interested in fatigue and neurasthenia, both as etiological factors in a wide variety of mental disorders and as symptoms of mental disorders (Berrios, 1990).

Interest in chronic fatigue increased in the 1980s. A number of studies of patients with debilitating fatigue have demonstrated an association between fatigue and the presence of psychiatric disorder (Lewis & Wessely, 1992). Studies in the community (Pawlikowska et al., 1994; Price et al., 1992), in primary care settings (David et al., 1990; Kroenke et al., 1988), and in tertiary care fatigue clinics (Manu et al., 1988) have demonstrated a significant relationship between fatigue and a variety of psychiatric disorders.

MODELS OF THE RELATIONSHIP OF PSYCHIATRIC SYMPTOMATOLOGY AND CFS

A number of models have been proposed for the relationship between psychiatric symptoms/diagnoses and CFS (Abbey & Garfinkel, 1991; Ray, 1991; Zubieta et al., 1994). Four of these models (Abbey & Garfinkel, 1991), which will be discussed in greater detail in the mood disorders section, include:

1. *The psychiatric disorder as primary.* In this model, the psychiatric disorder is felt to completely explain the clinical picture that is being incorrectly diagnosed as CFS. There are two variations of this model: (a) the psychiatric disorder is seen as the only condition; and (b) the psychiatric disorder is seen as having complicated the recovery from an illness of another etiology (e.g., infectious mononucleosis). In the second variation, the psychiatric disorder is felt to be of primary significance in the protracted debility the CFS patient is experiencing.

2. *The psychiatric disorder as secondary.* In this model, the psychiatric disorder develops secondary to CFS as (a) an organic mental syndrome secondary to pathophysiological changes associated with the still unspecified primary disease process; (b) a psychological response to having a poorly understood disorder that produces stress and distress and is transduced through the central nervous system, producing a psychiatric disorder.

3. *The psychiatric disorder occurring as a concurrent or coincidental disorder.* The psychiatric disorder occurs independently or as a covariate phenomenon and is of significance because it modifies or modulates the clinical presentation and course of CFS.

4. *The psychiatric disorder as an artifact.* This model proposes that, given that there is an overlap of symptoms between CFS and many psychiatric disorders, symptoms resulting from CFS are inappropriately attributed to a psychiatric disorder that does not in fact exist apart from these CFS symptoms.

THE PSYCHIATRIC STUDY OF CFS

A number of psychiatric diagnoses have been reported in research studies of samples of CFS patients and in case series or individual case reports. The following is a list of the most commonly reported diagnoses.

1. Mood disorders
   Major depressive episode
   Dysthymic disorder
2. Anxiety disorders
   Panic disorder
   Generalized anxiety disorder
3. Somatoform disorders
   Somatization disorder
   Undifferentiated somatoform disorder

The remainder of this chapter will review each of the diagnostic categories.

Mood Disorders: Major Depression and Dysthymia

The occurrence of mood disorders in patients with CFS has received the most study of all of the psychiatric diagnoses and has been the subject of theoretical papers and commentary. The relationship between mood disorders and CFS has also been the subject of the greatest controversy and concern to advocates of the CFS diagnosis because of fears that CFS would be dismissed as "only depression." This relationship is also the topic of most of the theoretical explorations of the relationship between psychiatric disorder and CFS (Abbey & Garfinkel, 1991; Ray, 1991). The first papers relating to psychiatric factors focused on depression in postinfectious neuromyasthenia (Salit, 1985), a condition that appears to be similar to CFS (Taerk et al., 1987), and in patients with chronic fatigue (Manu et al., 1988, 1989b). The results from both groups suggested that major depression and dysthymia were common diagnoses in these populations, that major depression was more common than dysthymia, and that the mood disorders were likely to have occurred prior to the onset of the CFS, thus appearing to be "an important precursor" (Manu et al., 1989b) or risk factor for the development or chronicity of an "organic illness in psychologically susceptible individuals" (Taerk et al., 1987). Subsequent research studies are summarized in Table 3.2. All studies have found relatively high rates of current and lifetime depressive disorders, although one study found that the rates were not higher than in the questionnaire and interview studies of general community samples (Hickie et al., 1990).

The significance of these findings with respect to the etiology of CFS and its natural course has spurred controversy. Unfortunately, the cross-sectional nature of the available data does not allow us to scientifically answer these questions. It is also important to note that more complex relationships may exist. For example, if CFS is the result of an independent viral entity, it is conceivable that the development of a sustained infection would be more likely to occur or persist in the depressed patient who may have abnormalities in immune function. Although the literature on immunity and major depression is equivocal (Abbey & Garfinkel, 1991; Hickie et al., 1990; Schleifer et al., 1989; Stein et al., 1991), there is evidence to support impairment in immune functioning in some subtypes of depression (see review in Hickie et al., 1990; Stein et al., 1991). One study reported that alterations in cell-mediated immunity were found to differ in prevalence and magnitude between CFS patients and patients with major depression (Lloyd et al., 1992). The importance of the hypothalamic–pituitary axis in both depression and CFS has been discussed (Demitrack, 1994; Demitrack et al., 1989, 1991, 1992; Ray, 1991; see also Chapter 4, in this volume). Other factors may also be important. For example, social adversity has been shown to influence the development of psychiatric disorders, and especially depressive illness (odds ratio 9:1 at 2 months and 11:9 at 6 months), in patients following glandular fever or an upper respiratory tract infection (Bruce-Jones et al., 1994). At 6 months after onset, social adversity was of much greater importance than any residual effect of the infection in producing such symptoms (Bruce-Jones et al., 1994).

Depression is often overlooked as a diagnosis in medically ill patients because health care providers feel that it is "understandable" and "appropriate" to be depressed when one has a chronic illness that is associated with multiple and significant losses in occupational, social, and interpersonal functioning such as those typically sustained by CFS patients. Nonetheless, recent research has demonstrated the importance of treating depression in the medically ill and in patients with medically unexplained symptoms (Abbey, in press; Rodin et al., 1991). In the past, psychiatric wisdom held that depression should be dichotomized into (1) "reactive depression," associated with external precipitants and not thought to require treatment, and (2) "endogenous depression," which appeared to arise spontaneously, could not be explained by external circumstance, and was thought to require treatment. More recently, it has been recognized that treatment is warranted whenever

TABLE 3.2. Studies of Depression in Chronic Fatigue Syndrome

Authors	Structured Psychiatric Interview and Diagnostic Criteria	Number of Fatigue Patients	1988 CDC Criteria	Percentage with Affective Illness before Fatigue	Percentage with Major Depression		
					Current MDE	Lifetime MDE	Over Course of Illness MDE
Taerk et al. (1987)	DIS DSM-III	24	NR	50%	NR	67%	54%
Wessely & Powell (1989)	SADS RDC	47	NR	43% "prior" psychiatric history	47%	NR	NR
Kruesi et al. (1989)	DIS DSM-III	28	100%	40% depression and anxiety prior to chronic fatigue	46% 55% of women 25% of men	21%	54%
Gold et al. (1990)	DIS DSM-III	26	23% retrospective assessment	50% MDE	42%	73%	NR
Hickie et al. (1990)	SCID-P DSM-III-R	48	NR	12.5% MDE	21% (45.8% during course of illness)	NR	46%
Katon et al. (1991)	DIS DSM-III-R	98	19% of sample	53%	15.3%	76.5%	45% simultaneous to onset,15% following onset
Wood et al. (1991)	PSE CATEGO	34	NR	20.6%	23.5%	NR	NR

Note: MDE, major depressive episode; DIS, Diagnostic Interview Schedule; DSM-III and DSM-III-R, Diagnostic and Statistical Manual, third edition and Third edition, revised (American Psychiatric Association); SADS, Schedule for Affective Disorders and Schizophrenia; RDC, Research Diagnostic Criteria; SCID-P, Structured Clinical Interview (psychiatric patient version) for DSM-III-R; PSE, Present State Examination; CATEGO, computerized diagnostic system for ICD-9 diagnoses; NR, not reported. Modified from Katon and Walker (1993) and Abbey (1994).

neurovegetative changes are present (e.g., alterations in sleep and appetite, impaired concentration, fatigue, anhedonia, dysphoria, or suicidality). Treatment may take the form of antidepressant pharmacotherapy or a specific psychotherapy targeted at major depression, such as interpersonal therapy (Klerman et al., 1984) or cognitive therapy (Beck et al., 1979). Psychiatrists involved in the care of the medically ill would say that anything less is akin to observing a patient brought to an emergency room with a fractured pelvis after a motor vehicle accident and commenting "Gee, that pelvic fracture sure makes sense; after all, she was hit by a truck! . . ." and then walking away without treating the patient (Cassem, N, personal communication).

A detailed discussion of the alternative hypotheses to explain the relationship of CFS and major depression is beyond the scope of this chapter (see Abbey & Garfinkel, 1991; Ray, 1991, for further review). Instead, the hypotheses will be summarized here.

1. *CFS as misdiagnosed major depression.* This hypothesis argues that CFS is either (a) an atypical manifestation of major depression in patients who preferentially focus on bodily rather than cognitive or affective symptoms of depression; or (b) the cause of prolonged disability and slowed recovery from a viral illness, rather than ongoing or persistent viral activity or viral reactivation. The hypothesis is supported by the overlap in epidemiology between CFS and major depression with respect to gender and age (Abbey & Garfinkel, 1991); is based on the clinical heterogeneity of major depression and the differential importance of somatic symptom presentation among patients with CFS (Abbey & Garfinkel, 1991); and argues that the abnormalities in cognitive and immune function characteristic of a subsample of CFS patients may be accounted for by major depression (Abbey & Garfinkel, 1991). The hypothesis also notes the importance of major depression in protracted recovery from trauma or infection, including work on chronic brucellosis, chronic influenza, and infectious mononucleosis (Imboden et al., 1959, 1961; Straus, 1988; Wessely et al., 1989; White, 1990). This hypothesis has anecdotal support among clinicians who have successfully "cured" some patients with "CFS" in 6 weeks with an antidepressant. A case example of CFS misdiagnosed as major depression is provided in Chapter 6 of this volume. We know, based on the treatment of a large number of CFS patients and their follow-up over a protracted period of time, that this scenario is the exception rather than the rule. More commonly, patients are seen who have had clearly documented evidence or presumptive evidence based on the clinical course of an infectious illness (e.g., infectious mononucleosis, cytomegalovirus, or hepatitis A) or trauma, and then have a protracted recovery characterized by prominent depressive symptomatology. Viral titers may show no ongoing active disease and yet the patient remains very disabled. In many cases, the patient has a treatable secondary depression that are impeding recovery.

2. *Major depression as a result of CFS.* This hypothesis argues that major depression results from CFS either as a form of organic mood disorder or as part of the psychological adjustment to having a debilitating disease that is poorly understood by physicians and is characterized by repeated experiences of delegitimation (Abbey & Garfinkel, 1991; Ware, 1994). The possibility that major depression occurs as an organic mood syndrome as the result of a neurotropic virus or centrally acting immune modulators (e.g., cytokines) is supported by the literature on the central nervous system effects of viruses (Abe, 1988; Cadie et al., 1976; Greenwood, 1987; Hendler, 1987; Hendler & Leahy, 1978; Lishman, 1987) and interferon (Adams et al., 1984; Denicoff et al., 1987; Mattson et al., 1983; Smedley et al., 1983). Recent research on the psychosocial adaptation to CFS has documented the often distressing responses of caregivers, family, friends, and coworkers to patients with CFS (Ware, 1992, 1994; Ware & Kleinman, 1992). The development of depressive symptoms or a depressive disorder would not be surprising for patients in this context.

3. *CFS and major depression as covariates.* CFS and major depression may be covariate phenomena arising from a shared underlying pathophysiology that, at present, has not been identified. For example, an infectious agent or toxin could produce major depression through activity on the central nervous system, and fatigue and the other symptoms of CFS through actions both centrally and in the periphery (Abbey & Garfinkel, 1991).

4. *Major depression as an artifactual diagnosis in patients with CFS.* This hypothesis argues that diagnoses of major depression in CFS samples are artifactual and represent an overlap of certain symptoms of major depression and CFS. It also argues that these symptoms are being inaccurately attributed to major depression. Investigators have tried to deal with this concern by analyzing data in such a way that symptoms that potentially overlap between major depression and CFS are both counted toward a diagnosis of major depression and eliminated from contributing to a diagnosis of major depression (Abbey & Garfinkel, 1991). When this type of analysis has been done, no significant difference in the rates of major depression has been documented (Kruesi et al., 1989; Wessely & Powell, 1989; Wood et al., 1991). If the finding was solely artifactual, a significant difference could be expected in the rates of major depression when using these two techniques (i.e., higher rates when overlapping symptoms are counted toward a major depression diagnosis, and lower rates when they are not counted).

One of the problems in assessing the relationship between major depression and CFS is that there is increasing evidence that both conditions are quite heterogeneous. Major depression is a heterogeneous diagnosis, and its phenomenology and biological correlates may vary depending on the severity and duration of depression, the subtype of depression (e.g., melancholic, psychotic, initial vs. recurrent episode), and the presence of nonaffective co-morbid psychiatric symptoms or diagnoses (Bech, 1992). Clinicians, and patients with CFS, recognize the heterogeneity among those with CFS in terms of severity, degree of disability, and duration of illness.

In conclusion, research has demonstrated the heterogeneity of both diagnostic categories and has emphasized the need for greater study of the phenomenology of both disorders (David et al., 1988; Ray, 1991). As Ray (1991, p. 6) has stated, "We should be cautious of implicitly reifying either CFS or depression, when these diagnostic categories are little more than summary descriptors of symptoms."

Anxiety Disorders

Panic disorder and generalized anxiety disorder, as defined by DSM-III-R, have been assessed in a number of research studies of psychiatric symptomatology in patients with CFS. These findings are summarized in Table 3.3. In those studies that have assessed these diagnoses, the point prevalence has been found to be higher than in community samples. The meaning of these findings remains unclear. As with major depression, a number of symptoms potentially overlap with CFS, and alternative hypotheses can be advanced to explain the findings. The intense, episodic, and somatic nature of panic disorder may result in a misinterpretation of the symptoms as evidence of a variety of medical disorders, including varying viral activity. It is important to note that a wide variety of pathophysiological mechanisms may be associated with the production of anxiety symptoms in individuals with medical disorders (Derogatis & Wise, 1989; Goldberg & Posner, 1993).

Somatoform Disorders

Somatization and the somatoform disorders remain poorly understood. Multiple etiological determinants have been postulated (Abbey, in press). The relationship between CFS and somatization disorder, specifically, and somatization and medically unexplained symptoms, more generally, has spurred considerable discussion. Research has persuasively demonstrated that the 1988 Centers for Disease Control criteria for CFS (Holmes et al., 1988), by requiring a large number of symptoms (i.e., eight), have inadvertently increased the risk that somatization disorder patients and patients with other psychiatric disorders will be recruited into CFS samples (Katon & Russo, 1992). The recent case definition (Fukuda et al., 1994) arrived at a consensus that a somatization disorder diagnosis did not exclude an individual from a CFS diagnosis. This view is controversial. The problems of diagnosing

TABLE 3.3. Studies of Anxiety Disorders in Chronic Fatigue Syndrome

Authors	Structured Psychiatric Interview and Diagnostic Criteria	Number of Fatigue Patients	1988 CDC Criteria	Percentage with Anxiety Diagnoses before Fatigue	Current Anxiety	Lifetime Anxiety
Taerk et al. (1987)	DIS DSM-III	24	NR	NR	NR	PD = 13% SPh = 25% Soc Ph = 4% (not different from control)
Wessely & Powell (1989)	SADS RDC	47	NR	NR	PhD = 4.3% GAD = 2.1%	NR
Kruesi et al. (1989)	DIS DSM-III	28	100%	32%	NR	PD = 17.9% SPh = 28.6%
Gold et al. (1990)	DIS DSM-III	26	23% retrospective assessment	NR	NR	NR
Hickie et al. (1990)	SCID-P DSM-III-R	48	NR	PD = 2%	PD = 6.3%	NR
Katon et al. (1991)	DIS DSM-III-R	98	19% of sample	NR	PD = 11.2% GAD = 17.3%	PD = 29.6% GAD = 30.6%
Wood et al. (1991)	PSE CATEGO	34	NR	5.8%	phobic anxiety neurosis = 11.8% generalized anxiety neurosis = 5.9%	NR

Note: PD, panic disorder; SPh, simple phobia; SocPh, social phobia; GAD, generalized anxiety disorder; DIS, Diagnostic Interview Schedule; SCID-P, Structured Clinical Interview (psychiatric patient version) for DSM-III-R; DSM-III, *Diagnostic and Statistical Manual*, third edition; SADS, Schedule for Affective Disorders and Schizophrenia; RDC, Research Diagnostic Criteria; PSE, Present State Examination; CATEGO, computerized diagnostic system for ICD-9 diagnoses; NR, not reported. Modified from Katon and Walker (1993) and Abbey (1994).

CFS in patients with somatization disorder are significant. Over time, it may become clearer which symptoms are part of the longer-standing somatization disorder and which symptoms may have developed de novo in the context of CFS. The most difficult scenario, both clinically and theoretically, is the question of diagnosing CFS in an adolescent who has already reported some medically unexplained symptoms, but has not had sufficient symptoms to warrant a somatization disorder or other somatoform disorder diagnosis. The somatoform disorders share a common feature of the "presence of physical symptoms that suggest a general medical condition (hence the term somatoform) and are not fully explained by a general medical condition, by the direct effects of a substance, or by another mental disorder" (American Psychiatric Association, 1994). Large-scale epidemiological studies of somatoform disorders have not been done, but they appear to be more common in medical settings (Abbey, in press). Somatoform disorders have received relatively little study in CFS samples apart from the diagnosis of somatization disorder.

Somatization disorder has been assessed in samples of patients with chronic fatigue (Manu et al., 1989a) and chronic fatigue syndrome (Hickie et al., 1990; Katon et al., 1991; Kruesi et al., 1989; Wessely et al., 1989; Wood et al., 1991). Somatization disorder, although uncommon in the community (e.g., 0.1%–2% lifetime prevalence), is overrepresented in clinical samples, especially in patients with chronic medical illnesses where the rate may be as high as 5% (Abbey, in press). Not unexpectedly, there appear to be increased rates of somatization disorder in patients with CFS (see Table 3.4). Among 100 patients presenting to a chronic fatigue clinic, 15 were diagnosed by the Diagnostic Interview Schedule (DIS) to have somatization disorder (Manu et al., 1989a). This group had a mean age of onset of 16.3 years for the somatization disorder and 23.5 years for fatigue, which had been present for an average of 19 years' duration. Symptoms reported more frequently by patients with somatization disorder included pain in the extremities, joint pain, other pain, shortness of breath, chest pain, blurred vision, muscle weakness or paralysis, and sexual indifference. In a larger cohort from the same group, somatization disorder was diagnosed using the DIS in 28% of 60 patients meeting the CDC criteria and in only 5% of fatigued controls age- and gender-matched from the same cohort. When abridged criteria for somatization (Escobar et al., 1987, 1989) were used, a much higher percentage of individuals were identified as demonstrating significant somatization—73% of the CFS subjects and 51% of controls when all symptoms were used, and 67% and 43% respectively when the abridged criteria did not include symptoms characteristic of CFS. Of note, 88% of the CFS patients meeting criteria for somatization disorder experienced significant functional somatic symptoms prior to the onset of the CFS, with the first symptom generally occurring in childhood.

TABLE 3.4. Studies of Somatization Disorder in Chronic Fatigue Syndrome

Authors	Structured Psychiatric Interview and Diagnostic Criteria	Number of Fatigue Patients	1988 CDC Criteria	Percentage with Somatoform Diagnoses before CFS	Current Somatization Disorder	Current Undifferentiated Somatoform Disorder
Taerk et al. (1987)	DIS DSM-III	24	NR	NR	NR	NR
Wessely & Powell (1989)	SADS RDC	47	NR	NR	15%	NR
Kruesi et al. (1989)	DIS DSM-III	28	100%	NR	10% if CFS symptoms excluded, 14.3% if included	NR
Gold et al. (1990)	DIS DSM-III	26	23 retrospective assessment	NR	NR	Increased rate of somatic symptoms on DIS—average of 9.7 symptoms
Hickie et al. (1990)	SCID-P DSM-III-R	48	NR	2.1%	0%	0%
Katon et al. (1991)	DIS DSM-III-R	98	19% of sample	NR	20% if CFS symptoms excluded, 46% if included	NR
Wood et al. (1991)	PSE CATEGO	34	NR	5.9%	5.9%	NR

Note: DIS, Diagnostic Interview Schedule; DSM-III and III-R, *Diagnostic and Statistical Manual*, third edition & third edition, revised (American Psychiatric Association); SADS, Schedule for Affective Disorders and Schizophrenia; RDC, Research Diagnostic Criteria; SCID-P, Structured Clinical Interview (psychiatric patient version) for DSM-III-R; PSE, Present State Examination; CATEGO, computerized diagnostic system for ICD-9 diagnoses; NR, not reported.

The relationship of reported food intolerance to somatization and somatization disorder has been studied in patients with chronic fatigue (Manu et al., 1993). In a sample of 200 patients, 27 (13.5%) reported intolerance to three or more foods. When compared with age- and gender-matched patients from the same sample, the food-intolerant groups reported more lifetime functional somatic symptoms (8.7 vs. 6.2) and a significantly higher prevalence of somatization disorders (33% vs. 7%). However, given that only 1 of the 27 patients with multiple food intolerance met the 1988 CDC criteria for CFS, it is difficult to extrapolate these findings to patients meeting the criteria.

Patients with conversion disorders presenting as CFS have been reported in the literature (Wessely & Powell, 1989) and anecdotally, but appear to be quite rare. These patients have been characterized by being in what they perceive as markedly overwhelming, highly personally charged situations that exceeded their coping capacities. These situations were heavily laden with dynamic meaning and were highly conflictual for the patient.

A controversial suggestion has been put forward by medical historian Edward Shorter: that CFS and chronic pain syndromes are common modern manifestations of conversion symptoms or conversion disorder. Shorter argues that conversion symptoms have moved from their 19th-century focus on the motor side of the nervous system to the sensory side of the nervous system because sensory symptoms are "more difficult to disprove medically" (Shorter, 1992, p. 285). He notes, "In addition to psychogenic pain, fatigue is the other great somatoform symptom of the end of the twentieth century" (1992, p. 300). As expected, this view has been actively challenged.

Substance Use Disorders

A number of individuals recovering from substance use disorders have markedly impaired energy and heightened fatigability. In part, this fatigue is related to sleep disturbance that may continue for months after the discontinuation of alcohol, benzodiazepines, or sedative hypnotics. At present, substance use within the preceding 2 years is considered to be an exclusionary criterion for the diagnosis of CFS (Fukuda et al., 1994).

Substance use disorders have received surprisingly little study in samples of patients with CFS or chronic fatigue. In a study of 100 patients attending a chronic fatigue clinic, 28 had a lifetime history of substance use (Kranzler et al., 1991)—a rate that exceeds the lifetime prevalence of 15% to 18% in community samples (Robins et al., 1984). Current substance abuse or dependence was described by 10 of 100 patients (Kranzler et al., 1991). Substance abuse disorders did not seem to influence the characteristics of chronic fatigue, although the coexistence of a substance use disorder was associated with a greater severity of depressive symptomatology. Only two studies report on data regarding substance use and abuse in patients with CFS or CFS-like conditions. A lifetime prevalence of alcohol abuse or dependence was reported by 10.7% of the CFS subjects in one sample (Kruesi et al., 1989) and a history of alcohol dependence prior to the onset of CFS was reported by 8% of CFS-like subjects (as defined by the Australian case definition criteria) and their relatives (Hickie et al., 1990). There are many anecdotal stories of physicians not taking an adequate substance abuse history and missing a primary substance use diagnosis. A case example is provided in Chapter 6 of this volume.

Seasonal Affective Disorder

Two cases of seasonal affective disorder that initially presented as CFS have been reported (Lam, 1991). Subsequently, seasonal symptom variation has been studied in one cohort of 73 patients with chronic idiopathic fatigue of whom 50 met CDC case definition criteria (Zubieta et al., 1994). Patients with chronic fatigue showed less seasonality in symptoms than did comparison groups of patients with major depression, atypical depression, and seasonal affective disorder (Zubieta et al., 1994). There were no significant differences between fatigue patients who showed high versus low seasonality in their symptomatology. Interestingly, women comprise 60% to 90% of individuals with a seasonal pattern to their depression, and it is unclear whether being a woman adds a specific risk for seasonality beyond that associated with the risk for recurrent major depressive disorder (American Psychiatric Association, 1994).

Eating Disorders

Patients with a primary eating disorder such as anorexia nervosa or bulimia nervosa have presented with physician or self-made diagnoses of CFS. Although, in the popular image, these patients are seen as being excessively active in order to burn calories, a number are, in fact, lethargic or fatigued. Fatigue, poor concentration, irritability, lability of mood, anxiety, and depression have been associated with prolonged caloric restriction such as occurs in anorexia nervosa (Garfinkel & Garner, 1982). Symptoms that could be attributed to CFS, such as fatigue, dizziness, and sleep difficulties, are among the most common physical symptoms observed with anorexics and bulimics (Garner & Garfinkel, 1985). Clinicians have also noted the difficulty in making a CFS diagnosis in the context of morbid obesity. The 1994 case definition criteria specifically exclude severely obese individuals with a body mass index of greater than 45 (Fukuda et al., 1994).

Obsessive–Compulsive Disorder

This disorder is characterized by the presence of either obsessions (i.e., recurrent, persistent, intrusive, unwanted thoughts that the individual tries to suppress or neutralize with other thoughts or actions, and which cause marked distress) or compulsions (i.e., repetitive behaviors or mental acts that the individual is driven to perform and that are aimed at reducing distress by preventing a dreaded event) (American Psychiatric Association, 1994). Enormous amounts of energy may be expended in carrying out compulsive behaviors or warding off obsessional thoughts. Simple activities such as going to the store may be extremely energy- and time-consuming for an individual with obsessive–compulsive disorder. For such an individual, the activity of leaving the house, which would be for most of us a 15-minute activity with minimal mental or physical strain, would require hours of preparation (e.g., prolonged bathing, checking that the stove is off, and making sure the door is locked), shopping would cause significant emotional distress (e.g., fears of contamination, fears of hurting someone with the shopping cart, fears of picking up a knife on sale in the store and stabbing others), and returning home would require lengthy decontamination behaviors or rituals. Patients with obsessive–compulsive disorder are usually ashamed of their behaviors and reluctant to spontaneously reveal them to clinicians, but when the appropriate questions are asked, they will typically answer truthfully.

Factitious Disorders and Malingering

Given the ongoing questions as to the nature of CFS and the lack of a diagnostic laboratory test, it is not surprising that there are concerns on the part of the disability insurance industry and government disability plans that CFS has become a "diagnosis of choice" for a number of patients with factitious disorders or malingering. There is an important distinction between these two diagnostic categories: although both are characterized by intentional symptom production, they differ with respect to the reason(s) for symptom production. Factitious disorders are defined by the intentional production of physical or psychological signs or symptoms, including subjective complaints for the unconscious purpose of assuming the sick role. This definition is in contrast to malingering, where there is intentional symptom production or reporting but the conscious goal of such behavior is external incentives. Most clinicians do not include these disorders within their differential diagnosis because they assume that patients are coming in good faith for help with symptoms that they have not intentionally produced. They more commonly enter this differential diagnosis when individuals are seen for medicolegal assessments or independent medical examinations with regard to disability insurance. As with the assessment of malingering with respect to other diagnoses, malingering should be suspected if there is "any combination of the following: (1) a medicolegal context of presentation; (2) a marked discrepancy between the person's claimed stress or disability and the objective findings; (3) lack of cooperation during the diagnostic evaluation and in complying with prescribed treatment regimen; (4) the presence of antisocial personality disorder" (American Psychiatric Association, 1994).

Factitious disorder by proxy, which is colloquially known as Munchausen by proxy (Meadow, 1977), is the diagnosis used when the fabrication of symptoms in order to elicit care is done by another person, usually by a mother to a child. Mothers have been reported, by several English pediatricians, to describe myalgic encephalomyelitis in their children in a manner consistent with factitious disorder by proxy (Harris & Taitz, 1989; MacDonald, 1989).

REFERENCES

Abe, K. Depression after each respiratory tract infection in an adolescent girl. *J Nerv Ment Dis* 1988; 176:573–574.

Abbey, SE, Garfinkel, PE. Chronic fatigue syndrome and depression: Cause, effect or covariate. *Rev Infect Dis* 1991; 13(Suppl 1):S73–S83.

Abbey, SE. Psychopharmacology and chronic fatigue syndrome. In Straus, S, ed., *Chronic fatigue syndrome.* New York: Marcel Dekker, 1994; 405–434.

Abbey, SE. Physical symptoms and somatoform disorders. In Rundell, J, Wise, M, eds., *American Psychiatric Press textbook of consultation-liaison psychiatry.* Washington, DC: American Psychiatric Press, 1996.

Adams, F, Quesada, JR, Gutterman, JU. Neuropsychiatric manifestations of human leukocyte interferon therapy in patients with cancer. *JAMA* 1984; 252:938–941.

American Psychiatric Association. *Diagnostic and statistical manual of mental disorders,* third edition, revised (DSM-III-R). Washington, DC: American Psychiatric Association, 1987.

American Psychiatric Association. *Diagnostic and statistical manual of mental disorders,* fourth edition. Washington, DC: American Psychiatric Association, 1994.

Bech, P. Symptoms and assessment of depression. In Paykel, ES, ed., *Handbook of affective disorders,* second edition, New York: Guilford Press, 1992; 3–14.

Beck, AT, Rush, AJ, Shaw, BF, Emery, G. *Cognitive therapy of depression.* New York: Guilford Press, 1979.

Berrios, GE. Feelings of fatigue and psychopathology: A conceptual history. *Compr Psychiatry* 1990; 31:140–151.

Bruce-Jones, WDA, White, PD, Thomas, JM, Clare, AW. The effect of social adversity on the fatigue syndrome, psychiatric disorders and physical recovery, following glandular fever. *Psychol Med* 1994; 24:651–659.

Cadie, M, Nye, FJ, Storey, P. Anxiety and depression after infectious mononucleosis. *Br J Psychiatry* 1976; 128:559–561.

Cohen-Cole, SA, Brown, FW, McDaniel, JS. Assessment of depression and grief reactions in the medically ill. In Stoudemire, A, Fogel, B, eds., *Psychiatric care of the medical patient*. New York: Oxford University Press, 1993; 53–70.

Craven, JL, Rodin, GM, Johnson, L, Kennedy, SH. The diagnosis of major depression in renal dialysis patients. *Psychosom Med* 1987; 49:482–492.

David, A, Pelosi, A, McDonald, E, Stephens, D, Ledger, D, Rathbone, R, Mann, A. Tired, weak, or in need of rest: Fatigue among general practice attenders. *Br Med J* 1990; 301:1199–1202.

David, AS, Wessely, S, Pelosi, AJ. Postviral fatigue syndrome: Time for a new approach. *Br Med J* 1988; 296:696–699.

Demitrack, MA. Chronic fatigue syndrome: A disease of the hypothalamic–pituitary–adrenal axis. *Ann Med* 1994; 26:1–5.

Demitrack, MA, Dale, JK, Gold, PW, Chrousos, GP, Straus, SE. Neuroendocrine abnormalities in patients with chronic fatigue syndrome. *Clin Res* 1989; 37:532A.

Demitrack, MA, Dale, JK, Straus, SE, Laue, L, Listwak, SJ, Kruesi, MJP, Chrousos, GP, Gold, PW. Evidence for impaired activation of the hypothalamic-pituitary-adrenal axis in patients with chronic fatigue syndrome. *J Clin Endo Metab* 1991; 73(6):1224–1234.

Demitrack, MA, Gold, PW, Dale, JK, Krahn, DD, Kling, MA, Straus, SE. Plasma and cerebrospinal fluid monoamine metabolism in patients with chronic fatigue syndrome: Preliminary findings. *Biol Psychiatry* 1992; 32:1065–1077.

Denicoff, KD, Rubinow, DR, Papa, MZ, Simpson, C, Seipp, CA, Lotze, MT, Change, AE, Rosenstein, D, Rosenberg, SA. The neuropsychiatric effects of treatment with interleukin-2 and lymphokine-activated killer cells. *Ann Int Med* 1987; 107:293–300.

Derogatis, LR, Wise, TN. *Anxiety and depressive disorders in the medical patient*. Washington, DC: American Psychiatric Press, 1989.

Endicott, J. Measurement of depression in patients with cancer. *Cancer* 1984; 53(Suppl 10):2243–2249.

Escobar, JI, Burnam, MA, Karno, M, Forsythe, A, Golding, JM. Somatization in the community. *Arch Gen Psychiatry* 1987; 44:713–718.

Escobar, JI, Manu, P, Matthews, D, Lane, T, Swartz, M, Canino, G. Medically unexplained physical symptoms, somatization disorder and abridged somatization: Studies with the Diagnostic Interview Schedule. *Psychiatric Dev* 1989; 3:235–245.

Fava, GA, Molnar, G. Criteria for diagnosing depression in the setting of medical disease. *Psychother Psychosom* 1987; 48:21–25.

Frasure-Smith, N, Lesperance, F, Talajic, M. Depression following myocardial infarction: Impact on 6-month survival. *JAMA* 1993; 270:1819–1825.

Fukuda, K, Straus, SE, Hickie, I, Sharpe, MC, Dobbins, JG, Komaroff, A, and the International Chronic Fatigue Syndrome Study Group. The chronic fatigue syndrome: A comprehensive approach to its definition and study. *Ann Int Med* 1994; 121(12):953–959.

Garfinkel, PE, Garner, DM. *Anorexia nervosa: A multidimensional perspective*. New York: Brunner/Mazel, 1982.

Garner, DM, Garfinkel, PE, eds., *Handbook of psychotherapy for anorexia nervosa and bulimia.* New York: Guilford Press, 1985.

Gold, D, Bowden, R, Sixbey, J, Riggs, R, Katon, WJ, Ashley, R, Obrigewitch, RM, Corey, L. Chronic fatigue: A prospective clinical and virologic study. *JAMA* 1990; 264(1):48–53.

Goldberg, RJ, Posner, DA. Anxiety in the medically ill. In Stoudemire, A, Fogel, B, eds., *Psychiatric care of the medical patient.* New York: Oxford University Press, 1993; 87–104.

Greenwood, R. Residual mental disorders after herpesvirus infections. In Kurstak, E, Lipowski, ZJ, Morozov, PV, eds., *Viruses, immunity and mental disorders.* New York: Plenum, 1987; 65–80.

Guze, SB. The need for toughmindedness in psychiatric thinking. *South Med J* 1970; 63:662–671.

Guze, SB. *Why psychiatry is a branch of medicine.* New York: Oxford University Press, 1992.

Harris, F, Taitz, LS. Damaging diagnoses of myalgic encephalitic in children. *Br Med J* 1989; 299:790.

Hendler, N. Infectious mononucleosis and psychiatric disorders. In Kurstak, E, Lipowksi, ZJ, Morozov, PV, eds., *Viruses, immunity and mental disorders.* New York: Plenum, 1987; 81–94.

Hendler, N, Leahy, W. Psychiatric and neurologic sequelae of infectious mononucleosis. *Am J Psychiatry* 1978; 135:842–844.

Hickie, I, Lloyd, A, Wakefield, D, Parker, G. The psychiatric status of patients with chronic fatigue syndrome. *Br J Psychiatry* 1990; 156:534–540.

Hickie, I, Silove, D, Hickie, C, Wakefield, D, Lloyd, A. Is there immune dysfunction in depressive disorders? *Psychol Med* 1990; 20:755–761.

Holmes, GP, Kaplan, JE, Gantz, NM, Komaroff, AL, Schonberger, LB, Straus, SE, Jones, JF, Dubois, RE, Cunningham-Rundlls, C, Pahwa, S, Tosato, G, Zegans, LS, Purtilo, DT, Brown, N, Schooley, RT, Brus, I. Chronic fatigue syndrome: A working case definition. *Ann Int Med* 1988; 108:387–389.

Imboden, JB, Canter, A, Cluff, LE. Convalescence from influenza: A study of the psychological and clinical determinants. *Arch Int Med* 1961; 108:115–121.

Imboden, JB, Canter, A, Cluff, LE, Trever, RW. Brucellosis: III. Psychological aspects of delayed convalescence. *AMA Arch Intern Med* 1959; 103:406–414.

Katon, W. The epidemiology of depression in medical care. *Int J Psychiatry Med* 1987; 17:93–112.

Katon, W, Buchwald, DS, Simon, GE, Russo, JE, Mease, PJ. Psychiatric illness in patients with chronic fatigue and those with rheumatoid arthritis. *J Gen Intern Med* 1991; 6:277–285.

Katon, W, Russo, J. Chronic fatigue syndrome criteria: A critique of the requirement for multiple physical complaints. *Arch Int Med* 1992; 152:1604–1609.

Katon, WJ, Walker, EA. The relationship of chronic fatigue to psychiatric illness in community, primary care and tertiary care samples. In Bock, GR, Whelan, J, eds., *Chronic fatigue syndrome,* Ciba Foundation Symposium 173. New York: John Wiley & Sons, 1993; 193–211.

Kennedy, SH, Kaplan, AS, Garfinkel, PE, Rockert, W, Toner, B, Abbey, SE. Depression in anorexia nervosa and bulimia nervosa: Discriminating depressive symptoms and episodes. *J Psychosom Res* 1994; 38:773–782.

Kleinman, A. *Patients and healers in the context of culture: An exploration of the borderland between anthropology, medicine and psychiatry.* Berkeley: University of California Press, 1980.

Klerman, GL, Weissman, MM, Rounsaville, BJ, Chevron, ES. *Interpersonal psychotherapy of depression.* New York: Basic Books, 1984.

Kranzler, HR, Manu, P, Hesselbrock, VM, Lane, TJ, Matthews, DA. Substance use disorders in patients with chronic fatigue. *Hosp Comm Psychiatry* 1991; 42:924–928.

Kroenke, K, Wood, DR, Mangelsdorff, AD, Meier, NJ, Powell, JB. Chronic fatigue in primary care: Prevalence, patient characteristics and outcome. *JAMA* 1988; 260:929–934.

Kruesi, MJP, Dale, J, Straus, SE. Psychiatric diagnoses in patients who have chronic fatigue syndrome. *J Clin Psychiatry* 1989; 50:53–56.

Lam, RW. Seasonal affective disorder presenting as chronic fatigue syndrome. *Can J Psychiatry* 1991; 36:680–682.

Lewis, G, Wessely, S. The epidemiology of fatigue: More questions than answers. *J Epid Comm Health* 1992; 46:92–97.

Lipkin, M. Psychiatry and medicine. In Kaplan, HI, Sadock, BJ, eds., *Comprehensive textbook of psychiatry/IV.* Baltimore: Williams & Wilkins, 1985; 1263–1277.

Lishman, WA. *Organic psychiatry: The psychological consequences of cerebral disorder,* second edition. Boston: Blackwell Scientific Publications, 1987.

Lloyd, A, Hickie, I, Hickie, C, Dwyer, J, Wakefield, D. Cell-mediated immunity in patients with chronic fatigue syndrome, healthy control subjects and patients with major depression. *Clin Exp Immunol* 1992; 87:76–79.

Lustman, PJ, Harper, GW, Griffith, LS, Clouse, RE. Use of the Diagnostic Interview Schedule in patients with diabetes mellitus. *J Nerv Ment Dis* 1986; 174:743–746.

MacDonald, TM. Myalgic encephalomyelitis by proxy. *Br Med J* 1989; 299:1030.

Manu, P, Lane, TJ, Matthews, DA. Somatization disorder in patients with chronic fatigue. *Psychosomatics* 1989a; 30:388–395.

Manu, P, Matthews, DA, Lane, TJ. The mental health of patients with a chief complaint of chronic fatigue: A prospective evaluation and follow-up. *Arch Int Med* 1988; 148:2213–2217.

Manu, P, Matthews, DA, Lane, TJ. Food intolerance in patients with chronic fatigue. *Int J Eating Dis* 1993; 13:203–209.

Manu, P, Matthews, DA, Lane, TJ, Tennen, H, Hesselbrock, V, Mendola, R, Affleck, G. Depression among patients with a chief complaint of chronic fatigue. *J Affect Dis* 1989b; 17:165–172.

Mattson, K, Niiranen, A, Iivanainen, M, Farkkila, M, Bergstron, L, Holsti, LR, Kauppinen, J-L, Cantell, K. Neurotoxicity of interferon. *Cancer Treat Rep* 1983; 67:958–961.

Meadow, R. Munchausen syndrome by proxy—the hinterland of child abuse. *Lancet* 1977; ii:343–345.

Pawlikowska, T, Chalder, T, Hirsch, SR, Wallace, P, Wright, DJM, Wessely, SC. Population based study of fatigue and psychological distress. *Br Med J* 1994; 308:763–766.

Popkin, MK, Callies, AL, Colon, EA. A framework for the study of medical depression: A practical approach to classifying depression in the medically ill. *Psychosomatics* 1987; 28:27–33.

Price, RK, North, CS, Wessely, S, Fraser, VJ. Estimating the prevalence of chronic fatigue syndrome and associated symptoms in the community. *Public Health Reports* 1992; 107:514–522.

Rabinbach, A. *The human motor: Energy, fatigue, and the origins of modernity.* New York: Basic Books, 1990.

Ray, C. Chronic fatigue syndrome and depression: Conceptual and methodological ambiguities. *Psychol Med* 1991; 21:1–9.

Robins, E, Guze, SB. Establishment of diagnostic validity in psychiatric illness: Its application to schizophrenia. *Am J Psychiatry* 1970; 126:983–987.

Robins, LN, Helzer, JE, Weissman, MM, Orvaschel, H, Gruenberg, E, Burke, JD, Jr., Regier, DA. Lifetime prevalence of specific psychiatric disorders in three sites. *Arch Gen Psychiatry* 1984; 41:949–958.

Rodin, G, Craven, J, Littlefield, C. *Depression in the medically ill.* New York: Brunner/Mazel, 1991.

Rodin, G, Voshart, K. Depression in the medically ill: An overview. *Am J Psychiatry* 1986; 143:696–705.

Salit, IE. Sporadic postinfectious neuromyasthenia. *Can Med Assoc J* 1985; 133:659–663.

Schleifer, SJ, Keller, SE, Bond, RN, Cohen, J, Stein, M. Major depressive disorder and immunity: Role of age, sex, severity and hospitalization. *Arch Gen Psychiatry* 1989; 46:81–87.

Shorter, E. *From paralysis to fatigue: A history of psychosomatic illness in the modern era.* New York: Free Press, 1992.

Silverstone, PH. Depression increases mortality and morbidity in acute life-threatening medical illness. *J Psychosom Res* 1990; 34:651–657.

Silverstone, PH. Measuring depression in the physically ill. *Int J Methods Psychiatric Res* 1991; 1:3–12.

Smedley, H, Katrak, M, Sikora, K, Wheeler, T. Neurological effects of recombinant human interferon. *Br Med J* 1983; 286:262–264.

Stein, M, Miller, AH, Trestman, RL. Depression, the immune system, and health and illness: Findings in search of meaning. *Arch Gen Psychiatry* 1991; 48:171–177.

Stoudemire, A, Fogel, BS. *Psychiatric care of the medical patient.* New York: Oxford University Press, 1993.

Straus, SE. The chronic mononucleosis syndrome. *J Infect Dis* 1988; 157:405–412.

Taerk, GS, Toner, BB, Salit, IE, Garfinkel, PE, Ozersky, S. Depression in patients with neuromyasthenia (benign myalgic encephalomyelitis). *Int J Psychiatry Med* 1987; 17:49–56.

Ware, NC. Suffering and the social construction of illness: The delegitimation of illness experience in chronic fatigue syndrome. *Med Anthro Quart* 1992; 6(4):347–461.

Ware, NC. An anthropological approach to understanding chronic fatigue syndrome. In Straus, S, ed., *Chronic fatigue syndrome.* New York: Marcel Dekker, 1994; 85–97.

Ware, NC, Kleinman, A. Culture and somatic experience: The social course of illness in neurasthenia and chronic fatigue syndrome. *Psychosom Med* 1992; 54:546–560.

Wessely, S, David, A, Butler, S, Chalder, T. Management of chronic (post-viral) fatigue syndrome. *J Roy Coll Gen Pract* 1989; 39:26–29.

Wessely, S, Powell, R. Fatigue syndromes: A comparison of chronic "postviral" fatigue with neuromuscular and affective disorders. *J Neurol Neurosurg Psychiatry* 1989; 52:940–948.

White, PD. Fatigue and chronic fatigue syndromes. In Bass, CM, ed., *Somatization: Physical symptoms and psychological illness.* Oxford: Blackwell Scientific Publications, 1990; 104–140.

Wood, GC, Bentall, RP, Gopfert, M, Edwards, RHT. A comparative psychiatric assessment of patients with chronic fatigue syndrome and muscle disease. *Psychol Med* 1991; 21:619–628.

Zubieta, JK, Engleberg, NC, Yargic, LI, Pande, AC, Demitrack, MA. Seasonal symptom variation in patients with chronic fatigue: Comparison with major mood disorders. *J Psychiatric Res* 1994; 28:13–22.

4

The Psychobiology of Chronic Fatigue: The Central Nervous System as a Final Common Pathway

Mark A. Demitrack, M.D.

C hronic fatigue syndrome is an illness that is formed, in large part, by the complex context in which it is diagnosed—namely, the relationship between the symptom experience of the patient and the conceptual frame of reference of the diagnosing clinician. Because of this relationship, the particular biological model(s) employed by the patient and physician to talk about the nature of the disease process can have a tremendous influence on diagnosis, treatment, and outcome. For both the patient and the physician, intolerance of ambiguity is high. If the physician is unable to provide a definitive diagnosis, supported by objective testing, the patient may become doubtful of the physician's clinical skill. As a result, the patient's anxiety about the nature of the disease process is likely to increase, often prompting consultation with a different clinician. To avoid this outcome, the physician may reject the patient first, by outright dismissal of the validity of the patient's reported symptoms. Alternatively, the physician may pursue more exotic and expensive laboratory testing, justifying the cost, not as a search for a definitive diagnostic result, but to assemble "corroborating disease markers."

Given these considerations, it may not be surprising that, in the contemporary literature on chronic fatigue syndrome, an infectious/inflammatory disease model has been held preeminent over all others. Many investigators have commented that such a model is more acceptable to both patient and physician, by positing a discrete, external cause for the illness, and hence minimizing the self-blame that may ensue with a more ambiguous (usually psychological) diagnostic model. Moreover, an infectious/inflammatory disease model provides an endless array of diagnostic tests and treatment interventions that may be utilized to monitor the course of the disease. In this type of model, the patient typically assumes the role of a passive recipient of diagnostic and therapeutic manipulation, and the physician's interventive posture is encouraged. The powerful allure of this explanatory model is underscored by its persistence despite indeterminate scientific evidence supporting its validity as the principal pathogenetic process underlying the onset and course of chronic fatigue syndrome. Wilson and colleagues (1994), in a recent longitudinal study of outcome in chronic fatigue syndrome, showed that one of the most powerful predictors of functional impairment, over time, was the strong conviction of a physical disease process at initial evaluation, often to the exclusion of consideration of psychological factors in the disease process. Other factors, such as measures of cell-mediated immunity, duration of illness, age at onset, premorbid psychiatric diagnosis, or trait neuroticism, did not predict outcome. This finding was consistent with an earlier report of treatment outcome (Sharpe et al., 1994).

It is my contention that the formulation of alternate models of disease pathogenesis for chronic fatigue syndrome is not only possible, but is imperative to a favorable outcome, if for no other reason than that exploring different illness models increases the repertoire of potentially available recuperative strategies for the patient. Research, such as the report by Wilson and coworkers, is consistent with the view that the clinical course of chronic fatigue syndrome is determined by multiple factors. Hence, unimodal linear disease models that foster a passive role for the patient in clinical diagnosis and treatment are inappropriate. A model of illness that proposes multiple interactive events in the development of the clinical symptoms is more consistent with actual experience. Such a model encourages the active involvement of the patient in his or her own recovery. Furthermore, emerging treatment results are demonstrating the efficacy of multidimensional approaches, often utilizing cognitive-behavioral treatment techniques (see Chapters 9–11, this volume).

The purpose of this chapter is to increase understanding of (1) the potential relevance of disturbances in the function of the central nervous system to the development of chronic fatigue syndrome, and (2) how consideration of these issues may help in the formulation of a more integrative model of this illness and its treatment. I will show that an integrative model provides a much more congenial framework, allowing the patient and clinician to explore and understand the role of psychological and behavioral factors in the precipitation and perpetuation of chronic fatigue syndrome. To accomplish this, I will survey the biological studies of chronic fatigue syndrome that exist in the peer-reviewed, published literature. Much of this initial work was fraught with methodological confounds (see Table 4.1) that are, thankfully, being addressed in current studies. The most common examples of these problems include the

TABLE 4.1. Methodological Confounds in Biological Studies of
Chronic Fatigue Syndrome: Important Questions for Consideration

- What are the hypotheses under study?
- Is the study design appropriate to test the hypothesis?
- Problems in subject characterization:
    What is the source of the subjects?
    Which chronic fatigue syndrome definition is being employed?
    Is the psychiatric diagnostic status being assessed? How?
    Are the psychiatric symptoms being assessed? How?
    What is the disability status?
    Are the gender and age of the subjects specified?
    Is there a family history of medical or psychiatric illness?
    Are the subjects medication-free? For how long?
    What are the patients' attitudes regarding disease cause?
    What are the patients' activity levels?
    Is the method of matching to comparison subjects specified?
- What clinical algorithm was employed to determine subject "caseness"?
- Which comparison groups were chosen? Why?
- What screening methods were used for the comparison subjects?
- If it was a biological study:
    Is the collection method detailed?
    Are the samples being run in a blinded fashion?
    What is the variability in the biological determination?
    What is known about the nature of this biological variable in other diseases?
    Is an appropriate distinction made between causation and association?

use of inappropriate comparison groups; the absence of a clear delineation of
medication-free status prior to study; the failure to systematically employ a
consensually agreed-on, published, operationalized case definition and a corresponding algorithm for its clinical validation; the failure to include appropriate
descriptions of the study subjects (e.g., age and gender, or other relevant descriptive variables that could conceivably confound the results). It is important
to keep these issues in mind when considering the potential implications of
these reports.

   Five principal domains of study are relevant to the theme of this chapter:
(1) immunology, (2) neuroendocrinology, (3) polysomnography, (4) neuroimaging, and (5) neurotransmitter function. The following questions should
be kept in mind as these areas of investigation are discussed.

- Are there any biological correlates of chronic fatigue syndrome that
  may distinguish it from psychiatric illnesses as they are currently
  understood?

- What are the implications of these studies with respect to diagnostic testing for this illness?
- What is the evidence for causal relationships between specific biological events and clinical symptoms of the illness?
- How may these research findings play a role in the clinical management of patients with chronic fatigue syndrome?
- Taken as a whole, would these data suggest that it is more reasonable to view chronic fatigue syndrome as a medical illness or a psychiatric illness?

IMMUNOLOGY

As I have already stated, an immunological and/or infectious model for the pathogenesis of chronic fatigue syndrome remains among the most popular conceptual frameworks for understanding this illness. A complete examination of this topic is beyond the scope of this chapter. Nevertheless, in this section, I will review several important lines of evidence that have been used to bolster this view. Chapter 7 provides a further discussion of the role of infections in the development of chronic fatigue syndrome, as do several other recent reviews of this topic (Lloyd et al., 1993b; Strober, 1994).

Chapter 1 noted that the view that persistent, unexplained fatiguing illnesses are etiologically related to specific infectious agents can be traced to the early portions of this century, in association with events such as the Los Angeles County Hospital epidemic and the Royal Free Hospital outbreak. Among the infectious agents that have been studied as putative etiological factors in the development of chronic fatigue syndrome, Epstein–Barr virus (EBV), a member of the herpes virus family, remains among the most notorious in contemporary medical practice. It is not unusual for patients and physicians to presume that specific patterns of EBV serology are definitive diagnostic tests for chronic fatigue syndrome. A discussion of some of the studies that have fueled an interest in this agent is worthwhile because these studies have also served as the principal entry point in contemporary research of immune function in this illness.

Epstein–Barr virus is now well known as the most common cause of infectious mononucleosis in humans. In addition, EBV is implicated in the development of certain lymphomas, and in nasopharyngeal carcinoma. Although the primary infection with this agent is frequently not clinically apparent, it has long been known that infectious mononucleosis is associated with a protracted course of clinical recuperation in a substantial number of individuals. For instance, in 1948, Isaacs published a description of 53 patients with clinically substantiated infectious mononucleosis whose illness subsequently evolved into a persistent clinical condition characterized by profound fatigue, along with exhaustion, aching of legs, weakness, depression, mild feverishness, and low blood pressure. The striking clinical presentation appeared at odds with the absence of remarkable laboratory data and the apparently normal physical examination.

In 1982, Martin Tobi and his colleagues renewed an interest in this clinical entity by publishing a case series of seven patients with an atypical illness characterized by "non-specific symptoms of malaise, low-grade fever . . . weight loss . . . emotional distress, gastrointestinal discomfort, and myalgia. . . ." The characteristic atypical lymphocytosis of acute infectious mononucleosis was not seen in most patients, and there was no evidence of immune deficiency. However, Tobi et al. observed the persistent elevation of the IgM antibody to the EBV viral capsid antigen (expected only during acute primary infection with EBV), and elevated levels of antibodies to the restricted component of the EBV early antigen. Although they speculated that reactivation of EBV was the cause of the clinical syndrome, they carefully noted that the illness may also have arisen from "an aberrant immune response to primary EBV infection . . . ," possibly an abnormality in cell-mediated immune regulation of EBV-infected B-cells.

Three subsequent reports appeared, adding to the interest in what was becoming referred to as the "chronic active EBV syndrome" or "chronic mononucleosis syndrome." None of these reports was able to confirm the persistently elevated IgM antiviral capsid antigen titers described by Tobi's group. Dubois and colleagues (1984) described 14 patients with disabling fatigue and malaise, low-grade afternoon fever, and various other nonspecific symptoms that had persisted for at least 6 months. These patients were also recruited on the basis of a negative heterophile antibody test, absent IgM anti-EBV viral capsid antigen antibodies, and elevated IgG antiviral capsid antigen, elevated antiearly antigen, and elevated antinuclear antigen antibody titers. A majority of the patients in Dubois's sample had evidence of variable mild deficiency of one or more immunoglobulin isotypes. Several patients showed minor abnormalities of T-cell subsets, but no patient demonstrated anergy to cutaneous testing for delayed hypersensitivity. Two larger case series subsequently appeared in the same issue of the *Annals of Internal Medicine*. Jones et al. (1985) reported on 44 patients with a "persistent, unexplained illness" characterized by profound fatigue, "nervous system symptoms," depression, pharyngitis, fever, lymphadenopathy, myalgias, and several other constitutional symptoms. Thirty-nine of the subjects showed evidence of persistent elevation of antibody titers to the viral capsid antigen, the early antigen, and/or the nuclear antigen of EBV. Antibody titers to the viral capsid antigen and the early antigen were significantly elevated in comparison to age-group matched controls. Other immunological studies included lymphocyte phenotype and functional analyses, and measurement of circulating interferon levels, none of which revealed consistent differences, or, more importantly, any differences suggestive of an acute infectious process. There was no notable relationship between the pattern or magnitude of the antibody profiles and the symptoms or course of the illness in the patients described.

In the same issue of the *Annals of Internal Medicine,* a related report by Straus and coworkers (1985) described a group of 31 patients referred for evaluation of chronic ill health, with prominent and easy fatigability, lasting more than 1 year after documented or presumed infectious mononucleosis. In 23 patients, serologic evidence of EBV exposure was confirmed, and these patients were studied in more detail. Serologic profiles to EBV antigens were apparently abnormal in 20 patients, with elevations in the viral capsid antigen or early antigens, and an absence of elevations in the late-appearing antigens. In general, cellular immunity was normal, but minor immune abnormalities were found in some patients, including the presence of circulating immune complexes, and evidence of persistent T-cell-mediated suppression of immunoglobulin synthesis (a phenomenon characteristic of resolving acute infectious mononucleosis). In both of these reports, the authors were cautious in their interpretation of the meaning of these findings, emphasizing the nonspecificity of the symptoms as well as the immune disturbances that were evident: "it is by no means certain, however, that Epstein–Barr virus either causes the syndrome or plays an ongoing role in its chronic manifestations . . ." (Straus et al., 1985). Further work was urged in elucidating what appeared to be wide variations of host response to a ubiquitous viral agent.

Despite these cautious beginnings, widespread use of EBV serologies took hold as a diagnostic marker for this entity. Several subsequent important, yet frequently ignored, studies examined the potential role for chronic active EBV infection as a cause for this syndrome, and for the diagnostic utility of EBV serological testing. Horwitz and colleagues (1985) provided an important initial observation when they noted that evidence of enhanced EBV activity (i.e., elevated early antigen and IgG viral capsid antigen antibodies) was detectable in asymptomatic individuals for as long as 104 months after an acute illness. In 1987, the Centers for Disease Control and Prevention (CDC) conducted a seroepidemiological study of a reported cluster of cases of an apparent mononucleosis-like illness that occurred in Incline Village, Nevada (Holmes et al., 1987). The results of their investigation confirmed that elevation in antibodies to various EBV antigens was evident in affected cases. They pointed out, however, that these antibody titers were not limited to EBV. Elevations to other herpes viruses, including cytomegalovirus and herpes simplex, and to measles virus, a nonherpes virus, were also noted. Furthermore, there was no threshold titer that could reliably distinguish cases from controls, and there was an alarmingly low reproducibility of the results of serological tests within and between laboratories.

In the same issue of the *JAMA*, a separate report confirmed the inability of the specific EBV antibody profile to discriminate cases of a putative "chronic active EBV infection" from simultaneously recruited clinic controls (Buchwald et al., 1987). In a subsequent work, Hellinger and colleagues (1988) specifically examined the usefulness of the persistent elevation of the EBV early antigen as a serological marker for chronic fatigue syndrome. They examined 30 patients with chronic fatigue syndrome, who also had elevated early antigen titers (i.e., $\geq 1:160$), and compared clinical, laboratory, and follow-up data between this group and an age- and sex-matched group of 30 patients with chronic fatigue syndrome but no elevations of early antigen antibodies. Hellinger et al. found no difference on any of the initial evaluation measures between groups. In 15 matched pairs of subjects from this subset, follow-up examination showed no difference in outcome based on the initial presence or absence of early antigen antibodies. In a review of these diagnostic issues, Merlin (1986) noted that "these tests do, to some extent, suggest an organic basis for the illness, but only in the most vague, and clinically most useless, sense—the percentage of ill persons who have abnormalities of these test results is greater than that of healthy persons . . . the tests do not, however, establish a diagnosis of chronic mononucleosis. . . ."

If the antibody results were not diagnostically specific, was there any evidence at all to support the hypothesis of active EBV replication in patients with this syndrome? Several pieces of evidence address this issue. Sumaya (1991) reported no increase in the rates of infectious EBV in throat washings from patients with chronic persistent fatigue, compared to healthy controls. Nor was there any increase in the burden of EBV-infected peripheral blood cells in these patients. Sumaya's research did, however, show a subtle increase in the rate of spontaneous proliferation of peripheral blood lymphocytes compared to healthy controls, but this rate was lower than that seen in patients with acute mononucleosis. This latter test presumably reflects a disruption in cellular immune surveillance, rather than an indication of active viral disease. In a well-designed, placebo-controlled treatment trial of intravenously and orally administered acylcovir, an antiviral agent with modest efficacy against actively replicating EBV, Straus and colleagues (1988) were unable to show any evidence of clinical efficacy. Indeed, they commented that clinical improvement was more likely to be accompanied by improvement in psychological state, rather than any change in immunological status. This latter treatment result is consistent with several other immunotherapies conducted in patients with chronic fatigue syndrome (Lloyd et al., 1990; Lloyd et al., 1993b; Peterson et al., 1990; see Chapter 12).

Other viral causes of chronic fatigue syndrome have been studied, including members of the retrovirus or enterovirus families, and other herpes viruses. Despite intensive scrutiny, it appears unlikely that a primary infectious cause for chronic fatigue syndrome will be demonstrated. At the present time, a role for infections as anything other than one of many different ill-ness-triggering events in chronic fatigue syndrome cannot be supported by the available data. Whether reactivated viral disease plays a role in the symptom presentation of chronic fatigue syndrome remains to be demonstrated. More recently, a shift of attention has occurred toward viewing immune disturbances themselves as crucial pathophysiological underpinnings for the symptoms of chronic fatigue syndrome. In the earliest reports of the putative role of the EBV in chronic fatigue syndrome, several authors cautiously alluded to the possibility that the apparently disturbed levels of EBV antibodies may be evidence of an abnormality in the host response to physiological challenge, rather than an indicator of a primary or reactivated chronic infection. This view has driven much of the more recent work in the area of immunological function in patients with chronic fatigue syndrome. A major conceptual impetus for these studies has been that many of the symptoms of chronic fatigue syndrome resemble the symptoms associated with an acute infectious state (i.e., feverishness, adenopathy, myalgias, arthralgias, and cognitive difficulties). Therefore, the reasoning has been that some evidence of persistence of this physiological state of chronic immune activation should be detectable in patients with this illness, and, further, that these disturbances should correlate with the symptoms of the disease.

Nearly all areas of immunological function have been examined, including gross measures of lymphocyte count, phenotypical and functional measures of T- and B-cell populations, measures of natural killer cell number and function, static and stimulated measures of cytokine secretion, monocyte activity, immunoglobulin class and subclass levels, and other immune indexes such as allergy and autoantibody production. What evidence is there to support the hypothesis of chronic fatigue as an immunologically mediated disease? It is generally agreed that immune abnormalities are indeed detectable in patients with chronic fatigue syndrome across a series of studies, largely in comparison with healthy normal individuals. Among the most reproducible findings have been alterations, usually reductions, in natural killer cell function and number (Calgiuri et al., 1987; Chao et al., 1991; Gold et al., 1990; Gupta & Vayuvegula, 1991; Ho-Yen et al., 1991; Kibler et al, 1985; Klimas et al., 1990; Masuda et al., 1994; Ojo-Amaize et al., 1994; Wemm & Trestman, 1991), evidence of T-cell activation as measured by cell surface phenotype (Gupta & Vayuvegula, 1991; Klimas et al., 1990; Landay et al., 1991; Straus et al., 1993), impaired cell-mediated immunity as demonstrated by cutaneous anergy (Lloyd et al., 1989; Lloyd et al., 1992), reduced lymphocyte proliferative responses to in vitro mitogen stimulation (Lloyd et al., 1992; Straus et al., 1993), altered in vitro stimulated cytokine release (Chao et al., 1991; Gold et al., 1990; Kibler et al., 1985; Klimas et al., 1990), and increased suppressor T-cell function (Straus et al., 1985; Tosato et al., 1985). Direct measures of circulating cytokines have revealed levels that are normal, increased, or decreased (Chao et al., 1990, 1991; Cheney et al., 1989; Heyes et al., 1992; Kibler et al., 1985; Linde et al., 1992; Lloyd et al., 1991; Straus et al., 1989). Immunoglobulin production, particularly components of the IgG class, has been reduced in several studies (DuBois et al., 1984; Lloyd et al., 1989).

Although immunological abnormalities are indeed evident in patients with chronic fatigue syndrome across a number of cell types and functional measures, the implications of these findings are not clear. No specific measure of immune function is evident in all patients, over all studies; hence, a characteristic immune defect for use as a clinical marker is not available. Most remarkable are the sheer range and diversity of the immune findings, with apparently contradictory results over several different immune endpoints. More than anything, this overall observation probably points to the heterogeneity of the populations under study, and the methodological complexity in the assay techniques employed in immunology research. To address these concerns, in much of the current research of the immunology of chronic fatigue syndrome, the methodological issues outlined in Table 4.1 are receiving increasing and more rigorous consideration. This attention will, it is hoped, reduce some of the previously ignored confounding influences, and enhance our understanding of any true disease-associated abnormalities.

Probably the most important conclusion regarding immune abnormalities in chronic fatigue syndrome is that a clear interpretation of their physiological significance is an even greater challenge than was initially appreciated. Aside from the diversity of the findings themselves, several considerations, derived from two converging lines of evidence, are of direct relevance to this point. First, the behavioral characteristics of patients with chronic fatigue syndrome are now known to be as complex as the immune findings. As is discussed elsewhere in this book, it is unlikely that these symptoms are merely a reaction to the somatic symptoms of the illness; more likely, they reflect intrinsic aspects of the disease process itself. The second major observation has come from studies of immune regulation in psychiatric disorders and various stress-related situations. Some of the same immune disturbances that were hoped to emerge as characteristic of chronic fatigue syndrome (e.g., impaired lymphocyte proliferative response to mitogens, reduced natural killer cell function, increased levels of circulating cytokines, and alteration in lymphocyte cell surface markers) may be seen in such diverse clinical situations as major depression (Kronfol, 1994; Maes et al., 1992, 1993), anorexia nervosa (Pomeroy et al., 1994), bereavement (Schleifer et al., 1987), psychological stress (Cohen et al., 1991; Glaser et al., 1991; O'Leary, 1990; Sheridan et al., 1994), or laboratory-altered mood states (Futterman et al., 1994). Moreover, non–illness-specific subject characteristics such as age, gender, quantity and quality of sleep, and activity patterns may have significant effects on immune function (Cannon, 1993;

Cannon et al., 1989; Fielding et al., 1993; Irwin et al., 1994). In other words, one could reasonably ask whether the immune disturbance causes the symptoms of chronic fatigue syndrome, whether they arise as a consequence of it, or whether the immune disturbances and symptoms of the illness are functionally unrelated but arise from some other behavioral or biological attribute of the illness.

These studies, and others, have been intrinsic to the development of the field of psychoneuroimmunology. Far from being physiologically distinct biological compartments, the immune and nervous systems share extensive interrelationships. These interactions may be direct—for example, by anatomic connections, such as the innervation of lymphoid tissue by nerve terminals of the autonomic nervous system—or they may act indirectly, via the humoral influence of nervous system products acting on the diverse array of peptide, neurotransmitter, and steroid receptors located on peripheral lymphocytes. The range of potential pathways of communication among these networks is staggering in its complexity (Figure 4.1).

In summary, it would appear that a more broadly framed view of the functional meaning of the immune abnormalities seen in chronic fatigue

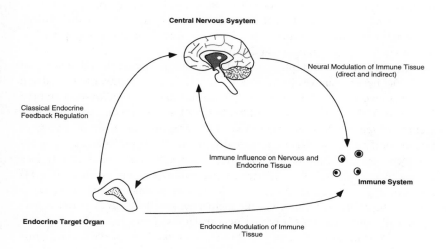

- Connections may be *structural* (e.g., hypophyseal portal system connecting hypothalamus and pituitary; autonomic nervous system innervation of spleen and lymphatic tissue) or *humoral* (e.g., endocrine regulation of lymphocyte function; cytokine modulation of neural tissues).
- Mediation of effect may be direct (e.g., ACTH stimulation of cortisol release) or indirect (e.g., brain modulation of immune function via cortisol secretion).

FIGURE 4.1. Schematic representation of the interaction of immune–nervous–endocrine systems.

syndrome should be proposed, a view that highlights the potential interaction among seemingly disparate behavioral and biological events within the individual. By placing these immunological findings in a wider context, the possibility that the changes seen in the peripheral immune system actually proceed from more proximate derangements in endocrine or central nervous system function must be introduced as a valid scientific question. In the next section, I consider the available data from neuroendocrine studies, which may suggest an answer to this question.

NEUROENDOCRINE STUDIES

Although chronic fatigue syndrome shares similarities with the symptoms of acute infectious states, and may indeed arise in the aftermath of an acute infection, the hypothesis that a persistent infectious state is present in the majority of patients with chronic fatigue syndrome is not tenable. Our group has previously commented that a unifying phenomenology for chronic fatigue syndrome can be proposed by noting that the *response to physical or psychological stress* is, more broadly, a hallmark characteristic of this condition (Demitrack, 1993; Demitrack & Greden, 1991b). Considered from this perspective, it is reasonable to ask whether there is any evidence that the principal biological machinery that coordinates the body's response to stress is impaired in patients with chronic fatigue syndrome.

In the coordinated physiological response to physical and emotional stress, the hypothalamic–pituitary–adrenal (HPA) axis is generally considered to play a pivotal role. Several aspects of the biochemical organization and the functional activity of this axis will be discussed in this section, and are represented in Figure 4.2. Regulation of the HPA axis involves a complex array of biochemical events occurring, principally, among the hypothalamus, the anterior pituitary, and the cortex of the adrenal gland (Swanson et al., 1983). Key among these biochemical signals are corticotropin-releasing hormone (CRH) and arginine vasopressin (AVP), peptide hormones whose major concentrations in the brain are localized in the medial parvocellular division of the paraventricular nucleus (PVN) of the hypothalamus. From the PVN, neuronal projections transport CRH and AVP to the external layer of the median eminence. Both peptides are widely distributed in other, extrahypothalamic locations, including the limbic system, cerebral cortex, midbrain areas, pons, and medulla. Acute stress results in the release of these peptides into the portal plexus, bathing the hormone-secreting cells of the anterior pituitary. Stimulation of specific receptors for CRH and AVP on the corticotroph cells of the anterior pituitary results in the release of adrenocorticotropic hormone (ACTH) into the systemic circulation, primarily effecting glucocorticoid release from the adrenal cortex. CRH and AVP act synergistically, with AVP

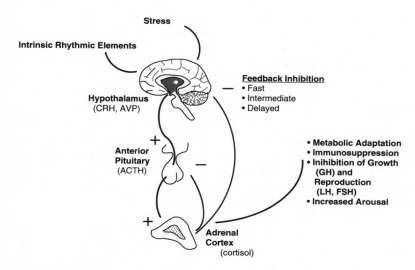

FIGURE 4.2. Hypothalamic–pituitary–adrenal axis: Principal functional connections.

causing a tremendous amplification of CRH-induced release of ACTH (Vale et al., 1983). Evidence supports a role for AVP in sustaining the activation of the HPA axis during chronic stress.

Complex short and long negative feedback circuits, primarily mediated by specific glucocorticoid receptors (the so-called Type I and Type II receptors), converge to terminate activation of the HPA axis (DeKloet et al., 1975). This negative feedback occurs along three principal time domains: fast (rate-sensitive) feedback, intermediate feedback, and delayed (genomic) feedback (Dallman et al., 1987). Fast feedback is responsive to the rate of the rise of circulating glucocorticoids, and occurs within minutes of activation of the axis; delayed feedback operates at a genomic level where the specific types of glucocorticoid receptors inhibit transcription of critical genes such as those for the precursor (POMC) peptides for ACTH biosynthesis, and those for CRH and AVP synthesis. The specific mechanisms underlying these modes of glucocorticoid negative feedback are unknown.

The particular suprahypothalamic biochemical signals that effect activation of hypothalamic CRH and AVP in response to stress are equally complex, involving both peptide- and monoamine-containing neural pathways (Herman et al., 1990). These pathways are usually redundant circuits, and are often composed of neuronal terminals that co-localize several peptide and nonpeptide elements. Less studied than these biochemical signals, but of equal importance, are several specific neural circuits that have regulatory effects on the HPA axis. These areas include the amygdala, hippocampus, septal area, cingulate cortex, and certain brainstem regions.

Finally, in addition to its stress-dependent activation, the HPA axis exhibits a pronounced spontaneous basal circadian rhythm. In humans, this circadian rhythm is entrained to the sleep/wake cycle (Krieger, 1979), with the trough of activity occurring in the evening and early night, and the peak in activity occurring just before waking. Intrinsic rhythmic elements in the suprachiasmatic nucleus appear to be the principal drive for the basal rhythm of the HPA axis. Any stress effects are then superimposed on this basal circadian rhythm. There is also evidence that the stress responsiveness and negative feedback regulation of the HPA axis vary across the day; hence, specific alterations in the timing, intensity, and duration of any stressor may result in widely varying patterns of HPA axis perturbation.

A seminal observation that heralded the modern era of biological psychiatry was that patients with major depression demonstrated a characteristic disruption of the normal diurnal rhythmicity of the pituitary–adrenal axis (Sachar et al., 1973). This disturbance involved an elevation of adrenal glucocorticoid output, usually seen as an earlier onset of the morning surge of the axis, in conjunction with enhanced cortisol secretion in the late afternoon. Aberrant feedback regulation of the axis was suggested by studies employing the synthetic glucocorticoid, dexamethasone (Carroll et al., 1976, 1981). In normal individuals, administration of dexamethasone in the late evening results in a sustained suppression of endogenous glucocorticoid production over the next 24 hours. In contrast, approximately two-thirds of hospitalized patients with major depression "escape" from the suppressive effects of dexamethasone earlier than normal, with a return of supranormal endogenous glucocorticoid secretion (Carroll et al., 1981). Over the past decade, detailed studies of the HPA axis have further refined an understanding of the biochemical events responsible for this finding. A model of HPA axis dysregulation, developed on the basis of this work, suggests that in some cases of major depression, there is an excessive central release of CRH, with the subsequent development of adrenal gland hypertrophy due to chronic overstimulation of the target organ. The specific mechanism(s) underlying this central activation, however, remains elusive. For instance, the relative contribution of absent feedback inhibition, intrinsic overproduction or impaired degradation of CRH, or sustained activation of the feed-forward biochemical and neural circuits driving the circadian rhythm of the axis is not completely understood.

In recent years, however, it has become increasingly apparent that the term "depression" may be considered to subsume a large collection of clinical conditions that are heterogeneous from both a psychological and a physiological perspective. The initial investigations of the neuroendocrine correlates of depression largely concerned the more classical, melancholic form of depression—namely, the form characterized by increased agitation, loss of sleep, loss of interest in all activities, persistent suicidal thoughts, and reduced appetite and libido. More recently, several alternative forms of depression-like syndromes that lack the features characteristic of the classical melancholic depression have been characterized. Of particular interest because of their overlap with the symptoms of chronic fatigue syndrome, these syndromes are usually dominated by reduced energy, reactive mood, and reversal of the typical pattern of vegetative features seen in classical depression. Examples of these syndromes include the depressive phase of manic-depressive illness, seasonal affective disorder (Rosenthal et al., 1984), "atypical" major depression (Quitkin et al., 1989), and the "depressive" syndromes seen in the context of certain endocrinopathies such as primary hypothyroidism and the postoperative state of Cushing's disease. Recent evidence suggests a pattern of HPA function in these syndromes, reflecting inappropriately normal or frankly reduced central nervous system activation of the axis (Joseph-Vanderpool et al., 1991; Kamilaris et al., 1987; Kling et al., 1991; Tomori et al., 1983).

Demitrack et al. (1991a) has suggested that one of the principal and specific features of the HPA axis disturbance in all of these conditions is a functional *deficit* in the release of hypothalamic CRH. This possibility is of interest because CRH serves not only as a principal stimulus to the HPA axis, but also as a behaviorally active neurohormone whose central administration to animals and nonhuman primates induces signs of physiological and behavioral arousal, including activation of the sympathetic nervous system (Brown et al., 1982), hyperresponsiveness to sensory stimuli (Swerdlow et al., 1986), and increased locomotion (Sutton et al., 1982). Hence, a relative or absolute deficiency of hypothalamic CRH could contribute to the profound lethargy and fatigue that are inherent characteristics of these "atypical" depressive syndromes and of chronic fatigue syndrome, either through direct effects on the central nervous system or, indirectly, by causing a relative glucocorticoid deficiency. Although this is an attractive model, it should be emphasized that, to date, the assessment of CRH activity in these patient groups is inferential, based primarily on peripheral pituitary–adrenal responses to hormonal challenge. Furthermore, the direct measurement of CRH in these patients has involved lumbar cerebrospinal fluid determinations, which may merely reflect cortical or spinal sources of CRH, and not direct functional CRH activity in the PVN. Because the behavioral effects of CRH listed above are produced at disparate sites within the central nervous system, there is no reason to presume that a functional deficit of CRH in the PVN is associated with similar reductions of CRH activity in limbic or cortical locations.

Could a relative glucocorticoid deficiency contribute to the symptoms of chronic fatigue syndrome? A review of the clinical features of chronic fatigue syndrome shows considerable overlap with the symptoms seen in patients with glucocorticoid deficiency. One of the principal symptoms of glucocorticoid deficiency is debilitating fatigue. An abrupt onset of fatigue, precipitated by a stressor, arthralgias, myalgias, feverishness, adenopathy, postexertional fatigue, exacerbation of allergic responses, and disturbances in mood and sleep is also characteristic of glucocorticoid insufficiency (Baxter & Tyrell, 1981). Notably, these symptoms are often seen in the relatively rare syndrome of partial or subclinical adrenal insufficiency, which may only be detectable by ACTH stimulation or other endocrine testing in patients who fail to show the symptoms of classical Addison's disease. Of particular relevance to the immunological data presented in the previous section of this chapter, glucocorticoids represent the most potent endogenous immunosuppressive compounds. Hence, our group has suggested that some of the reported immune disturbances in patients with chronic fatigue syndrome may also reflect the immune activation that might be expected to accompany a mild or relative glucocorticoid deficiency. In this regard, animal research has shown that a defect in the responsiveness of the HPA axis to immune mediators confers a risk for the development of inflammatory disease (Sternberg et al., 1989a, 1989b). Furthermore, in humans, withdrawal from hypercortisolemic states has been associated with the exacerbation of autoimmune thyroiditis (Takasu et al., 1990), as well as the development of myalgias, arthralgias, muscle weakness (Dixon & Christy, 1980), and even severe fibromyalgia (Disdier et al., 1991).

The phenomenological similarity of chronic fatigue syndrome to some forms of depression and depression-like illnesses, in addition to the biochemical considerations outlined above, has lent further interest toward an examination of the specific neuroendocrine characteristics of fatigued patients (see Table 4.2). Several early studies add to this interest. In 1981, Poteliakhoff reported that subjects with both acute and chronic fatigue states showed reductions in plasma cortisol compared to nonfatigued individuals, along with altered circadian variation in capillary resistance and eosinophil counts. These results are particularly intriguing because they suggest that even mild decrements in circulating glucocorticoids may be associated with measurable physiological changes. In a report of benign myalgic encephalomyelitis (an illness essentially identical to chronic fatigue syndrome) employing the dexamethasone suppression test, only 1 of 16 subjects showed evidence of glucocorticoid nonsuppression, a remarkably low percentage (Taerk et al., 1987). In our own work, we have shown that patients with chronic fatigue syndrome demonstrate a novel defect in HPA function characterized by a reduction in the 24-hour excretion of urine-free cortisol, and a reduction in evening basal plasma cortisol (Demitrack et al., 1991a). This hypocortisolism is accompanied by an impaired reactivity of the HPA axis to provocative challenge with either ACTH or ovine CRH. We have argued that these

TABLE 4.2. Summary of Neuroendocrine Studies in Patients with Chronic Fatigue or Chronic Fatigue Syndrome

Study	Subjects	Results
Poteliakhoff (1981)	*Exp. 1:* 25 patients with chronic fatigue (> 1 month); 25 age- and sex-matched healthy controls; *Exp. 2:* 22 subjects with acute (same day) fatigue; 28 healthy, nonfatigued controls	Lower plasma cortisol levels in individuals with chronic fatigue; increased evening eosinophil counts in individuals with acute fatigue, in conjunction with a modest attenuation of diurnal capillary resistance; increased self-rated life stress in fatigued subjects
Demitrack et al. (1991a)	30 patients with chronic fatigue syndrome; 72 age- and sex-matched healthy controls	Reduced 24-hour urine-free cortisol excretion; reduced basal evening plasma total and free cortisol; impaired adrenal response to maximal ACTH stimulation; blunted ACTH response to CRH, but elevated evening ACTH levels
Bakheit et al. (1992)	15 patients with postviral fatigue syndrome; 13 age- and sex-matched healthy controls; 13 patients with primary depression	Increased buspirone-stimulated prolactin release in postviral fatigue patients compared to either of the control groups
Bakheit et al. (1993)	9 patients with postviral fatigue syndrome; 8 age- and sex-matched healthy controls	In response to either water loading or water deprivation, there was a lack of correlation between AVP levels and serum or urine osmolality in patients with postviral fatigue; low basal AVP levels were seen in fatigue subjects; increased total body water
Bearn et al. (1995)	9 patients with chronic fatigue syndrome; 10 healthy controls	In response to insulin-induced hypoglycemia, fatigued patients showed blunted prolactin responses and a trend toward lower growth hormone responses; during D-fenfluramine challenge, patients with fatigue showed enhanced ACTH responses

results are most consistent with a mild, centrally mediated reduction in HPA axis function in patients with chronic fatigue syndrome, an observation that contrasts sharply with the sustained hypercortisolism seen in classical, melancholic depression.

As noted in Chapter 1, fibromyalgia is a clinical syndrome that shares a remarkable symptom similarity to chronic fatigue syndrome. In light of the neuroendocrine findings associated with chronic fatigue syndrome, it is of interest that in fibromyalgia, 5% to 35% of patients in various studies showed abnormal suppression to dexamethasone (Ferraccioli et al., 1990; Hudson et al., 1984). Furthermore, McCain and Tilbe (1989) reported that patients with fibromyalgia have reduced 24-hour urine-free cortisol excretion and a loss of the diurnal fluctuation of glucocorticoid levels. More recently, Griep and colleagues (1993) reported exaggerated ACTH but blunted cortisol response to exogenous administration of CRH and to insulin-induced hypoglycemia. Crofford and her associates (1994) have also shown that patients with fibromyalgia have reduced 24-hour urine-free cortisol levels and an impaired response to ovine CRH challenge, suggestive of reduced central drive to the HPA axis.

How might an impairment in the activation of the HPA axis arise? Although there is no definitive answer to this question, several recent reports have begun to shed light on some potential answers. As described previously, among the many influences regulating the activity of the HPA axis are several neurotransmitter and neuropeptide compounds. For instance, peripherally directed AVP serves as an important ACTH secretagogue. When present in conjunction with CRH, there is a marked synergism of these two neuropeptides upon the resultant release of ACTH (Vale et al., 1983). Interestingly, Bakheit and coworkers have reported that patients with postviral fatigue syndrome show a reduction in basal AVP levels, along with an apparent reduction in the release of AVP during water deprivation challenge (Bakheit et al., 1993). Therefore, it is attractive to hypothesize that the impaired reactivity of the HPA axis may arise in part from an array of neuroendocrine events—in this case, a reduction in CRH secretion and/or an inadequate accompanying level of peripherally directed AVP. Among other neurochemical influences on the HPA axis, the monoamine neurotransmitters have recently been studied in a series of preliminary reports. Our group has noted that cerebrospinal fluid levels of the principal monoamine neurotransmitter metabolites—homovanillic acid, 5-hydroxyindoleacetic acid (5-HIAA), and 3-methoxy-4-hydroxyphenylglycol (MHPG) (from dopamine, serotonin, and norepinephrine, respectively)—are normal. However, plasma concentrations of these same compounds reveal a subtle reduction in circulating MHPG and a twofold increase in the serotonin metabolite, 5-HIAA (Demitrack et al., 1992). This latter observation, suggesting a disruption in the metabolism of serotonin, is of interest given the results of two more recent reports that have examined the activity of serotonin receptor function via the administration of specific neuropharmacological probes. Bakheit and colleagues (1992) noted that the prolactin response to buspirone (a serotonin 1A receptor agonist) was markedly increased in patients with chronic fatigue syndrome, and argued that the sensitivity of serotonin receptors was increased. Such a postsynaptic supersensitivity would be consistent with a reduction in central serotonergic activity. If reduced central serotonin function were present, this would provide an attractive pathophysiological explanation for the putative reduction in central CRH activity, because serotonin serves as a potent stimulus to the HPA axis. However, using a different, more selective serotonin receptor ligand (D-fenfluramine), Bearn and coworkers (1995) were unable to confirm this observation, finding, instead, a blunting of the prolactin rise in response to challenge with this pharmacological probe.

The studies reviewed in this section provide further evidence suggesting the complexity of the biological events that accompany chronic fatigue syndrome. In response to the question posed at the end of the previous section, these data are also consistent with the view that the immune findings in patients with chronic fatigue syndrome may arise from more proximate pathophysiological events in the central nervous system.

POLYSOMNOGRAPHY

Among the principal features in the clinical presentation of chronic fatigue syndrome is disturbed sleep. Research suggests that abnormal sleep, in the form of daytime tiredness, unrefreshing or fragmented sleep, insomnia, or hypersomnia, is present in the majority of all patients. In some instances, the sleep disturbance may be so striking that clinical polysomnography may be justified.

Aside from determining the presence or absence of a formal sleep disorder, there are several reasons why the study of sleep physiology is of interest in chronic fatigue syndrome. First, the sleep EEG of several major psychiatric illnesses—in particular, major depression—is well characterized in the literature. In major depression, several characteristic polysomnographic abnormalities may be seen, including a disruption in sleep continuity, a decrease in the latency to onset of the first rapid eye movement (REM) period, an increase in REM density, and a reduction in the amounts of stages 3 and 4 sleep (Buysse & Kupfer, 1990). More recently, it has been appreciated that many of these abnormalities do not have diagnostic specificity, but may be driven by biological events that are shared among a number of psychiatric disorders.

The second reason why the study of sleep physiology is of interest to understanding the physiology of chronic fatigue syndrome comes from work in the related clinical entity, fibromyalgia. In 1975, Moldofsky and colleagues reported a novel sleep abnormality characterized by the intrusion of high-frequency alpha waves upon the slower delta waves normally seen in non-REM sleep. Indeed, in one study, the group showed that patients with a postinfectious fatigue syndrome of greater than 6 months' duration also showed this non-REM sleep anomaly (Whelton et al., 1992). As described above, this pattern is quite different from that seen in primary psychiatric disorders. Although the specific cause for this sleep disturbance is unknown, central nervous system factors are strongly implicated, at least in part.

The third reason why an understanding of sleep physiology may be particularly relevant to the study of chronic fatigue syndrome is that several physiological systems appear to have an intimate connection to the integrity of normal sleep. Of particular interest, in light of the material presented in the previous sections, are the effects of the immune and endocrine systems. For instance, several cytokines are known to have sleep-promoting properties, which may be functionally separable from their well-known pyretic actions. In animals, Kruger and his colleagues have shown that interleukin-1α and β, tumor necrosis factor, and interferon-α are somnogenic, leading to a substantial increase in non-REM or slow-wave sleep during acute challenge (Krueger et al., 1990). In humans, Moldofsky and associates have shown that plasma interleukin-1 activity increases during sleep (Moldofsky et al., 1986). A specific relationship between immune function and slow-wave sleep in human disease states is suggested by recent observations of a group of asymptomatic, HIV-infected men (Norman et al., 1992). Their sleep EEG shows a distortion of the non-REM/REM cycles across the night, with an apparent sustained activity of slow-wave sleep during the second half of the night, when it should normally be declining. Whether such putative immune system–sleep cycle interactions are relevant to the sleep of patients with chronic fatigue syndrome is unknown.

With respect to the interaction of endocrine events and sleep, it is well known that the circadian rhythm of adrenocortical activity is synchronized with the sleep wake cycle, with the largest portion of adrenocortical output occurring during the second half of the sleep period. Several studies have demonstrated alterations in cortisol output when sleep is denied or deliberately fragmented throughout the day (Follenius et al., 1992; Weitzman et al., 1973, 1983). In a study comparing the sleep EEG and cortisol secretory profiles in 22 healthy individuals, Kupfer and colleagues (1983) noted that the length of the non-REM sleep period between the first and second REM periods was inversely associated with cortisol secretion during the night. This time interval was also positively correlated with the time of the normal cortisol rise that occurs prior to awakening. More recent work has suggested that the reduction in cortisol secretion during the early part of the night may be due, in part, to changes in the sensitivity of the HPA axis to the effects of glucocorticoid negative feedback inhibition, so that the early morning cortisol rise emerges from a relative decrease in feedback sensitivity of the axis during the second half of the night (Spath-Schwalbe et al., 1991, 1992).

The interaction of sleep and the activity of the HPA axis may also be demonstrated in other ways. For example, exogenous administration (Born et al., 1989; Gillin et al., 1972) or disease-related alteration of any of the principal biochemical constituents of the HPA axis—namely, CRH, ACTH, or glucocorticoids—may lead to disruption of the normal architecture of nocturnal sleep. When patients with Addison's disease are taken off hormonal replacement therapy, there is no change in REM sleep characteristics; however, there is a substantial increase in stages 3 and 4 sleep and in the proportion of time spent in slow-wave sleep (Gillin et al., 1974). Similarly, in normal individuals treated with the cortisol synthesis inhibitor, metyrapone, there is a significant increase in stage 4 and delta sleep in the night immediately following metyrapone administration (Gillin et al., 1974). In contrast to the glucocorticoid-deficient Addison's patient, individuals with Cushing's syndrome demonstrate impaired sleep continuity, along with a reduction in stage 4 sleep and no change in the amount of time spent in REM sleep (Shipley et al., 1992). Whether these effects arise as a direct response of brain sleep centers to the alterations in glucocorticoid secretion, or from feedback effects on hypothalamic CRH or pituitary ACTH secretion, is unknown.

In light of the neurotransmitter data discussed in the previous section, it is worth noting that several other neurobiological events are known to affect sleep physiology. Among these events is the activity of the monoamine neurotransmitter, serotonin. In general, serotonin appears to promote slow-wave sleep activity while probably decreasing overall REM activity (Wauquier & Dugovic, 1990). Whether the putative disturbances in serotonin metabolism noted above reflect an actual disruption of serotonin activity that may result in altered sleep physiology in patients with chronic fatigue syndrome remains to be determined.

Several studies of sleep and its polysomnographic features have been conducted in patients with chronic fatigue syndrome (see Table 4.3). In the work by Krupp and colleagues (1993), there was a high prevalence of polysomnographically diagnosed sleep disorders in a group of 16 patients who met the CDC case definition for chronic fatigue syndrome. In a separate study, Buchwald and her group (1994) noted that at least 81% of a sample of 59 patients with chronic fatigue syndrome had one or more sleep disorders diagnosed by an overnight sleep EEG study. These two studies provide important information about the clinical assessment of patients with a presenting complaint of chronic fatigue, emphasizing that the diagnosis of formal sleep disorders may often go unnoticed in this patient group. A thorough sleep history is an essential part of the clinical workup for this illness. When symptoms are strongly suggestive of a primary sleep disorder, formal overnight sleep studies

TABLE 4.3. Summary of Polysomnography Studies in Patients with Chronic Fatigue Syndrome

Study	Subjects	Results
Whelton et al. (1992)	14 patients with chronic fatigue syndrome; 12 healthy age- and sex-matched controls	Patients showed reduced sleep efficiency, increased levels of alpha rhythm intrusion in non-REM sleep, decreased percentage of REM sleep
Krupp et al. (1993)	16 patients with chronic fatigue also reporting prominent sleep complaints	Majority of subjects (62.5%) showed a diagnosable sleep disorder (e.g., periodic limb movement disorder, excessive daytime sleepiness, apnea, narcolepsy)
Morriss et al. (1993)	12 patients with chronic fatigue syndrome; 12 healthy age-, sex-, and weight-matched controls	Patients reported increased time in bed, but showed reduced sleep efficiency; seven patients had a diagnosable sleep disorder, and this group had greater functional disability than the remaining patients
Buchwald et al. (1994)	59 patients with chronic fatigue selected for the prominence of their sleep complaints	A majority (81%) of patients had a diagnosable sleep disorder, most commonly sleep apnea (44%), and idiopathic hypersomnia (12%)
Manu et al. (1994)	30 consecutive clinic patients with chronic fatigue	Eight patients (26%) showed alpha rhythm intrusion into non-REM sleep, and ten patients (33%) were diagnosed with a sleep disorder (e.g., sleep apnea, periodic limb movements, or narcolepsy)

may be appropriate. However, the implications of these findings for the pathophysiology of chronic fatigue syndrome, *per se,* are confounded by the fact that the patients included in each sample were selected based on the prominence of specific sleep complaints in their initial clinical evaluation.

In another study, by Morriss and coworkers (1993), which did not select patients on the basis of their sleep history, a group of 12 patients with chronic unexplained fatigue had an overall reduction in sleep efficiency, and a majority of the subjects met criteria for a formal sleep disorder. However, there was no evidence for any other disturbance of sleep architecture. Our group (Zubieta et al., 1993) has provided a preliminary report of overnight sleep EEG activity compared among 4 groups: 16 individuals with chronic fatigue syndrome, 17 inpatients with major depression, 17 never-hospitalized outpatients with major depression, and 17 healthy controls. We observed a striking increase in the amount of time spent in stage 4 and in delta sleep in patients with chronic fatigue syndrome, when compared to either of the depressed-patient groups or to the healthy controls. In addition, patients with chronic fatigue syndrome did not show a reduction in REM latency or any increase in REM activity and density, as was seen in the two patient groups with major depression. On the other hand, the chronic fatigue patients showed an increase in sleep latency and a reduction in sleep efficiency comparable to that seen in the two depressed comparison groups. Interestingly, none of the sleep studies performed to date has documented the non-REM sleep anomaly previously described in patients with fibromyalgia (Manu et al., 1994). Whether this represents a true pathophysiological distinction between otherwise clinically similar entities, or simply sample heterogeneity, is unclear.

The reasons for the differences between the study of Morriss and coworkers and our own work are not readily apparent, but they may relate to the inevitable issue of population heterogeneity, complicated possibly by the use of two different operational definitions for chronic fatigue syndrome. Further studies will be of interest. However, it is intriguing that the observation of a possible increase in slow-wave sleep forms a coherent physiological framework when considered in light of the sleep–immune system–endocrine system effects discussed above. These data also underscore the contention that the immune abnormalities described previously cannot be considered in isolation.

NEUROIMAGING STUDIES

Direct anatomical or functional evidence of brain abnormalities in patients with chronic fatigue syndrome would certainly provide the most compelling support for central nervous system involvement in this disease. Few neuroimaging studies of chronic fatigue syndrome have been performed to date. These studies, which are summarized in Table 4.4, are discussed briefly in this section.

In one of the first major reports on neuroimaging (Buchwald et al., 1992), a series of 144 patients with a chronic fatiguing illness, descriptively similar to chronic fatigue syndrome, underwent magnetic resonance imaging (MRI). In 78% of the patients, foci of high-signal intensity were found on

TABLE 4.4. Summary of Neuroimaging Studies in Patients with
Chronic Fatigue Syndrome

Study	Subjects	Results
Buchwald et al. (1992)	114 patients with chronic fatigue syndrome; 41 age- and sex-matched controls	Foci of high-signal intensity seen on T2-weighted MRI scans in 78% of patients compared with 21% of controls
Ichise et al. (1992)	60 patients with chronic fatigue syndrome; 14 controls	Significant decrease in cortical/cerebellar regional cerebral blood flow in patients as measured with ^{99m}Tc-HMPAO SPECT scan; principal areas of brain involvement included frontal (63% of cases), temporal (35%), parietal (53%), and occipital (38%) lobes
Natelson et al. (1993)	52 patients with chronic fatigue syndrome; 52 age- and sex-matched neurological controls	In patients with chronic fatigue syndrome, significant increase in percentage (27% vs. 2%) of abnormal scans (foci of high-signal intensity seen on T2-weighted scans [$n = 9$], or ventricular or sulcal enlargement [$n = 5$])
Schwartz et al. (1994a)	16 patients with chronic fatigue syndrome; 15 age-matched controls (MRI); 14 age-matched controls (SPECT)	Foci of high-signal intensity seen on T2-weighted MRI scans was seen in 50% of patients compared with 20% of controls (NS); SPECT scans showed perfusion abnormalities in 81% of patients and 21% of controls ($p < .01$); SPECT abnormalities resolved with clinical improvement, MRI abnormalities did not
Schwartz et al. (1994b)	45 patients with chronic fatigue syndrome; 27 patients with AIDS dementia complex; 14 patients with unipolar depression; 38 healthy controls	Perfusion defects were similar in distribution and number in chronic fatigue syndrome and depressed patients, and greater than those seen in controls
Goldstein et al. (1995)	33 patients with either chronic fatigue or chronic fatigue syndrome; 26 patients with major depression; 19 healthy controls	Significant reduction in global cerebral blood flow measured by ^{133}Xe in both patient groups; more prominent right dorsal frontal and temporal lobe perfusion impairment with ^{99m}Tc-HMPAO SPECT scan in chronic fatigue syndrome compared with depression

T2-weighted scan images. These foci consisted of punctate areas, or areas of patchy intensity. The abnormalities were most often detected in the subcortical white matter, and typically appeared to correlate with the clinical symptoms reported by the patients. In several individuals for whom studies were repeated over time, the abnormalities appeared to persist, even after resolution of the symptoms. Although the percentage of abnormal scans in this study was a notable contrast (21% of the controls had positive scans), the interpretation of the findings was confounded by several issues. For instance, although most of the patients appeared to meet the subsequently published clinical criteria for chronic fatigue syndrome, the possibility that an alternative neurodegenerative disease was present in a subset of the group could not be excluded. Indeed, symptoms that are not typical of most individuals with chronic fatigue syndrome, such as primary seizures, profound ataxia, and transient paresis, were seen. Also, the reading of the scans was not performed blindly, nor were they read on the same machine as the controls' scans. The fact that the abnormalities persisted, despite clinical improvement in several individuals also raises questions about the functional meaning of the findings.

Ichise and colleagues (1992) published the first report of a functional imaging technique in chronic fatigue syndrome, namely regional cerebral blood flow using ^{99m}Tc-hexamethylpropyleneamine oxime (HMPAO) single-photon emission computed tomography (SPECT). In a comparison of 60 patients with chronic fatigue syndrome and 14 healthy controls, the patients with chronic fatigue syndrome showed reduced global regional cerebral blood flow. Eighty percent of the fatigue sample showed reduced blood flow in at least one or more regions, most commonly the left basal ganglia, left superomedial frontal lobe, left superoposterior frontal lobe, right superomedial frontal lobe, and right anteroinferior frontal lobe. The investigators commented that, although differences were apparent, no unique anatomical profiles were noted in the patients with chronic fatigue syndrome. Certain confounds limit the conclusions to be drawn from these data, including the lack of specification of the psychiatric assessment of the study subjects, and the fact that several patients were taking antidepressants at the time of the study.

Natelson and colleagues (1993) have recently reported the results of magnetic resonance imaging studies in a group of 52 patients meeting the CDC case criteria for chronic fatigue syndrome, as compared to 52 age- and sex-matched neurological controls. Twenty-seven percent (14 patients) in the chronic fatigue group had scans that were read as abnormal, compared with only one of the control scans. The majority of the scans revealed multiple small areas of abnormal increased signal intensity in cerebral white matter, most often in the area of the corona radiata. Interestingly, when the depression ratings of 12 of the subjects with abnormal scans were compared to an age- and sex-matched subset of the fatigued subjects whose scans were normal, the subjects with abnormal scans showed a nonsignificant trend toward higher depression scores. On subsequent clinical follow-up, three of the fatigue subjects developed neurological symptoms and laboratory findings suggestive of multiple sclerosis (two subjects) or Behçet's disease. Excluding these subjects, the study yielded a significantly higher rate of positive scans in the fatigued sample. Although the functional meaning of these results was not clear, the overall prevalence of abnormal scans, though still greater than in a control population, was much lower than that reported by Buchwald and coworkers (1992).

In a comparison of magnetic resonance imaging and SPECT scanning, Schwartz and colleagues (1994a) have examined the correspondence between these two methods of anatomical and functional neuroimaging, respectively. They examined the MRI and SPECT scans of a group of 16 patients with chronic fatigue syndrome, for whom these studies were performed within a 10-week period. The results were compared to a group of age- and sex-matched healthy controls. Although the patients reportedly had no previous medical or psychiatric disease, current psychiatric symptoms were not specified. In 50% of the patients, abnormalities were noted on magnetic resonance imaging. These abnormalities were similar to previous reports, consisting of small foci of increased T2 signal, located in the white matter. Principal areas involved included the centrum semiovale, corona radiata, internal capsule, periventricular region, subcortical white matter, and basal ganglia. Unlike the previous reports, there was no significant difference between the percentage or number of abnormalities in the patients when compared to the healthy controls (20% abnormal). In contrast, SPECT abnormalities were present in 81% of the patient scans, and only 21% of the healthy controls, a significant difference. The principal areas of involvement in the patients who differed from the controls included the lateral frontal cortex, the lateral temporal cortex, and the basal ganglia. SPECT scanning revealed more evidence of abnormality than the MRI scanning technique. There was little anatomic correspondence between the SPECT and MRI scans. In four patients, SPECT scans were repeated over a 6-month interval; fewer perfusion defects were noted in the three patients who showed clinical improvement. The MRI scans did not change with time in any of the subjects. Overall correspondence of the imaging abnormalities with specific clinical features was not observed.

In their companion report, the same group (Schwartz et al., 1994b) compared SPECT images in a group of 45 patients with chronic fatigue syndrome to three other subject groups: 27 patients with AIDS dementia complex, 14 patients with unipolar depression, and 38 healthy controls. The age and gender matchings among groups were significantly different, the chronic fatigue sample being predominantly younger and female. In contrast, the AIDS dementia patients were largely young males, and the depressed and normal groups, although largely female, were considerably older than the chronic fatigue syndrome or AIDS dementia groups. Furthermore, several of the depressed subjects were receiving antidepressant medications at the time of study. Nevertheless, several abnormalities were described. The study showed significantly more defects among all of the patient groups compared to the healthy controls. Comparable numbers of defects were seen in the chronic fatigue and depressed groups, but the AIDS dementia patients had a significantly greater number of defects than the chronic fatigue sample. The investigators also noted that the midcerebral uptake index was significantly lower in the chronic fatigue and AIDS dementia groups than in either the depressed or healthy control samples. No specific information was given regarding the relationship between the functional imaging studies and any measures of clinical symptomatology.

Goldstein and colleagues (1995) have also reported the results of SPECT scanning in patients with chronic fatigue syndrome, compared to depressed patients and healthy controls. In their report, regional cerebral blood flow was determined using ^{133}Xe, and brain perfusion abnormalities were quantified using ^{99m}Tc-HMPAO, as in the previous reports. The study samples included 33 patients with chronic fatigue syndrome, who were all over age 45; 16 of these patients also met clinical critieria for major depression. The comparison groups included a medication-free group of 26 patients with unipolar major depression, and two groups of healthy, elderly community controls. The age and gender matching revealed a slightly lower age and slightly greater preponderance of women in the chronic fatigue sample. Regional cerebral blood flow was reduced in both the chronic fatigue syndrome and depressed subject samples when compared to healthy controls. Perfusion defects, upon SPECT imaging, were seen, in both the chronic fatigue and depressed samples, in the frontal and temporal lobes. The results appeared more prominent in the right hemisphere for the chronic fatigue sample, but left hemispheric abnormalities were more evident in the depressed sample. No relationship was apparent between the depressed and nondepressed chronic fatigue subjects.

Functional and structural brain imaging studies support the hypothesis that central nervous system disturbances are more evident in patients with chronic fatigue syndrome than in healthy individuals. However, this work must clearly be regarded as preliminary. Indeed, several caveats should be noted in the interpretation of these findings beyond the general statement in the first sentence of this paragraph. It is striking, for example, that none of the later studies confirmed the substantially high prevalence of magnetic resonance imaging abnormalities seen in the report by Buchwald and colleagues (1992). As noted, this may relate most directly to the inherent problem of population heterogeneity in these studies. Because these scans were collected on a large clinical sample that was generated prior to the development of the CDC case definition and before the complexities of the behavioral confounds were appreciated, this sample may not be representative of currently described patients with chronic fatigue syndrome. The observation by Natelson's group that three of their subjects appeared to develop other, nonchronic fatigue syndrome disease states also addresses these diagnostic concerns, and emphasizes the need to avoid premature diagnostic closure in routine clinical practice. Also of note is the fact that several of the studies were not able to adequately match the age or gender of their sample groups. The influence of these variables on the interpretation of the results is unclear. Furthermore, as pointed out by Ichise, the results do not represent unique functional or anatomic profiles, sharing apparent similarities with either neurodegenerative or central nervous system inflammatory diseases and with major psychiatric disorders. More detailed behavioral descriptions will be necessary in future work. These studies, as emphasized by Dr. Komaroff in Chapter 7, do not indicate any usefulness of these techniques in routine clinical practice. Even with these issues considered, the results highlight the observation that central nervous system disturbances are present in chronic fatigue syndrome.

CONCLUSIONS

Mechanic (1993) has noted that "it is essential to differentiate the scientific study of chronic fatigue syndrome from its management in routine practice." The data summarized in this section emphasize this point by noting that the pragmatic experience of chronic fatigue syndrome extends far beyond the itemization of its specific biological correlates. A general conclusion of the research studies reviewed here would suggest that it is unlikely that biological descriptors alone will ultimately allow a categorical delineation of chronic fatigue syndrome as a discrete entity. However, it is equally appropriate to note that this is not the same as saying that chronic fatigue syndrome does not exist. It does exist, though its development may be conceptualized as the complex unfolding of the particular life experiences and adaptive capabilities, physiological and behavioral, in an affected individual.

A major challenge that confronts clinical research into the biology of chronic fatigue syndrome, therefore, is the task of distinguishing the intrinsic biological or behavioral attributes of the individual, which may increase susceptibility to develop the clinical syndrome or perpetuate it once it is present, from the biological changes that may arise as a consequence of behavioral changes emerging during the illness. These considerations are necessary for a thorough integration of the pathophysiological meaning of the data presented in this chapter. A hypothetical schematic of these issues is depicted in Figure 4.3. The studies reviewed here provide compelling data to suggest that patients with chronic fatigue syndrome should be regarded as a heterogeneous group of individuals with a variety of infectious and/or noninfectious antecedent events contributing to the development of their illness.

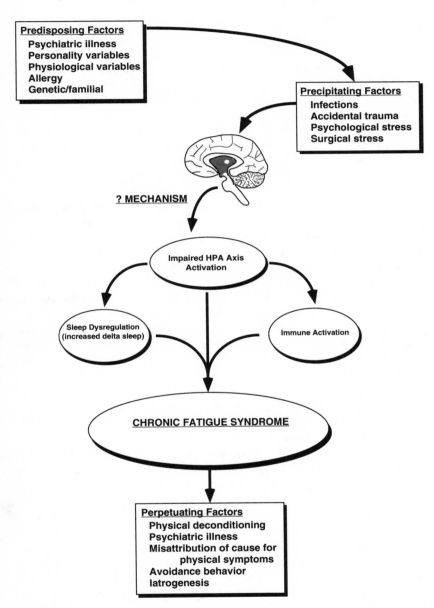

FIGURE 4.3. Chronic fatigue syndrome as a central nervous system–mediated disease.

Given the available information, it seems unreasonable to presume a unidimensional illness model in which patients with chronic fatigue syndrome represent a discrete disease with a singular cause. Instead, a more useful formulation would propose that this illness is more appropriately analogous to several complex medical conditions, such as hypertension, where many direct and indirect factors (some of which may be psychological) lead to the development of the observable clinical syndrome.

This type of illness model rejects a unitary etiological event to explain the condition (i.e., the chronic infectious model), and emphasizes the importance of shared pathophysiological processes, and the interactive relation among many potentially disparate factors (i.e., biological events coupled with maladaptive coping strategies). It may be difficult, if not impossible, to elucidate all of the causal interactions among these factors, and the consequent sequence of pathophysiological events, with complete surety. However, given what is currently known about the functional organization of the physiological systems that have been investigated in chronic fatigue syndrome, it seems reasonable to propose the sequence of events depicted in Figure 4.3 as a tentative model. Hence, acquired factors such as cumulative life stress, psychiatric illness, or an intrinsic deficit in HPA axis reactivity may render the individual incapable of mounting an adequate response to an acute stressor (infectious or otherwise). As a consequence, a relative or absolute reduction of adrenal glucocorticoids ensues, resulting in the loss of some or all of the counterregulatory effects of the HPA axis normally called into play in response to stress. Sustained activation of the immune response or an increase in delta sleep time then arises as a secondary biological consequence of the primary impairment in central nervous system-mediated stress responsiveness. Whether any of these biological events actually relates to the observable clinical symptoms of chronic fatigue syndrome remains to be shown.

There are several useful consequences of considering the development of chronic fatigue syndrome in this fashion. Most importantly, it broadens the field of clinical view for both patient and clinician. The illness is no longer seen as merely the result of a specific, reflexive, biological response induced by a putative disease agent. Instead, symptoms may also be brought about and/or shaped by the adaptive and maladaptive responses employed by the patient, or others in the patient's environment. In other words, it becomes relevant to examine factors such as the psychological or social context in which the illness emerges, the specific coping strategies employed by the patient, or the particular disease models employed by the patient and physician to account for the confusing array of symptoms seen in this illness. If the patient and physician maintain a rigid view of the illness as solely due to a specific exogenous agent or the involuntary physiological response of the patient, recuperation may be stymied. Data exist to support the view that these "perpetuating" factors may be of even greater relevance than change in any specific biological parameter. For instance, in a follow-up study of patients presenting with chronic fatigue to an infectious disease clinic, Sharpe and colleagues (1994) observed that greater functional impairment was associated with factors such as the patient's belief in a viral cause for the illness, the limiting of exercise, the patient's membership in a self-help organization, and any current emotional disorder. Similarly, Cope and coworkers (1994) examined the predictors of the development of chronic fatigue in the aftermath of a diagnosis of "viral illness" on a visit to a general practitioner. Among the "host factors" relevant to the development of fatigue was the tendency to attribute common symptoms to physical disorder, rather than to psychological factors, or to normal bodily events. They commented that "this presentation conceals emotional distress from the physician and shapes the subsequent interaction. . . ."

Placing the biological events of the illness in a broad-based, interactive framework expands the range of potential therapeutic options available for the patient and the physician to use in the management of the illness, and appropriately discourages the utilization of repeated and expensive diagnostic interventions. Later chapters in this book will address these treatment issues in greater depth—for example, the rational use of pharmacotherapy (e.g., antidepressants and nonsteroidal anti-inflammatory medications) to target specific symptoms (e.g., depressed or anxious mood, or diffuse musculoskeletal pain). In Chapters 9 and 10, the use of cognitive-behavioral therapy is addressed. In this approach, the consequences of specific, potentially maladaptive behaviors, such as excessive sleep, or prolonged physical activity are examined with the collaboration of the patient. With thoughtful collaborative exploration, it can often be demonstrated that these behaviors can have important and disabling symptomatic consequences.

REFERENCES

Bakheit, AM, Behan, PO, Dinan, TG, Gray, CE, O'Keane, V. Possible upregulation of hypothalamic 5-hydroxytryptamine receptors in patients with post-viral fatigue syndrome. *Br Med J* 1992; 304(6833):1010–1012.

Bakheit, AM, Behan, PO, Watson, WS, Morton, JJ. Abnormal arginine vasopressin secretion and water metabolism in patients with postviral fatigue syndrome. *Acta Neurol Scand* 1993; 87(3):234–238.

Baxter, JD, Tyrell, JB. The adrenal cortex. In Felig, P, Baxter, JD, Broadus, AE, Frohman, LA, eds., *Endocrinology and metabolism*. New York: McGraw-Hill, 1981;385–510.

Bearn, JA, Allain, T, Coskeran, P, Munro, N, Butler, J, McGregor, A, Wessely, S. Neuroendocrine responses to D-fenfluramine and insulin-induced hypoglycemia in chronic fatigue syndrome. *Biol Psychiatry,* 1995 Feb 15; 37(4):245–252.

Born, J, Spath-Schwalbe, E, Schwakenhofer, H, Kern, W, Fehm, HL. Influences of corticotropin-releasing hormone, adrenocorticotropin, and cortisol on sleep in normal man. *J Clin Endo Metab* 1989; 68(5):904–911.

Brown, MR, Fisher, LA, Spiess, J, Rivier, C, Rivier, J, Vale, W. Corticotropin-releasing factor: Actions on the sympathetic nervous system and metabolism. *Endocrinology* 1982; 111:928–931.

Buchwald, D, Cheney, PR, Peterson, DL, Henry, B, Wormsley, SB, Geiger, A, Ablashi, DVM, Salahuddin, SZ, Saxinger, C, Biddle, R, Kikinis, R, Jolesz, FA, Folks, T, Balanchandran, N, Peter, JB, Gallo, RC, Komaroff, AL. A chronic illness characterized by fatigue, neurologic and immunologic disorders, and active human herpes virus type 6 infection. *Ann Int Med* 1992; 116:103–113.

Buchwald, D, Pascualy, R, Bomardier, C, Kith, P. Sleep disorders in patients with chronic fatigue. *Clin Inf Dis* 1994; 18(suppl 1):S68–S72.

Buchwald, D, Sullivan, JL, Komaroff, AL. Frequency of "chronic active Epstein–Barr virus infection" in a general medical practice. *JAMA* 1987; 257(17): 2303–2307.

Buysse, DJ, Kupfer, DJ. Diagnostic and research applications of electroencephalographic sleep studies in depression: Conceptual and methodological issues. *J Nerv Ment Dis* 1990; 178(7):405–414.

Calgiuri, M, Murray, C, Buchwald, D, Levine, H, Cheney, P, Peterson, D, Komaroff, AL, Ritz, J. Phenotypic and functional deficiency of natural killer cells in patients with chronic fatigue syndrome. *J Immunol* 1987; 139:3306–3313.

Cannon, JG. Exercise and resistance to infection. *J Appl Physiol* 1993; 74(3): 973–981.

Cannon, JG, Fielding, RA, Fiatarone, MA, Orencole, SF, Dinarello, CA, Evans, WJ. Increased interleukin 1 beta in human skeletal muscle after exercise. *Am J Physiol* 1989; 257(2 Pt 2):R451–455.

Carroll, BJ, Curtis, GC, Mendels, J. Neuroendocrine regulation in depression: I. Limbic system-adrenocortical dysfunction. *Arch Gen Psychiatry* 1976; 33:1039–1044.

Carroll, BJ, Feinberg, M, Greden, JF, Tarika, J, Albala, AA, Haskett, RF, James, NM, Kronfol, Z, Lohr, N, Steiner, M, de Vigne, JP, Young, E. A specific laboratory test for the diagnosis of melancholia: Standardization, validation, and clinical utility. *Arch Gen Psychiatry* 1981; 38(1):15–22.

Chao, CC, Gallagher, M, Phair, J, Peterson, PK. Serum neopterin and interleukin-6 levels in chronic fatigue syndrome. *J Inf Dis* 1990; 162:1412–1413.

Chao, CC, Janoff, EN, Hu, S, Thomas, K, Gallagher, M, Tsang, M, Peterson, PK. Altered cytokine release in peripheral blood mononuclear cell cultures from patients with the chronic fatigue syndrome. *Cytokine* 1991; 3:292–298.

Cheney, PR, Dorman, SE, Bell, DS. Interleukin-2 and the chronic fatigue syndrome. *Ann Int Med* 1989; 110:321.

Cohen, S, Tyrrell, DA, Smith, AP. Psychological stress and susceptibility to the common cold. *N Engl J Med* 1991; 325(9):606–612.

Cope, H, David, A, Pelosi, A, Mann, A. Predictors of chronic "postviral" fatigue. *Lancet* 1994; 344:864–868.

Crofford, LJ, Pillemer, SR, Kalogeras, KT, Cash, JM, Michelson, D, Kling, MA, Sternberg, EM, Gold, PW, Chrousos, GP, Wilder, RL. Hypothalamic–pituitary–adrenal axis perturbations in patients with fibromyalgia. *J Rheumatol* 1994 Nov; 37(11):1583–1592.

Dallman, MF, Akana, SF, Cascio, ES, Darlington, DN, Jacobson, L, Levin, N. Regulation of ACTH secretion: Variations on a theme of B. *Rec Prog Horm Res* 1987; 43:113–173.

DeKloet, R, Wallach, G, McEwen, BS. Differences in corticosterone and dexmethasone binding to rat brain and pituitary. *Endocrinology* 1975; 76:598–609.

Demitrack, MA. Chronic fatigue syndrome: A disease of the hypothalamic–pituitary–adrenal axis? *Ann Med* 1993; 26(1):1–5.

Demitrack, MA, Dale, JK, Straus, SE, Laue, L, Listwak, SJ, Kruesi, MJP, Chrousos, GP, Gold, PW. Evidence for impaired activation of the hypothalamic–pituitary–adrenal axis in patients with chronic fatigue syndrome. *J Clin Endo Metab* 1991a; 73(6):1224–1234.

Demitrack, MA, Gold, PW, Dale, JK, Krahn, DD, Kling, MA, Straus, SE. Plasma and cerebrospinal fluid monoamine metabolites in patients with chronic fatigue syndrome: Preliminary findings. *Biological Psychiatry* 1992; 32:1065–1077.

Demitrack, MA, Greden, JF. Chronic fatigue syndrome: The need for an integrative approach. *Biological Psychiatry* 1991b; 30(8):747–752.

Disdier, P, Harle, J-R, Brue, T, Jaquet, P, Chambourlier, P, Grisoll, F, Weiller, P-J. Severe fibromyalgia after hypophysectomy for Cushing's disease. *Arthr and Rheum* 1991; 34(4):493–495.

Dixon, RB, Christy, NP. On the various forms of corticosteroid withdrawal syndrome. *Am J Med* 1980; 68(2):224–230.

DuBois, RE, Seeley, JK, Brus, I, Sakamoto, K, Ballow, M, Harada, S, Bechtold, TA, Pearson, G, Purtilo, DT. Chronic mononucleosis syndrome. *S Med J* 1984; 77(11):1376–1382.

Ferraccioli, G, Cavalieri, F, Salaffi, F, Fontana, S, Scita, F, Nolli, M, Maestri, D. Neuroendocrinologic findings in primary fibromyalgia (soft tissue chronic pain syndrome) and in other chronic rheumatic conditions (rheumatoid arthritis, low back pain). *J Rheum* 1990; 19:869–873.

Fielding, RA, Manfredi, TJ, Ding, W, Fiatarone, MA, Evans, WJ, Cannon, JG. Acute phase response in exercise: III. Neutrophil and IL-1 beta accumulation in skeletal muscle. *Am J Physiol* 1993; 265(1 Pt 2):R166–72

Follenius, M, Brandenberger, G, Bandesapt, JJ, Libert, JP, Ehrhart, J. Nocturnal cortisol release in relation to sleep structure. *Sleep* 1992; 15(1):21–27.

Futterman, AD, Kemeny, ME, Shapiro, D, Fahey, JL. Immunological and physiological changes associated with induced positive and negative mood. *Psychosom Med* 1994; 56:499–511.

Gillin, JC, Jacobs, LS, Fram, DH, Snyder, F. Acute effect of a glucocorticoid on normal human sleep. *Nature* 1972; 237:398–399.

Gillin, JC, Jacobs, LS, Snyder, F, Henkin, RI. Effects of decreased adrenal corticosteroids: Changes in sleep in normal subjects and patients with adrenal cortical insufficiency. *Electroencephal Clin Neurophysiol* 1974; 36:283–289.

Glaser, R, Pearson, GR, Jones, JF, Hillhouse, J, Kennedy, S, Mao, H, Kiecolt-Glaser, JK. Stress-related activation of Epstein–Barr virus. *Brain Behav Immunity* 1991; 5:219–232.

Gold, D, Bowden, R, Sixbey, J, Riggs, R, Katon, WJ, Ashley, R, Obrigewitch, RM, Corey, L. Chronic fatigue: A prospective clinical and virologic study. *JAMA* 1990; 264(1):48–53.

Goldstein, JA, Mena, I, Jouanne, E, Lesser, I. The assessment of vascular abnormalities in late life chronic fatigue syndrome by brain SPECT: Comparison with late life major depressive disorder. *J Chronic Fatigue Synd* 1995; 1(1):55–79.

Griep, EN, Boersma, JW, deKloet, ER. Altered reactivity of the hypothalamic–pituitary–adrenal axis in the primary fibromyalgia syndrome. *J Rheum* 1993; 20:469–474.

Gupta, S, Vayuvegula, B. A comprehensive immunological analysis in chronic fatigue syndrome. *Scand J Immunol* 1991; 33:319–327.

Hellinger, WC, Smith, TF, Van Scoy, RE, Spitzer, PG, Forgacs, P, Edson, RS. Chronic fatigue syndrome and the diagnostic utility of antibody to Epstein–Barr virus early antigen. *JAMA* 1988; 260(7):971–973.

Herman, JP, Wiegand, S, Watson, SJ. Regulation of basal corticotropin releasing hormone and arginine vasopressin mRNA expression in the paraventricular nucleus: Effects of selective hypothalamic deafferentation. *Endocrinology* 1990; 127:2408–2417.

Heyes, MP, Saito, K, Crowley, J, Davis, LE, Demitrack, MA, Der, M, Kruesi, MJP, Lackner, A, Larsen, SA, Lee, K, Leonard, H, Martin, A, Markey, SP, Milstein, S, Mouradian, MM, Pranzatelli, MR, Quearry, BJ, Rapoport, JL, Salazar, A, Smith, M, Straus, SE, Sunderland, T, Swedo, S, Tourtellotte, WW. Quinolinic acid and kynurenine pathway metabolism in inflammatory and non-inflammatory neurological disease. *Brain* 1992; 115:1249–1273.

Holmes, GP, Kaplan, JE, Stewart, JA, Hunt, B, Pinsky, PF, Schonberger, LB. A cluster of patients with a chronic mononucleosis-like syndrome: Is Epstein–Barr virus the cause? *JAMA* 1987; 257(17):2297–2302.

Horwitz, CA, Henle, W, Henle, G, Rudnick, H, Latts, E. Long-term serological follow-up of patients for Epstein–Barr virus after recovery from infectious mononucleosis. *J Inf Dis* 1985; 151(6):1150–1153.

Ho-Yen, DO, Billington, RW, Urquhart, J. Natural killer cells and the post viral fatigue syndrome. *Scand J Infect Dis* 1991; 23(6):711–716.

Hudson, JI, Pliner, LF, Hudson, MS, Goldenberg, DL, Melby, JC. The dexamethasone suppression test in fibrositis. *Biol Psychiatry* 1984; 19:1489–1493.

Ichise, M, Salit, IE, Abbey, SE, Chung, D-G, Gray, B, Kirsh, JC, Freedman, M. Assessment of regional cerebral perfusion by ^{99}Tc-HMPAO SPECT in chronic fatigue syndrome. *Nuc Med Comm* 1992; 13:767–772.

Irwin, M, Mascovich, A, Gillin, JC, Willoughby, R, Pike, J, Smith, TL. Partial sleep deprivation reduces natural killer cell activity in humans. *Psychosom Med* 1994; 56:493–498.

Isaacs, R. Chronic infectious mononucleosis. *Blood* 1948; 3:858–861.

Jones, JF, Ray, G, Minnich, LL, Hicks, MJ, Kibler, R, Lucas, DO. Evidence for active Epstein–Barr virus infection in patients with persistent, unexplained illnesses: Elevated anti-early antigen antibodies. *Ann Int Med* 1985; 102(1):1–7.

Joseph-Vanderpool, JR, Rosenthal, NE, Chrousos, GP, Wehr, TA, Skwerer, R, Kasper, S, Gold, PW. Abnormal pituitary–adrenal responses to oCRH in patients with seasonal affective disorder: Clinical and pathophysiological implications. *J Clin Endo Metab* 1991; 72(6):1382–1387.

Kamilaris, TC, DeBold, CR, Pavlou, SN, Island, DP, Hoursandis, A, Orth, DN. Effect of altered thyroid hormone levels on hypothalamic–pituitary–adrenal function. *J Clin Endo Metab* 1987; 65(5):994–999.

Kibler, R, Lucas, DO, Hicks, MJ, Poulos, BT, Jones, JF. Immune function in chronic active Epstein–Barr virus infection. *J Clin Immunol* 1985; 5:46–54.

Klimas, NG, Salvato, FR, Morgan, R, Fletcher, MA. Immunological abnormalities in chronic fatigue syndrome. *J Clin Microbiol* 1990; 28:1403–1410.

Kling, MA, Roy, A, Doran, AR, Calabrese, JR, Rubinow, DR, Whitfield, HJ, Jr, May, C, Post, RM, Chrousos, GP, Gold, PW. Cerebrospinal fluid immunoreactive CRH and ACTH secretion in Cushing's disease and major depression: Potential clinical implications. *J Clin Endo Metab* 1991; 72(2):260–271.

Krieger, DT. Rhythms in CRH, ACTH and corticosteroids. *Endo Rev* 1979; 1:123.

Kronfol, Z. Immune function in depression and anxiety. In den Boer, J, Sitsen, JM, eds., *Handbook of Depression and Anxiety: A Biological Approach.* New York: Marcel Dekker, 1994; 515–527.

Krueger, JM, Obal, F, Opp, M, Toth, L, Johannsen, L, Cady, AB. Somnogenic cytokines and models concerning their effects on sleep. *Yale J Biol Med* 1990; 63:157–172.

Krupp, LB, Jandorf, L, Coyle, PK, Mendelson, WB. Sleep disturbance in chronic fatigue syndrome. *J Psychosom Res* 1993; 37(4):325–331.

Kupfer, DJ, Bulik, CM, Jarrett, DB. Nighttime plasma cortisol secretion and EEG sleep—are they associated? *Biol Psychiatry* 1983; 10:191–199.

Landay, AL, Jessop, C, Lennette, ET, Levy, JA. Chronic fatigue syndrome: Clinical condition associated with immune activation. *Lancet* 1991; 338(8769):707–712.

Linde, A, Andersson, B, Svenson, SB, Ahrne, H, Carlsson, M, Forsberg, P, Hugo, H, Karstorp, A, Lenkei, R, Lindwall, A, et al. Serum levels of lymphokines and soluble cellular receptors in primary Epstein–Barr virus infection and in patients with chronic fatigue syndrome. *J Infect Dis* 1992; 165(6):994–1000.

Lloyd, AR, Hickie, I, Brockman, A, Dwyer, J, Wakefield, D. Cytokine levels in serum and cerebrospinal fluid in patients with chronic fatigue syndrome and control subjects. *J Infection* 1991; 164:1023–1024.

Lloyd, AR, Hickie, I, Brockman, A, Hickie, C, Wilson, A, Dwyer, J, Wakefield, D. Immunologic and psychologic therapy for patients with chronic fatigue syndrome: A double-blind, placebo-controlled trial. *Am J Med* 1993a; 94(2): 197–203.

Lloyd, AR, Hickie, I, Hickie, C, Dwyer, J, Wakefield, D. Cell-mediated immunity in patients with chronic fatigue syndrome, healthy control subjects and patients with major depression. *Clin Exp Immunol* 1992; 87(1):76–79.

Lloyd, AR, Hickie, I, Wakefield, D, Boughton, C, Dwyer, J. A double-blind, placebo controlled trial of intravenous immunoglobulin therapy in patients with chronic fatigue syndrome. *Am J Med* 1990; 89:561–568.

Lloyd, AR, Wakefield, D, Boughton, CR, Dwyer, JM. Immunological abnormalities in the chronic fatigue syndrome. *Med J Austral* 1989; 151:122–124.

Lloyd, AR, Wakefield, D, Hickie, I. Immunity and the pathophysiology of chronic fatigue syndrome. In *Chronic fatigue syndrome,* Ciba Foundation Symposium, 1993b; 173:176–192.

Maes, M, Bosmans, E, Meltzer, HY, Scharpe, S, Suy, E. Interleukin-1β: A putative mediator of HPA axis hyperactivity in major depression? *Am J Psychiatry* 1993; 150(8):1189–1193.

Maes, M, Lambrechts, J, Bosmans, E, Jacobs, J, Suy, E, Vandervorst, C, de Jonckheere, C, Minner, B, Raus, J. Evidence for a systemic immune activation during depression: Results of leucocyte enumeration by flow cytometry in conjunction with monoclonal antibody staining. *Psychol Med* 1992; 22:45–53.

Manu, P, Lane, TJ, Matthews, DA, Castriotta, RJ, Watson, RK, Abeles, M. Alphadelta sleep in patients with a chief complaint of chronic fatigue. *S Med J* 1994; 87(4):465–470.

Masuda, A, Nozoe, SI, Matsuyama, T, Tanaka, H. Psychobehavioral and immunological characteristics of adult people with chronic fatigue and patients with chronic fatigue syndrome. *Psychosom Med* 1994; 56(6):512–518.

McCain, GA, Tilbe, KS. Diurnal hormone variation in fibromyalgia syndrome: A comparison with rheumatoid arthritis. *J Rheumatol* 1989 (suppl); 16:154–157.

Mechanic, D. Chronic fatigue syndrome and the treatment process. In *Chronic fatigue syndrome,* Ciba Foundation Symposium, 1993; 173:318–327.

Merlin, TL. Chronic mononucleosis: Pitfalls in the laboratory diagnosis. *Human Path* 1986; 17(1):2–8.

Moldofsky, H, Lue, FA, Eisen, J, Keystone, E, Gorczynski, RM. The relationship of interleukin-1 and immune functions to sleep in humans. *Psychosom Med* 1986; 48(5):309–318.

Moldofsky, H, Scarisbrick, P, England, R, Smythe, H. Musculoskeletal symptoms and nonREM sleep disturbance in patients with "fibrositis syndrome" and healthy subjects. *Psychosom Med* 1975; 37:341–351.

Morriss, R, Sharpe, M, Sharpley, AL, Cowen, PJ, Hawton, K, Morris, J. Abnormalities of sleep in patients with the chronic fatigue syndrome. *BMJ* 1993; 306(6886):1161–1164.

Natelson, BH, Cohen, JM, Brassloff, I, Lee, HJ. A controlled study of brain magnetic resonance imaging in patients with the chronic fatigue syndrome. *J Neurol Sci* 1993; 120(2):213–217.

Norman, SE, Chediak, AD, Freeman, C, Kiel, M, Mendez, A, Duncan, R, Simoneau, J, Nolan, B. Sleep disturbances in men with asymptomatic human immunodeficiency virus (HIV) infection. *Sleep* 1992; 15(2):150–155.

Ojo-Amaize, EA, Conley, EJ, Peter, JB. Decreased natural killer cell activity is associated with severity of chronic fatigue immune dysfunction syndrome. *Clin Inf Dis* 1994; 18(suppl 1):S157–S159.

O'Leary, A. Stress, emotion, and human immune function. *Psychol Bull* 1990; 108(3):363–382.

Peterson, PK, Shepard, J, Macres, M, Schenck, C, Crosson, J, Rechtman, D, Lurel, N. A controlled trial of intravenous immunoglobulin G in chronic fatigue syndrome. *Am J Med* 1990; 89:554–560.

Pomeroy, C, Eckert, E, Hu, S, Eiken, B, Mentink, M, Crosby, RD, Chao, CC. Role of interleukin-6 and transforming growth factor-b in anorexia nervosa. *Biol Psychiatry* 1994; 36:836–839.

Poteliakhoff, A. Adrenocortical activity and some clinical findings in acute and chronic fatigue. *J Psychosom Res* 1981; 25:91–95.

Quitkin, FM, McGrath, PJ, Stewart, JW, Harrison, W, Wager, SG, Nunes, E, Rabkin, JG, Tricamo, E, Markowitz, J, Klein, DF. Phenelzine and imipramine in mood reactive depressives: Further delineation of the syndrome of atypical depression. *Arch Gen Psychiatry* 1989; 46(9):787–793.

Rosenthal, NE, Sack, DA, Gillin, JC, Lewy, AJ, Goodwin, FK, Davenport, Y, Mueller, PS, Newsome, DA, Wehr, TA. Seasonal affective disorder: A description of the syndrome and preliminary findings with light therapy. *Arch Gen Psychiatry* 1984; 41(1):72–80.

Sachar, EJ, Hellman, L, Roffwarg, HP, Halpern, FS, Fukush, DK, Gallagher, TF. Disrupted 24 hour patterns of cortisol secretion in psychotic depressives. *Arch Gen Psychiatry* 1973; 28:19–24.

Schleifer, SJ, Keller, SE, Stein, M. Conjugal bereavement and immunity. *Isr J Psychiatry Relat Sci* 1987; 24(1-2):111–123

Schwartz, RB, Garada, BM, Komaroff, AL, Tice, HM, Gleit, M, Jolesz, FA, Holman, BL. Detection of intracranial abnormalities in patients with chronic fatigue syndrome: Comparison of MR imaging and SPECT. *Amer J Roentgen* 1994a; 162:935–941.

Schwartz, RB, Komaroff, AL, Garada, BM, Gleit, M, Doolittle, TH, Bates, DW, Vasile, RG, Holman, BL. SPECT Imaging of the brain: Comparison of findings in patients with chronic fatigue syndrome, AIDS dementia complex, and major unipolar depression. *Amer J Roentgen* 1994b; 162:943–951.

Sharpe, M, Hawton, K, Seagroatt, V, Pasvol, G. Follow up of patients presenting with fatigue to an infectious diseases clinic. *BMJ* 1994; 305:147–152.

Sheridan, JF, Dobbs, C, Brown, D, Zwilling, B. Psychoneuroimmunology: Stress effects on pathogenesis and immunity during infection. *Clin Microbiol Rev* 1994; 7(2):200–212.

Shipley, JE, Schteingart, DE, Tandon, R, et al. EEG sleep in Cushing's disease and Cushing's syndrome: Comparison with patients with major depressive disorder. *Biol Psychiatry* 1992; 32:146–155.

Spath-Schwalbe, E, Gofferje, M, Kern, W, Born, J, Fehm, HL. Sleep alters nocturnal ACTH and cortisol secretory patterns. *Biol Psychiatry* 1991; 29:575–584.

Spath-Schwalbe, E, Scholler, T, Kern, W, Fehm, H, Born, J. Nocturnal adrenocorticotropin and cortisol secretion depends on sleep duration and decreases in association with spontaneous awakening in the morning. *J Clin Endo Metab* 1992; 75:1431–1435.

Sternberg, EM, Hill, JM, Chrousos, GP, Kamilaris, T, Listwak, SJ, Gold, PW, Wilder, RL. Inflammatory mediator-induced hypothalamic–pituitary–adrenal activation is defective in streptococcal cell wall arthritis-susceptible rats. *Proc Natl Acad Sci USA* 1989a; 86:2374–2378.

Sternberg, EM, Young, WS, III, Bernardini, R, Calogero, AE, Chrousos, GP, Gold, PW, Wilder, RL. A central nervous system defect in biosynthesis of corticotropin-releasing hormone is associated with susceptibility to streptococcal cell wall-induced arthritis in lewis rats. *Proc Natl Acad Sci USA* 1989b; 86:4771–4775.

Straus, SE, Dale, JK, Peter, JB, Dinarello, CA. Circulating lymphokine levels in the chronic fatigue syndrome. *J Infect Dis* 1989; 160:1085–1086.

Straus, SE, Dale, JK, Tobi, M, Lawley, T, Preble, O, Blaese, RM, Hallahan, C, Henle, W. Acyclovir treatment of the chronic fatigue syndrome: Lack of efficacy in a placebo-controlled trial. *N Engl J Med* 1988; 319(26):1692–1698.

Straus, SE, Fritz, S, Dale, J, Gould, B, Strober, W. Lymphocyte phenotype analysis suggests chronic immune stimulation in patients with chronic fatigue syndrome. *J Clin Immunol* 1993; 13(1):30–40.

Straus, SE, Tosato, G, Armstrong, G, Lawley, T, Preble, OT, Henle, W, Davey, R, Pearson, G, Epstein, J, Brus, I. Persisting illness and fatigue in adults with evidence of Epstein–Barr virus infection. *Ann Int Med* 1985; 102(1):7–16.

Strober, W. Immunological function in chronic fatigue syndrome. In Straus, SE, ed., *Chronic fatigue syndrome,* New York: Marcel Dekker, 1994; 207–237.

Sumaya, CV. Serologic and virologic epidemiology of Epstein–Barr virus: Relevance to chronic fatigue syndrome. *Rev Inf Dis* 1991; 13(Suppl 1):S19–S25.

Sutton, RE, Koob, GF, LeMoal, M, Rivier, J, Vale, W. Corticotropin-releasing factor produces behavioural activation in rats. *Nature* 1982; 297:331–333.

Swanson, LW, Sawchenko, PE, Rivier, J, Vale, WW. Organization of ovine corticotropin-releasing factor immunoreactive cells and fibers in the rat brain. An immunohistochemical study. *Neuroendocrinology* 1983; 36:165–186.

Swerdlow, NR, Geyer, MA, Vale, WW, Koob, GF. Corticotropin-releasing factor potentiates acoustic startle in rats: Blockade by chlordiazepoxide. *Psychopharmacology* (Berlin) 1986; 88:147–152.

Taerk, GS, Toner, BB, Salit, IE, Garfinkel, PE, Ozersky, S. Depression in patients with neuromyasthenia (benign myalgic encephalomyelitis). *Int J Psychiatry Med* 1987; 17(1):49–56.

Takasu, N, Komiya, I, Nagasawa, Y, Asawa, T, Yamada, T. Exacerbation of autoimmune thyroid dysfunction after unilateral adrenalectomy in patients with Cushing's syndrome due to an adrenocortical adenoma. *N Engl J Med* 1990; 322(24):1708–1712.

Tobi, M, Morag, A, Ravid, Z, Showers, I, Feldman-Weiss, V, Michaeli, Y, Ben-Chetrit, E, Shalit, M, Knobler, H. Prolonged atypical illness associated with serological evidence of persistent Epstein–Barr virus infection. *Lancet* 1982; 9:61–64.

Tomori, N, Suda, S, Tozawa, F, Demura, H, Shizume, K, Mouri, T. Immunoreactive corticotropin-releasing factor concentrations in cerebrospinal fluid from patients with hypothalamic–pituitary–adrenal disorders. *J Clin Endo Metab* 1983; 56(6):1305–1307.

Tosato, G, Straus, SE, Henle, W, Pike, SE, Blaese, RM. Characteristic T cell dysfunction in patients with chronic active Epstein–Barr virus infection (chronic infectious mononucleosis). *J Immunol* 1985; 134:3082–3088.

Vale, W, Vaughan, J, Smith, M, Yamamoto, G, Rivier, J, Rivier, C. Effects of synthetic ovine corticotropin-releasing factor, glucocorticoids, catecholamines, neurohypophysial peptides, and other substances on cultured corticotropic cells. *Endocrinology* 1983; 113:1121–1131.

Wauquier, A, Dugovic, C. Serotonin and sleep-wakefulness. In Whitaker-Azmitia, PM, Peroutka, SJ, eds., *The neuropharmacology of serotonin.* New York: Annals of the New York Academy of Science, 1990; 600:447–459.

Weitzman, ED, Nogeire, C, Perlow, M, et al. Effects of a prolonged 3-hour sleep–wake cycle on sleep stages, plasma cortisol, growth hormone and body temperature in man. *J Clin Endo Metab* 1973; 38:1018–1030.

Weitzman, ED, Zimmerman, JC, Czeisler, CA, Ronda, J. Cortisol secretion is inhibited during sleep in normal man. *J Clin Endo Metab* 1983; 56:352–358.

Wemm, KM, Jr, Trestman, RL. The effects of a laboratory stressor on natural killer cell function in chronic fatigue syndrome patients [letter]. *Psychosomatics* 1991; 32(4):470–471.

Whelton, CL, Salit, I, Moldofsky, H. Sleep, Epstein–Barr virus infection, musculoskeletal pain, and depressive symptoms in chronic fatigue syndrome. *J Rheumatol* 1992; 19:939–943.

Wilson, A, Hickie, I, Lloyd, A, Hadzi-Pavlovic, D, Boughton, C, Dwyer, J, Wakefield, D. Longitudinal study of chronic fatigue syndrome. *Br Med J* 1994; 308:756–759.

Zubieta, JK, Demitrack, MA, Shipley, JE, Engleberg, NC, Eiser, A, Douglass, A. *Sleep EEG in chronic fatigue syndrome: Comparison with major depression.* Presented at the annual meeting of the Society for Biological Psychiatry, San Francisco, May, 1993.

II
ASSESSMENT

5

Neuropsychological Assessment of Patients with Chronic Fatigue Syndrome

Jordan Grafman, Ph.D.

One of the cardinal complaints of patients with chronic fatigue syndrome (CFS) is impaired cognition. Komaroff has reported that 50% to 85% of CFS patients in published studies claim that their cognitive functioning is impaired (Komaroff, 1993). Despite the frequency of this complaint, only a few peer-reviewed neuropsychological studies of CFS patients have been published. These studies have been remarkably varied in their assessment techniques, subject selection methods, and conclusions.

In this chapter, I note those aspects of CFS that could conceivably lead to neuropsychological deficits. More detailed coverage of this topic can be found elsewhere (Grafman, 1995; Grafman et al. 1991). The chapter then reviews all published neuropsychological studies of CFS patients at the time of writing. The review is followed by suggestions for a neuropsychological assessment targeted to the CFS patient. The chapter concludes with some comments about the value of neuropsychological assessment in CFS.

CHARACTERIZATION OF THE NEUROLOGY OF CFS

The objective neurological examination of CFS patients is typically completely normal, although patients may report problems with strength, sleep, balance, cognition, and mood (Bock & Whelan, 1993; Dawson & Sabin, 1993). Only a few reports have given more precise information regarding neurological findings in CFS (see Grafman et al., 1991, for a review). CFS rarely presents with objective changes in muscle functions or with hard neurological symptoms or signs (Holmes et al., 1988). Between 10% and 20% of CFS patients have an abnormal Romberg test, and 15% to 25% of CFS patients demonstrate an impaired tandem gait (Komaroff, 1993). Magnetic resonance imaging (MRI) studies of CFS patients are controversial. For example, one recent study indicated that 70% of the CFS patients associated with an outbreak of the disorder in Lake Tahoe, Nevada, had punctate bright signals on their MRIs (Buchwald et al., 1992). Such nondiagnostic MRI abnormalities appear to resemble the hyperintensities reported in leukoariosis. On the other hand, in the NIH CFS patients reported on below, no patient had a positive MRI finding (S. Straus, personal communication). A few metabolic imaging studies have been attempted with CFS patients. For example, several recent studies using single photon emission computed tomography (SPECT) found abnormalities in the basal ganglia and cortex in CFS patients (Ichise et al., 1992; Wessely, 1993).

Pharmacological treatment is generally ineffective in CFS unless targeted to ameliorate mood state abnormality (Goodnick & Sandoval, 1993; Straus et al., 1988). Nevertheless, because many CFS patients tend to improve over time and do not show any significant progressive neurological deterioration, CFS should not be portrayed as a neurodegenerative disorder.

Although the illness has been labeled chronic fatigue syndrome, no obvious markers of central fatigue are available, although some promising leads are currently being explored (Brasil-Neto et al., 1993; Chalder et al., 1993). The presence of neurological findings in some CFS patients and imaging studies suggesting brain dysfunction require the neuropsychologist to be especially careful in interpreting the results of neuropsychological testing in CFS patients.

THE NEUROPSYCHOLOGICAL EVALUATION

Neuropsychological evaluations are an integral part of the clinical neuroscience workup of most patients with neurological and psychiatric disorders. Neuropsychological evaluations provide the referral source with clinical and quantitative information about the patients' cognitive processes and mood state. The standard neuropsychological evaluation typically examines motor coordination and strength, simple sensory functions, general intellectual functioning, information processing speed, attention, language, perception, reasoning and problem-solving, memory, mood state, and personality. Interpretation is usually based on test profile analysis. The neuropsychological evaluation may be conducted by a trained technician, student-in-training, research assistant, or licensed psychologist. Clinical neuropsychologists interpreting the test results should have, at a minimum, specialized training as postdoctoral fellows in a clinical neuropsychology program.

The neuropsychological evaluation of CFS patients can be useful as an aid in interpreting their neurological complaints and in estimating symptom progression or rate of patient recovery (Grafman et al., 1991; Schluederberg et al., 1991, 1992). The neuropsychological evaluation is particularly important when a diagnosis is one of exclusion, as it is with CFS, to establish a neuropsychological baseline by which subsequent clinical fluctuations could be judged.

NEUROPSYCHOLOGICAL FINDINGS IN CFS

Self-Report

Forty years ago, chronic brucellosis challenged many investigators to identify the cause(s) of the symptoms of nervousness and difficulty in concentrating that were frequently reported by patients. Eventually, an objective study of these patients by Imboden and his colleagues (Imboden et al., 1959) found no evidence of cognitive deficits. Whether the neuropsychological symptoms of CFS will meet a similar fate is as yet unknown.

In CFS, as previously noted, up to 85% of patients will complain of impaired cognition. Until recently, these problems had not been recorded systematically. Grafman et al. (1993) investigated patient self-report of cognitive status by mailing out surveys to a sample of CFS patients who were being followed at the National Institutes of Health. About two-thirds of the patients returned the forms. No relationship was found between selected laboratory findings and severity of self-reported symptoms. A large proportion of CFS patients complained about verbal memory and mood state changes, whereas problems in perceptual, linguistic, spatial, and nonverbal memory functions were rarely endorsed. The memory complaints of these CFS patients were occasionally so severe that they could be compared to those reported by patients with amnesia. Although indicating that their current memory and mood state impairment was upsetting, the respondents reported that during the worst period of their illness, their memory and mood state problems were even more severe. Using a Beck Depression Inventory total score of 15 as a clinical cutoff for depression, more than 50% of the sample were currently depressed, whereas up to 90% of the sample had been depressed during the worst period of their illness. Women had more complaints than men. There was a strong correlation between the degree of depression and the severity of memory complaints. The complaints were certainly serious enough to merit an objective neuropsychological evaluation.

Issues Regarding the Neuropsychological Evaluation

The issue of whether the symptoms of CFS are caused by concurrent affective disease has emerged as a polarizing and confounding issue in studies of neuropsychological function in CFS (see other chapters in this volume). Most published studies have shown a higher proportion of mood state changes and psychiatric diagnoses in CFS than in the population at large. It is known, for example, that depression may affect the cognitive processes that demand more "effort" (e.g., some free-recall or executive function tasks) (Weingartner & Silberman, 1987). In this case, the cognitive deficits reported or found in CFS could be secondary to a primary psychiatric disorder (Demitrack et al., 1992; Ray et al., 1992; Wessely, 1993). An alternative possibility is that the mood state changes arise from the social and physical limitations imposed on patients by their illness. A third possibility is that depression and cognitive deficits co-occur and are the result of single or multiple central nervous system lesions or dysfunctions (Grafman et al., 1991).

Some patients who are initially considered to have CFS may, in fact, be misdiagnosed and actually have another disorder that affects the central nervous system, such as multiple sclerosis or a definable acute viral infection (Durack & Street, 1991; Grafman et al., 1991; Kachuck & Weiner, 1993; Katon & Russo, 1992).

There is even evidence that colds and flus may acutely and selectively affect cognitive performance. The element that separates CFS patients from patients with known neurological and viral illnesses is the chronicity of their neuropsychological complaints in conjunction with negative neurological and physical findings.

Many CFS patients may be experiencing sleep disturbance (Morriss et al., 1993). Testing any patient after a night of little sleep would result in a poorer-than-expected performance on cognitive tests.

Neuropsychological Studies

The first published neuropsychological study of CFS was from a Toronto group. Altay et al. studied 21 subjects diagnosed with postinfectious neuromyasthenia who also met CFS criteria (Altay et al., 1990). Seventeen of the 21 subjects were women. The average age of the subjects was 36 years, and most had an undergraduate college degree. The subjects were administered the following tests: the Trail Making Test A and B (measures attention and the ability to shift concepts); the Digit Symbol Subtest of the Wechsler Adult Intelligence Scale–Revised (WAIS-R [measures speed of information processing and short-term memory]); the Similarities Subtest from the WAIS-R (measures verbal reasoning and concept formation); and the Shipley Institute of Living Scale (measures vocabulary knowledge and abstract reasoning). The results were compared with the most recently revised normative data available on each test, matched for age. The results demonstrated that the CFS subjects performed at or above the age-matched normative sample despite the fact that 20 of the 21 subjects in this study felt that they performed quite poorly and were nowhere near their premorbid standard.

In contrast, Riccio et al. (1992) found significant abnormalities in memory in a sample of CFS patients they studied. Nine patients (median age was 30; 4 females) who fulfilled the operational criteria for a diagnosis of myalgic encephalomyelitis (ME) were compared to a matched control group on a set of neuropsychological and psychiatric tests. ME is defined by profound physical and mental fatigue along with a variety of other symptoms including neuromuscular, cardiovascular, and gastrointestinal complaints. The criterion to be diagnosed with ME focuses more on neurological symptoms than the criterion for CFS, but, in many respects, the patients appear to present with a similar illness profile (Wessely, 1990). All the patients reported problems in concentrating prior to the testing.

Subjects were assessed with the (1) National Adult Reading Test; (2) WAIS-R; (3) Wechsler Memory Scale ([WMS] measures various aspects of verbal and nonverbal memory); (4) Sentence Verification Test (measures speeded semantic processing); (5) Letter and Category Verbal Fluency Tests (requires subjects to generate as many words as they can within 1 minute that begin with a specific letter or belong to a specific semantic category); (6) Grooved Pegboard Test (evaluates fine motor coordination); (7) Wisconsin Card Sorting Test ([WCST] measures concept formation and shifting); (8) Trailmaking Test A and B; (9) Present State Examination ([PSE] a standardized psychiatric interview); (10) Hospital Anxiety and Depression Questionnaire; (11) State–Trait Anxiety Scale; (12) Profile of Mood States; (13) Illness Behavior Questionnaire; and (14) Eysenck Personality Questionnaire.

The ME patients had a significantly lower score on the WMS subtest that measures story memory, and a modest decline in paired-associate learning when compared to the matched control group. No other significant differences emerged from the neuropsychological comparisons. No substantial differences between groups were found on the psychiatric interview or objective personality inventories. In their conclusion, Riccio et al. argued that the isolated deficits they observed in their patients were caused by central nervous system dysfunction.

Smith (Smith, 1992a, 1992b; Smith et al., in press), in examining self-report of cognitive deficits in a sample of 232 ME patients, found that they reported a higher level of cognitive complaints than controls but that their complaints largely reflected their degree of psychopathology as estimated by objective inventories. Smith went on to study differing subsets of these patients on a variety of performance measures. He found that ME patients were substantially slower than controls (409 < 253 ms, respectively) on a simple and a five-choice visual serial response time task. The ME patients were also shown a spatial pattern that is known to induce visual discomfort and illusions. The ME patients were more likely than controls to report visual illusions and dizziness after observing the pattern. In a task that required subjects to visually search for a target among distractors, ME patients were slower and less accurate than controls. On the Stroop Color–Word Test (which requires selective attention and inhibition of competing information), ME patients performed more slowly and were more prone to distraction from competing stimuli than controls. Thus, the ME patients experienced problems across a wide range of visual processing tasks.

In a story memory task, ME patients were poorer than controls in recalling both gist and detailed information. Smith found no difference between ME patients and controls on a digit span test. ME patients demonstrated a problem in learning words from a list on the early trials, but by the later trials, overall recall was similar to controls. On a word recognition test, ME patients developed a yes strategy in saying whether words were seen before or not thus, they had a large number of correct answers and a very large number of false alarms. The number of false alarms was so large, in fact, that Smith commented that their performance was similar to Korsakoff patients who have a rather profound organic amnesia.

On a sentence verification task (requiring semantic processing speed), ME patients completed fewer items than controls. ME patients also produced fewer words on a verbal fluency test. It is important to note that the number of subjects completing each task varied and that no significance levels were reported. The pattern of visual processing and memory deficits held whether patients were viewed as mildly or severely affected.

Krupp et al. found that neuropsychological differences between CFS patients ($n = 45$) and controls disappeared when self-report of depression was adjusted for (Krupp et al., 1992).

DeLuca et al. (1993) studied 12 CFS patients on the Paced Auditory Serial Addition Test (PASAT), which measures information processing speed and divided attention. CFS patients had significantly worse scores than controls on this task but performed similarly to a comparison group of MS patients. Beck Depression Inventory scores were not correlated with CFS patient performance on the PASAT.

Sandman et al. (1993) studied 39 CFS patients along with depressed patients and a normal control group on a set of neuropsychological and memory tests. Seventy percent of their CFS patients had fibromyalgia. The report did not indicate the proportion of females in their samples or whether they were matched for education level. There were no between-group differences on any of the neuropsychological tests. The CFS patients demonstrated slower response times, and impaired cued-recall (as opposed to their normal free-recall) and working memory. The CFS patients also tended to overestimate their memory abilities. Neither mood state nor personality was assessed in this study. Sandman et al. concluded that limbic system dysfunction caused CFS patients to experience memory deficits. In fact, Sandman et al. went so far as to compare the memory deficits to those seen in patients with Herpes Simplex Encephalitis (HSE). In contradiction to the speculation of Sandman et al., most patients with HSE are severely impaired on free-and cued-recall tests, and are generally much more impaired than the CFS patients they studied.

McDonald et al. (1993) reported the results of a brief cognitive screening of patients with chronic fatigue. The report did not clarify whether these patients met the CDC criteria. The sample was obviously mixed because at least one of the patients described had suffered previously from poliomyelitis and would ordinarily have been excluded from CDC definition-based studies. Fifty of the 65 patients studied were female. Their results indicated that 72% of the sample would have met ICD-9 psychiatric classification criteria for various forms of depression. There was a correlation between the subjective belief of cognitive impairment and the presence of depression. The degree of fatigue was correlated with cognitive performance. McDonald et al. also found that CFS patients performed poorly on a cued-recall task, but they noted that the patients' performance rapidly improved to normal over several trials.

The studies reviewed so far provide a confusing picture of the cognitive status of CFS patients. Some studies find normal to near-normal cognitive status in CFS patients or can account for the mild neuropsychological deficits on the basis of severity of depression. Several of the studies mainly found memory deficits. One study with British ME patients identified delays in visual information processing speed and response times, in addition to memory deficits. Did these disparate results arise because the subject samples were not comparable among studies? All of the samples seem to involve relatively young, mostly female, well-educated subjects who met either the CFS or ME criteria that describe similar but not necessarily identical cohorts. Yet, until the Centers for Disease Control and Prevention publish the results of their descriptive surveillance study, which is intended to better characterize CFS, some caution needs to be exercised when generalizing from one sample of patients with CFS (or ME) to others.

The National Institutes of Health (NIH) Studies

CFS patients predominantly complain about problems in concentration, memory, and mood (Grafman et al., 1993; Katon & Russo 1992; Smith et al., in press). If their concentration is impaired, it might be expected that designing a study that would require CFS subjects to keep their attention focused for several hours would exacerbate their concentration problems. Our first study was designed to examine this simple hypothesis.

For this study, we adapted a well-known paradigm that requires sustained attention (Scheffers et al., 1992). In this task, subjects are asked to look at a computer monitor and determine when a target letter appears among a set of distractor letters. The target and distractors may remain similar over all of the trials, or they may change: targets from previous trials or totally new items may be the distractors. This task requires both controlled processing (when the target and distractor relations shift) or relatively automatic processing (when the target and distractor relations remain the same). In our adaptation, subjects were required to press a key as quickly as possible when they saw a target (targets were not present on all trials). In addition, the patients' event-related brain evoked potentials (ERP) during their performance were recorded. The event-related brain potential is a sensitive measure of "central/cognitive processing time" and is independent of response execution. This measurement allows for a subtle evaluation of the integrity of brain mechanisms involved in the perception of, and reasoning about, stimuli. Both the latency and amplitude of the various event-related brain potentials can be measured and, when altered, have different implications for brain functions.

Besides the main attention task described above, a standard visual "oddball" task was administered in which the subject had to respond with a key press when a target stimuli appeared. The target stimuli can appear with different probabilities—the one most often used is the 20% probability that led investigators to describe this task as the oddball. This task was administered briefly before and after the main attention task. The whole testing session took approximately 4 hours. Of particular interest was whether there would be observeable objective changes in test performance, response times (rt), or ERPs over the 4-hour test period.

The results were unexpected. The study showed that there were no overall between-group differences in performance accuracy, ERP latency, or ERP amplitude on any of the tasks. Performance and ERP similarities were maintained across the 4-hour session. Interestingly, despite normal performance accuracy and ERPs, the CFS patients' response times were significantly slower than controls in both tasks. These rt differences were not exacerbated across the 4-hour session. Furthermore, patients complained during the session (despite normal accuracy and central processing times) and the following day about how tired the testing had made them.

These results suggest that, under some conditions, CFS patients can adequately attend selectively to information over a long period of time—even when the information is presented rapidly and requires sustained focused attention. The results also show that the brain mechanisms required for this attentiveness appear to be normally operating (but see Prasher et al., 1990, for a contrary finding). Brain wave measures of motor preparation were not collected and, therefore, no clear explanation for the observed delayed response times or for the severity of the patients' complaints (in light of their adequate performance accuracy) is possible.

Given the patients' other major complaints about memory and problem-solving, a second study was done to evaluate the memory and reasoning capacity of CFS patients (Grafman et al., 1993). Twenty CFS patients and 17 normal volunteers were studied. Although the study focused on memory measures, tests of planning, response time, and intellectual capacity were also included. Two "Tower" planning tasks were selected because they represented different difficulty levels in planning. Thus, this battery not only measured those domains of cognition noted by CFS patients to be taxing, but included measures known to be sensitive to "subcortical dementia," such as time perception, response speed, and planning. A more detailed description of these tests (and all others mentioned in this chapter), except where noted, is available in Grafman et al., 1993 or Lezak, 1983.

All patients and controls demonstrated excellent effort and motivation during the evaluation. As in the first study, all of the patients remarked that the examination was tiring. Some patients complained of debilitating fatigue only on the day following the completion of the evaluation.

The study showed no significant between-group differences in performance on tests of intelligence, response time, planning, time perception, or problem-solving, with two exceptions: (1) the CFS patients demonstrated greater variability than the controls in the timing of their tapping on a Time Clock task, $F(1,33) = 4.62$, $p < .03$, although the overall mean tapping times of the CFS patients and controls were similar; and (2) CFS patients solved *more* problems than did the controls on the Tower of London task, $F(1,33) = 4.04$, $p < .05$, but tended to make more errors in correctly solving the Tower of London problems, $F(1,30) = 7.38$, $p < .01$.

Several different components of memory functioning were evaluated. There were no between-group differences on the digit span task, indicating that short-term memory span was intact in the CFS group. There were also no between-group differences in retrieval of category exemplars, suggesting that at least some aspects of semantic memory search and retrieval were intact. The CFS patients also demonstrated normal reaction times (in contrast to their response times during the ERP study) and visuomotor procedural learning.

Despite normal functioning on these memory measures, CFS patients had a significantly lower average score than controls on the General Memory Index of the WMS, $F(1,34) = 5.05$, $p < .03$, suggesting that some aspects of their current memory functioning were impaired. Specific subtest raw-score comparisons revealed that the CFS patients were only impaired on the immediate, $(F(1,34) = 5.94, p < .02)$, and delayed, $(F(1,34) = 5.15, p < .02)$, visual reproduction subtests, which required the subject to reproduce complex geometric designs. Other subtests—requiring attention and orientation, immediate and delayed verbal cued- and free recall, and nonverbal recognition memory—were all performed within normal limits. On two measures of free and incidental recall (from the Experimental Paired-Associates and Hasher Frequency tasks), CFS patients' recall and judgment were similar to those of the controls. On the first of two experimental stories, the CFS patients recalled as many story idea units as did the controls. However, following the second story, patients recalled significantly fewer idea units than did controls, $F(1,33) = 15.26, p < .0004$. Furthermore, on the Experimental Paired-Associates Test, CFS patients recalled fewer words in the cued-retrieval condition than did controls, $F(1,35) = 4.81, p < .03$.

Thus, CFS patients appeared to have generally normal memory functioning; yet, paradoxically, they demonstrated specific difficulties in recalling information under conditions of greater semantic structure and context (e.g., cued as opposed to free recall, and recall of story propositions as opposed to isolated words) and in reproducing geometric designs. This result is the opposite of the common finding in which normal subjects *and* patients with various types of central nervous system impairments are generally helped by increasing stimulus structure (as seen in story memory or cued-recall tasks). Correlational analysis was not particularly helpful in identifying associations between other variables (e.g., age, education, degree of fatigue, or mood state) and the memory test scores in the CFS patients, although verbal IQ was significantly correlated with the number of propositions retrieved on story two ($r = .46$), suggesting that the general verbal skills of these patients were partially responsible for their poorer performance.

Test results showed no significant differences in the number of depressive symptoms reported by the CFS patients and controls on the Beck Depression Inventory. Scores from an examiner rating scale showed that about one-quarter of the CFS patients tested demonstrated mild to moderately impaired attention and memory in their interactions with the examiner. As expected, CFS patients reported being significantly more fatigued on the day of testing than controls, $F(1,30) = 46.37, p < .0001$. Their fatigue on the testing day was compatible with their general level of fatigue throughout the illness. However, there were no differences between the level of preillness fatigue in the CFS patients and the current level of fatigue in the controls. Furthermore, there was no relationship between any of these fatigue measures and cognitive performance in the CFS group.

This neuropsychological evaluation demonstrated that CFS patients may have selective deficits in memory processing arising against a background of relatively normal cognitive functioning. Curiously, the CFS patients had greater problems recalling material when the material or retrieval measure was the most structured. There was no relationship between performance on these specific memory measures and mood state, fatigue level, age, or education, although verbal intelligence was correlated with story memory performance. Furthermore, the study was unable to replicate their previously reported problems in visual processing and attention.

Although this sample of CFS patients was similar to other samples reported in the literature, in terms of illness profile, severity, and disability, the subjects were, nevertheless, able to come to the NIH and participate in extensive evaluations. Such testing might reflect the optimal performance of CFS patients rather than the more disabling symptoms that would force patients to remain at home rather than be tested (Wood et al., 1992).

Several other aspects of cognitive functioning in CFS patients, including selective attention and the ability of CFS patients to accurately predict the level of their subsequent cognitive performance, are currently being examined. Also under analysis is the performance of over 480 subjects who participated in the Centers for Disease Control and Prevention surveillance study of CFS on a neuropsychological screening battery. This latter analysis should provide valuable information regarding the range of cognitive functioning in the CFS population.

Summary of Neuropsychological Studies

In summarizing the results of the few neuropsychological studies so far published, some general observations can be made. A majority of CFS patients will have marked complaints of cognitive deficits, particularly in the domains of memory, attention and concentration, and problem solving. A majority of patients will also have marked complaints of emotional distress. In some studies, the severity of the cognitive and mood-state complaints tends to be correlated. Objective neuropsychological testing does not substantiate the severity of the cognitive complaints of CFS patients. However, some areas of cognitive deficit emerge with memory, attention, and response speed problems most frequently identified. The severity of the objectively recorded cognitive deficits ranges from mild to severe, although most deficits fall into the mild range. Some evidence shows that CFS patients have more difficulty remembering well-structured as opposed to loosely structured information. On the other hand, CFS patients' performance remains normal on many tests of memory and cognitive processing. In some instances, covarying for the level of depression removed the between-group differences in cognitive performance that had existed.

THE TARGETED
NEUROPSYCHOLOGICAL ASSESSMENT

The neuropsychological complaints of CFS patients must be addressed by trained neuropsychologists. Therefore, the standard neuropsychological screening evaluation for CFS should include tasks that focus on memory, attentional processes, response times, and problem-solving. Some attempt to estimate premorbid cognitive abilities would be useful, given that CFS patients are generally premorbidly bright and, thus, currently obtained scores that are simply compared to a normative sample may underestimate the true level of their deficit. Some personality scales measuring anxiety, depression, somatization, and level of fatigue and its effect on interpersonal functioning should also be included (in part, to assess concurrent mood state or the possibility of malingering, Franzen et al., 1990). A scale that measures the cognitive complaints of CFS patients should be used in conjunction with their objective test performance. A careful mood state and personality evaluation can help account for some of the confounding variables (e.g., decreased effort or alertness due to a depressive disorder) that may affect performance on cognitive tasks. Table 5.1 lists some of the domains and types of tests potentially useful in the examination of CFS patients. When possible, a formal psychiatric diagnostic interview should be conducted with each patient by a trained examiner. Because the patient may have cycles of fatigue, testing can be scheduled to either optimize test performance or to assess the patient when he or she is fatigued.

There are several possible explanations for the impaired cognitive performance in CFS patients. For example, CFS could involve lesions or dysfunction in one or more subcortical brain structures (e.g., hypothalamic-pituitary dysfunction, Demitrack et al., 1991, 1992) that are, in turn, partially responsible for the instantiation of the specific cognitive processes that patients complain are being impaired (e.g., memory or speed of information processing). On the other hand, CFS, as a chronic but non-neurological illness, could lead to a reactive psychiatric disorder, such as depression, that would then affect the effort patients would make on specific cognitive tasks. The cognitive deficits in CFS could also represent an exaggerated behavioral response, in certain personalities, to a "normally" occurring fluctuation in immune system regulation due to increased stress induced by problems in interpersonal or professional relationships (Abbey & Garfinkel, 1991; Lane et al., 1991; White, 1990). Neuropsychological deficits are surely not proof of CNS dysfunction or lesions. Because of the diagnostic dilemma posed by CFS patients and the current lack of hard neurological signs, it will be an interesting challenge for the neuropsychologist to interpret their test results. In addition, studying patients whose illness is characterized by a persistent

TABLE 5.1. A Neuropsychological Test Battery for CFS

Intelligence

A test of global intellectual ability

Reasoning and Problem Solving

Measure of concept formation   Measure of planning
Measure of analogical reasoning   Measure of "feeling of knowing"

Attention

Measure of sustained attention   Measures of selected and divided attention

Memory

Measures of working memory   Measures of learning
Measures of recall and recognition   Measures of implicit memory and
                                         automatic processing

Response Time

Measures of motor speed and   Measures of simple and choice response
  coordination   times

Mood State and Personality

Measure of fatigue   Measure of somatization
Measure of personality traits   Measures of depression and anxiety
Measure of self-report of cognitive   Psychiatric interview
  status

Note: The evaluation of CFS patients should target specfic domains of cognitive functioning. Specific tests for each domain can be identified in Lezak (1983).

fatigue (occasionally in the absence of a confirmed psychiatric disorder/history) can help neuropsychologists understand the effects of peripheral and central fatigue on specific cognitive functions—an unresolved issue in interpreting the results of a neuropsychological evaluation that may last several hours.

CONCLUSIONS

Chronic fatigue syndrome is a diagnostic entity that eludes a single etiological description (Daugherty et al., 1991; Dawson & Sabin, 1993; Durack & Street, 1991; Holmes et al., 1988; Levine et al., 1992; Peterson et al., 1991; Schluederberg et al., 1991, 1992), but it is accepted as a medical illness by general physicians (Denz-Penhey & Murdoch, 1993). Studies to date, in general, have only revealed relatively minor cognitive problems in patients. These problems lie in the domains of memory and attention, and are occasionally related to the degree of mood state changes as reported by the patient. To date, studies indicate that the severity of impairment in attention and memory as reported by the CFS patient exceeds their objective performance.

Neuropsychological testing should be done in conjunction with a comprehensive medical diagnostic workup (Demitrack & Greden, 1991) that is targeted to evaluate whether the patient meets the CDC CFS criteria. Currently, and unfortunately, these criteria are not strictly adhered to but instead depend on the hospital, region, or country where the diagnosis is made (Scheffers et al., 1992; Schluederberg et al., 1991, 1992).

Regardless of the comparisons of CFS to neurasthenia, or the words of pundits who dismiss CFS as nothing more than a "yuppie disease" or a euphamism for a psychiatric diagnosis, these patients present with cognitive complaints that require the involvement of trained neuropsychologists for assessment. The inclusion of a neuropsychological evaluation in the medical workup for CFS will surely lead to improved sensitivity, if not specificity, and characterization of the disabling neurological and behavioral symptoms so often reported by patients with this disorder.

ACKNOWLEDGMENTS

Thanks go to Kim Clark for her help in testing the CFS patients. I would also like to thank Steve Straus and Janet Dale for referring their CFS patients for neuropsychological studies. The National Institute for Neurological Disorders and Stroke provided the resources that enabled us to carry out our studies. Portions of this chapter are taken from Grafman (1995).

REFERENCES

Abbey, SE, Garfinkel, PE. Neurasthenia and chronic fatigue syndrome: The role of culture in the making of a diagnosis. *Am J Psychiatry* 1991; 148(12): 1638–1646.

Altay, HT, Toner, BB, Brooker, H, Abbey, SE, Salit, IE, Garfinkel, PE. The neuropsychological dimensions of postinfectious neuromyasthenia (chronic fatigue syndrome): A preliminary report. *Int J Psychiatry Med* 1990; 20(2):141–149.

Bock, GR, Whelan, J, ed. *Chronic fatigue syndrome,* Ciba Foundation Symposium 173. New York: John Wiley & Sons, 1993.

Brasil-Neto, JP, Pascual-Leone, A, Valls-Sole, J, Cammarota, A, Cohen, LG, Hallett, M. Postexercise depression of motor evoked potentials: A measure of central nervous system fatigue. *Experimental Brain Res* 1993; 93:181–184.

Buchwald, D, Cheney, PR, Peterson, DL, Henry, B., Wormsley, SB, Geiger, A, Ablashi, DV, Salahuddin, SZ, Saxinger, C, Biddle, R, Kikiuis, R, Jolesz, FA, Folks, T, Balachandrau, N, Peter, JB, Gallo, RC, Komaroff, AL. A chronic illness characterized by fatigue, neurologic and immunologic disorders, and active human herpesvirus type 6 infection. *Ann Int Med* 1992; 116(2):103–113.

Chalder, T, Berelowitz, G, Pawlikowska, T, Watts, L, Wessely, S, Wright, D, Wallace, EP. Development of a fatigue scale. *Psychosom Res* 1993; 37(2):147–153.

Daugherty, SA, Henry, BE, Peterson, DL, Swarts, RL, Bastien, S, Thomas, RS. Chronic fatigue syndrome in northern Nevada. *Rev Infect Dis* 1991; 13(Supplement 1):S39–S44.

Dawson, DM, Sabin, TD, eds. *Chronic fatigue syndrome*. Boston: Little, Brown, & Company, 1993.

DeLuca, J, Johnson, SK, Natelson, BH. Information processing efficiency in chronic fatigue syndrome and multiple sclerosis. *Arch Neurology* 1993; 50(3):301–304.

Demitrack, MA, Dale, JK, Straus, SF, Laue, L, Listwak, SJ, Kruesi, MJP, Chrousos, GP, Gold, PW. Evidence for impaired activation of the hypothalamic–pituitary–adrenal axis in patients with chronic fatigue syndrome. *J Clin Endocrin Metab* 1991; 73(6):1224–1234.

Demitrack, MA, Gold, PW, Dale, JK, Krahn, DD, Kling, MA, Straus, SE. Plasma and cerebrospinal fluid monoamine metabolism in patients with chronic fatigue syndrome: Preliminary findings. *Biol Psychiatry* 1992; 32:1065–1077.

Demitrack, MA, Greden, JF. Chronic fatigue syndrome: The need for an integrative approach. *Biol Psychiatry* 1991; 30(8):747–752.

Denz-Penhey, H, Murdoch, JC. General practitioners acceptance of the validity of chronic fatigue syndrome as a diagnosis. *N Zealand Med J* 1993; 106 (April 14; 953):122–124.

Durack, DT, Street, AC. Fever of unknown origin—reexamined and redefined. *Curr Clin Top Infect Dis* 1991; 11(35):35–51.

Franzen, MD, Iverson, GL, McCracken, LM. The detection of malingering in neuropsychological assessment. *Neuropsychol Rev* 1990; 1(3):247–279.

Goodnick, PJ, Sandoval, R. Psychotropic treatment of chronic fatigue syndrome and related disorders. *J Clin Psychiatry* 1993; 54(1):13–20.

Grafman, J. Neuropsychological features of chronic fatigue syndrome. In Straus, S, ed., *Chronic fatigue syndrome*. New York: Marcel Dekker, 1995.

Grafman, J, Johnson, RJ, Scheffers, M. Cognitive and mood-state changes in patients with chronic fatigue syndrome. *Rev Infect Dis* 1991; 13(Supplement 1):S45–S52.

Grafman, J, Schwartz, V, Dale, JK, Scheffers, M, Houser, C, Straus, SE. Analysis of neuropsychological functioning in patients with chronic fatigue syndrome. *J Neurol Neurosurg Psychiatry* 1993; 56(6):684–689.

Holmes, GP, Kaplan, JE, Gantz, NM, Komaroff, AL, Schonberger, LB, Straus, SE, Jones, JF, Dubois, RE, Cunningham-Rundles, C, Pahwa, S, Tosato, G, Zegans, LS, Purtilo, DT, Brown, N, Schooley, RT, Brus, I. Chronic fatigue syndrome: A working case definition. *Ann Int Med* 1988; 108(3):387–389.

Ichise, M, Salit, IE, Abbey, SE, Chung, DG, Gray, B, Kirsh, JC, Freedman, M. Assessment of regional cerebral perfusion by 99 Tcm-HMPAO SPECT in chronic fatigue syndrome. *Nuclear Med Comm* 1992; 13:767–772.

Imboden, JB, Canter, A, Cluff, LB, Trever, RW. Brucellosis: III. Psychological aspects of delayed convalescence. *Arch Int Med* 1959; 103(3):406–414.

Kachuck, NJ, Weiner, LP. Viral infection and the chronic fatigue syndrome. *Curr Neurol,* 289–324. St. Louis: Mosby–Year Book, 1993.

Katon, W, Russo, J. Chronic fatigue syndrome criteria: A critique of the requirement for multiple physical complaints. *Arch Intern Med* 1992; 152(8):1604–1609.

Komaroff, AL. Clinical presentation of chronic fatigue syndrome. *Chronic fatigue syndrome,* Ciba Foundation Symposium 173. New York: John Wiley & Sons, 1993; 43–61.

Krupp, L, Sliwinski, MJ, Doscher, C, Jandorf, L, Burns, L, Coyle, PK. *Fatigue, mood, and cognitive functions in chronic fatigue syndrome (CFS) and multiple sclerosis (MS).* Albany Conference on Chronic Fatigue Syndrome. Albany, New York, 1992.

Lane, TJ, Manu, P, Matthews, DA. Depression and somatization in the chronic fatigue syndrome. *Am J Med* 1991; 91(4):335–344.

Levine, PH, Jacobson, S, Pocinki, AG, Cheney, P, Peterson, D, Connelly, RR, Weil, R, Robinson, SM, Ablashi, DV, Salahuddin, SZ, Pearson, GR, Hoover, R. Clinical, epidemiologic, and virologic studies in four clusters of the chronic fatigue syndrome. *Arch Intern Med* 1992; 152(8):1611–1616.

Lezak, M. *Neuropsychological assessment.* New York: Oxford University Press, 1983.

McDonald, E, Cope, H, David, A. Cognitive impairment in patients with chronic fatigue: A preliminary study. *J Neurol Neurosurg Psychiatry* 1993; 56(7):812–815.

Morriss, R, Sharpe, M, Sharpley, AL, Cowen, PJ, Hawton, K, Morris, J. Abnormalities of sleep in patients with the chronic fatigue syndrome. *Br Med J* 1993; 306(May 1 (6886)):1161–1164.

Peterson, PK, Schenck, CH, Sherman, R. Chronic fatigue syndrome in Minnesota [see comments]. *Minn Med* 1991; 74(5):21–26.

Prasher, P, Smith, A, Findley, L. Sensory and cognitive event-related potentials in myalgic encephalomyelitis. *J Neurol Neurosurg Psychiatry* 1990; 53(3):247–253.

Ray, C, Weir, WRC, Cullen, S, Phillips, S. Illness perception and symptom components in chronic fatigue syndrome. *J Psychosom Res* 1992; 36(3):243–256.

Riccio, M, Thompson, C, Wilson, B, Morgan, DJ, Lant, AF. Neuropsychological and psychiatric abnormalities in myalgic encephalomyelitis: A preliminary report. *Br J Clin Psychol* 1992; 31(2):111–120.

Sandman, CA, Barron, JL, Nackoul, K, Goldstein, J, Fidler, F. Memory deficits associated with chronic fatigue immune dysfunction syndrome. *Biol Psychiatry* 1993; 33(8–9):618–623.

Scheffers, MK, Johnson, RJ, Grafman, J, Dale, JK, Straus, SE. Attention and short-term memory in chronic fatigue syndrome patients: An event-related potential analysis. *Neurology* 1992; 42(9):1667–1675.

Schluederberg, A, Straus, SE, Grufferman, S. Considerations in the design of studies of chronic fatigue syndrome. *Rev Infect Dis* 1991; 13(Supplement 1):S1–S140.

Schluederberg, A, Straus, SE, Peterson, P, Blumenthal, S, Komaroff, AL, Spring, SB, Landay, A, Buchwald, D. Chronic fatigue syndrome research: Definition and medical outcome assessment. *Ann Int Med* 1992; 117(4):325–331.

Smith, AP. Chronic fatigue syndrome and performance. In Smith, AP, Jones, DM, eds., *Handbook of human performance.* London: Academic Press, 1992a.

Smith, AP. Cognitive changes in myalgic encephalomyelitis. In Jenkins, R, Mowbray, J, eds., *Post-viral fatigue syndrome*. London: John Wiley & Sons, 1992b.

Smith, AP, Behan, PO, Bell, W, Millar, K, Bakheit, M. Behavioral problems associated with the chronic fatigue syndrome. *Br J Psychol,* in press.

Straus, SE, Dale, JK, Tobi, M, Lawley, T, Preble, O, Blaese, RM, Hallahan, C, Henle, W. Acyclovir treatment of the chronic fatigue syndrome: Lack of efficacy in a placebo-controlled trial. *N Engl J Med* 1988; 319:1692–1698.

Weingartner, H, Silberman, E. Cognitive changes in depression. In Post, R, Ballenger, J, eds., *Neurobiology of mood disorders*. Baltimore: Williams & Wilkins, 1987.

Wessely, S. Old wine in new bottles: Neurasthenia and "ME." *Psychol Med* 1990; 20(1):35–53.

Wessely, S. The neuropsychiatry of chronic fatigue syndrome. In Dawson, DM, Sabin, TD, eds., *Chronic fatigue syndrome,* Ciba Symposium 173. New York: John Wiley & Sons, 1993; 229–237.

White, PD. Fatigue and chronic fatigue syndromes. *Somatization: Physical symptoms and psychological illness*. London: Blackwell Scientific Publications, 1990; 104–140.

Wood, C, Magnello, ME, Sharpe, MC. Fluctuations in perceived energy and mood among patients with chronic fatigue syndrome. *J Roy Soc Med* 1992; 85(4): 195–198.

6

Psychiatric Assessment of Patients with Chronic Fatigue Syndrome

Susan E. Abbey, M.D.
Mark A. Demitrack, M.D.

All patients presenting with chronic fatigue syndrome (CFS) require an assessment of psychiatric symptomatology. This assessment should include a review of symptoms of the diagnoses most commonly associated with CFS and a mental status examination to evaluate general appearance, behavior, mood, neurovegetative changes of depression, and suicidality. A basic psychiatric assessment should be done in *all* patients assessed by primary care practitioners and tertiary care CFS specialists for a diagnosis of CFS. A subgroup of patients will require further evaluation by a psychiatrist, psychologist, or neuropsychologist for diagnostic clarification when symptoms are atypical or the case is complex. For a cognitive therapy or cognitive-behavioral therapy rehabilitation program, a more comprehensive psychiatric and psychosocial assessment is typically needed (see Chapter 10, this volume). This chapter will review the components of the psychiatric assessment of the patient presenting with CFS, discuss a variety of assessment strategies and tools, and examine the problems inherent in conducting psychiatric assessments in individuals with medical diagnoses characterized by symptoms that may be confounded with the somatic symptoms of psychiatric disorders.

THE SOCIOCULTURAL CONTEXT OF THE PSYCHIATRIC ASSESSMENT OF PATIENTS PRESENTING WITH CHRONIC FATIGUE SYNDROME

The psychiatric assessment of the patient with CFS must be understood within the broader sociocultural context of CFS (Abbey & Garfinkel, 1990, 1991; Wessely, 1990). The study of the psychiatric aspects of CFS reminds us of the ongoing stigmatization of psychiatric disorders and the pejorative and damaging attributions given to individuals with psychiatric diagnoses. Psychiatric symptomatology continues to be seen as being under the voluntary control of the individual; thus, symptoms are associated with blame. The ongoing Cartesian dualism of mind and body has also resulted in the unfortunately still widespread opinion that "organic" disorders are "real" and that psychiatric disorders are "imaginary" at best and "fake" at worst. Psychiatric disorders still are seen by many as being equivalent to lying, faking, or malingering and are thought to result from moral laxity or a failure of will. This position is made clear in the media with titles announcing research discoveries about possible viral etiologies for the syndrome. For example, one headline announced: "Virus Research Doctors Prove Shirkers Really Are Sick." This thinking leads to an attitude, among many patients, that has been summarized as "the only good psychiatrist is the one who returns the patient to the internist or family doctor saying, 'This is not my field; there is nothing I can do'" (Wessely, 1989).

GOALS OF THE PSYCHIATRIC ASSESSMENT

1. *Case definition.* Psychiatric diagnoses such as psychotic disorders (schizophrenia, bipolar affective disorder, and psychotic depression), melancholic depression, substance use disorders, and eating disorders must be excluded if a patient is to meet the current case definition criteria for CFS (Fukuda et al., 1994; see Chapter 1, this volume).

2. *Identifying treatable psychiatric disorders in patients meeting the case definition for CFS.* The assessment of psychiatric symptomatology in patients meeting the case definition criteria opens the possibility for treatment that can substantially improve the individual's quality of life. Appropriate treatment should be instituted when symptoms are of a number and severity to meet psychiatric diagnostic criteria. Recognizing the presence of a somatoform disorder assists the clinician in planning further investigations and treatments so as to minimize iatrogenic complications and commence a treatment program that will be of the most benefit to the patient (Abbey, in press).

3. *Identifying primary psychiatric disorders misdiagnosed as CFS.* Patients with self- or physician diagnoses of CFS may actually be suffering from a misdiagnosed or undiagnosed primary psychiatric disorder. Highly effective treatments now exist for the mood and anxiety disorders that may be misdiagnosed as CFS. These patients can be helped in short periods of time with pharmacotherapy or focused psychotherapy, and protracted periods of dysfunction and disability may be averted.

4. *Effective rehabilitation.* Effective rehabilitation programs are founded on comprehensive psychiatric and psychosocial assessments to rule out mood disorders that require treatment prior to commencing rehabilitation, and to identify psychiatric and psychosocial factors that must be taken into account in treatment planning. The importance of untreated mood disorders in patients who refuse treatment or drop out of treatment has been described (Butler et al., 1991; Wessely et al., 1991). Detailed psychosocial assessments are necessary in order to develop appropriate cognitive and cognitive-behavioral interventions for patients with CFS. Specific assessment issues related to the development of cognitive-behavioral interventions are described by Sharpe (see Chapter 10, this volume).

PROBLEMS ASSOCIATED WITH DIAGNOSING PSYCHIATRIC DISORDERS IN PATIENTS WITH MEDICAL ILLNESSES

Somatic symptoms that are used to diagnose depression (e.g., sleep and appetite disturbance, low energy, increased fatigability) are frequent in patients with a variety of medical disorders (Rodin et al., 1991). The problems, both practical and theoretical, in sorting out the etiology of such symptoms has been discussed at length earlier in this volume (see Chapter 3).

PROBLEMS IN ASSESSING PSYCHIATRIC SYMPTOMATOLOGY IN PATIENTS WITH CFS

The assessment of psychiatric symptomatology is complicated by a number of factors, including (1) underreporting of symptoms secondary to the sociocultural context of CFS; (2) temporal sequencing of symptoms related to the retrospective nature of symptom reports; (3) incomplete symptom reporting because of patients' etiologic assumptions regarding CFS as the basis for symptoms, and thus not reporting them to a psychiatrist doing a psychiatric review of symptoms; (4) possible mismatch between the patients' subjective symptoms or lack thereof and the clinician's "objective" assessment. Problems related to temporal sequencing of symptoms and nonreporting due to differing etiologic assumptions are well known to the consultation-liaison psychiatrist assessing patients with medical comorbidities. Problems related to a mismatch between subjective and objective symptoms are common in a variety of other disorders at the interface of medicine and psychiatry.

THE MISDIAGNOSIS OF PRIMARY PSYCHIATRIC DISORDERS AS CFS

Clinicians performing assessments of individuals with physician or self-diagnosis of CFS not uncommonly diagnose a primary psychiatric disorder that has been mistakenly diagnosed as CFS. The misdiagnosis of primary emotional disorders as physical illness has been described and is of just as much concern as the reverse type of error because it precludes people from receiving effective treatment (Stewart, 1990). An accurate diagnosis opens the door to specific, effective treatments, although it may be experienced as more stigmatizing by the patient. It is important to aggressively treat patients whose primary psychiatric disorders are eminently treatable (e.g., major depression or panic disorder). For those individuals who are invested in CFS as a diagnosis, it may be counterproductive to engage in a debate as to the etiology of their symptomatology. Effort should be made to encourage them to accept treatments that are widely used in the management of CFS. Examples of the misdiagnosis of primary psychiatric disorders as CFS are discussed in the following case vignettes. These examples are not meant to undermine the validity of the CFS diagnosis but rather to draw attention to the importance of the misdiagnosis of conditions that have specific, efficacious treatments, in contrast to CFS, where there is no single effective treatment and symptom control and rehabilitation are the goals of therapy.

THE ASSESSMENT PROCESS

A number of differences exist between standard outpatient psychiatric assessment procedures and the assessment process in the patient with CFS. The examiner must be cognizant of the reluctance and fear that many patients bring to the process and of the ongoing stigmatization of psychiatric evaluation. The assessment process can be broken down into three major phases: (1) engage the patient in the assessment process; (2) satisfy yourself that treatable medical illnesses have been excluded; and (3) assess for a range of psychopathology. Always tailor the assessment to the concerns and the physical and psychiatric symptomatology of the individual patient.

Engage the Patient in the Assessment Process

Physicians must elicit and openly address patients' concerns about psychiatric assessment. This discussion should be done in primary care, tertiary care, and psychiatric referral settings. In the latter, it is important to know what the patient understands about the reasons for psychiatric referral and what is anticipated to be the results of such an assessment. Unfortunately, primary care practitioners and specialists continue to have difficulty in facilitating patient acceptance of psychiatric referral, and this difficulty may result in the patients' arriving in the psychiatrist's office with a distorted view of the psychiatric assessment process. Several recent publications have discussed how the internist may facilitate referrals to psychiatry (Burszatjn & Barsky, 1985; Smith, 1991). It is important for the physician to convey the "normativeness" of psychiatric referral in patients with complex medical illnesses associated with significant dysfunction, disability, and uncertain prognosis. Most patients are willing to accept a psychiatric referral when they see it as benefiting their doctor in treatment planning or as one component of a multidisciplinary treatment approach. Patients are understandably reluctant to follow through with an assessment that they perceive as being a means of their physician's withdrawing from care or "dumping" or "disposing" of them, or when they perceive the physician as devaluing their suffering and labeling it as "all in the head."

The majority of patients come to psychiatrists with a variety of misconceptions about or negative attitudes toward psychiatry and psychiatrists. This attitude may be informed by negative personal or family experiences with psychiatry. However, many patients' odd ideas about psychiatry have been derived from the media, especially films and television, where psychiatrists are often stereotyped as "crazy," "incompetent," "evil," or sexually inappropriate (Gabbard & Gabbard, 1989). The stereotype of psychiatric treatment as being limited to the analytic couch and the silent analyst remains all too common among the general public. The recent attention given to inappropriate therapist–patient sexual conduct is also of concern to many patients. It is helpful to address these concerns in a direct, nondefensive manner and to provide explanation or reassurance as needed.

Patients must have the time to tell their story in their own way. For most CFS patients, this translates into a necessity of focusing on their physical symptoms and their illness course as a prelude to discussing their life stressors, coping strategies, psychosocial adjustment, and psychiatric symptomatology. The assessment of CFS patients typically requires more than one session. Additional sessions are necessary because of the need to allow adequate time to review the medical aspects of the syndrome and because patients are often more willing to discuss psychologically meaningful themes as they become more comfortable with the psychiatrist and develop a positive therapeutic alliance.

A variety of techniques have been described to assist in evaluating patients who are reluctant to be assessed. These techniques have been described in reviews of psychiatric assessment (Taylor, 1993) and in the literature on the assessment of patients with functional somatic symptoms and those who are somatically focused (Creed & Guthrie, 1993; Sharpe et al., 1992). The importance of a conversational tone and a nonjudgmental atmosphere cannot be underestimated. When the appropriate tone and atmosphere are combined with supportive statements, the patient is put at ease and there is an increased likelihood of obtaining a more complete assessment (Taylor, 1993). The interview should begin with questioning the patient about his or her understanding of the purpose of the assessment and the expected results. The patient should be asked about the reason given for the referral and about any concerns regarding the assessment. Although many patients initially indicate that these are not important issues for them, when concerns are presented as "normal" and "common" in patients seen with CFS, they are often very forthcoming in describing their many concerns, including worries that their physician is "getting rid of" them, does not believe they are truly distressed or sick, or sees their problem as "all in the head." Similarly, many patients will raise these issues later in the course of the interview, as they feel increasingly comfortable with the examiner.

The examiner may facilitate the process by reading whatever documentation accompanies the referral letter and by indicating to the patient a familiarity with CFS and experience in dealing with it. The clinician can reassure the patient that psychiatric symptomatology and psychiatric disorders are common comorbid occurrences with a variety of illnesses, including CFS, and that in many cases psychiatric treatment may lead to a substantial improvement in quality of life.

Sufficient time must be set aside for the assessment. In contrast to standard outpatient psychiatric assessments, where 45 to 50 minutes is adequate, most CFS assessments require either two sessions or one extended session, to give patients enough time to tell their story in their own way. An interview should begin with giving the patient the opportunity to recount the course of the illness and the most troublesome current symptoms. It is helpful to get an estimate of the person's energy level, and, although somewhat artificial and arbitrary, the use of a visual analog scale from 0% to 100% can be very helpful. Patients are asked to use the scale to describe their level of energy prior to becoming ill, at the worst period during their illness, on a "bad day" now, on a "better or not-so-bad day" in recent weeks, and on the day of the assessment.

Empathizing with the patient's difficult situation and with the losses associated with the illness facilitates the CFS patient's storytelling. The distant "analytic" stance, in which the examiner is unresponsive so as not to contaminate the interview, is extremely counterproductive in this patient population as well as in other medical populations. Patients need to know that the interviewer is truly hearing their stories. Withholding empathic or supportive comments can only be experienced negatively: the examiner will be seen as either not listening or not appreciating the seriousness of the patients' condition, or as being an unkind, unfeeling, cold "jerk."

Satisfy Yourself That Treatable Medical Illnesses Have Been Excluded

Ensure that patients with CFS have had an adequate medical workup and that appropriate screening evaluations have been done (see Chapters 6 and 7, this volume). Despite the expectation that these steps would have been completed prior to a psychiatric referral, many patients seen in consultation by mental health professionals have not received a complete basic medical investigation (e.g., thyroid function testing has not been done or antinuclear antibodies have not been measured despite significant joint and muscle symptoms). Psychiatrists have the advantage of knowing what "sick" looks like, and their intuition, based on their experience as physicians, may lead them to question whether another, potentially treatable, underlying process needs to be investigated. Similarly, over the course of working with a patient, if there is a change in symptoms or if a new symptom pattern emerges and is of concern, further medical evaluation should be undertaken. Many patients involved in CFS rehabilitation programs have, during the course of treatment or follow-up, developed definitive symptoms of rheumatoid arthritis, multiple sclerosis, or cancer.

Assess for a Range of Psychopathology

A number of psychiatric disorders may complicate the course of CFS or may be mistakenly diagnosed as CFS. The assessment of all patients should include a review of symptoms for mood disorders, anxiety disorders, somatization disorder, and substance use. Criteria for other diagnoses, such as eating disorders, should be reviewed when clinically indicated. The technical challenge for the interviewer is one of evaluating (a) affect and cognition in the context of somatic symptomatology, and (b) the quality and implications of somatic symptoms that may be characteristic of CFS but may also be part of other medical or psychiatric disorders.

The key components of history taking are shown in Table 6.1, and the mental status examination is shown in Table 6.2. There may be a mismatch between a patient's objective appearance (i.e., well-groomed, without the usual stigmata of chronic illness) and subjective reports. This mismatch has been a

TABLE 6.1. Key Components of Psychiatric History Taking in the CFS Patient

- Details of syndrome onset
  - Acute or gradual
  - Initiating events (e.g., infection, trauma, surgery, or life stress)
- Course of illness
  - Duration to date
  - Pattern of illness (e.g., slow improvement or "roller-coaster")
- Symptoms experienced
  - Which symptoms?
  - How frequently do they occur?
  - How severe are they?
  - Do they produce dysfunction or impairment?
- Current degree of function and dysfunction/impairment
  - A useful technique is to go hour-by-hour through a typical "bad" day and, depending on the patient's current status a "not so bad," "better," or "good" day
  - Attempt to specify types of physical and mental activity and their duration
  - Itemize activities that are avoided
  - Ability to socialize
  - Sexual functioning
  - Sources of pleasure
- Impact of illness on important relationships
- Current social supports—instrumental and emotional support
- Review of psychiatric symptomatology
- Medical review of systems for evidence of other medical illnesses
- Psychosocial context of the illness at syndrome onset and currently
  - Psychosocial stressors (positive and negative)
  - Psychosocial buffers or protective factors
- Coping style
  - Coping styles/techniques being used to deal with CFS
  - Most difficult life circumstance prior to this illness and how the patient coped with it
- Past personal psychiatric history
- Family medical and psychiatric history

frequent (and mistaken) cause for discounting patients and devaluing their suffering. Greg Fisher, in recounting his own experiences as a CFS sufferer, noted, "I'm afraid that many people because of their unfamiliarity with CFS and its often unobservable symptoms tend to see me as either a hypochondriac or malingerer . . . my illness will always seem more like a crutch, masking deep psychological problems, than a cry of pain caused by a very real sickness" (Fisher, 1987). The assessment of mood may be complicated by the patient's

TABLE 6.2. Mental Status Examination of the Patient with CFS

- Appearance and behavior
- Mood and affect
- Major themes of conversation
- Thought form and content

- Perceptual abnormalities
- Screening cognitive examination
- Assessment of suicidality

TABLE 6.3. DSM-IV Diagnostic Criteria for Major
Depressive Disorder

A. Five (or more) of the following symptoms have been present during the same
2-week period (most of the day, nearly every day) and represent a change from
previous functioning: at least one of the symptoms is either (1) depressed mood
or (2) loss of interest or pleasure.

Note: Do not include symptoms that are clearly due to a general medical condition, or mood-incongruent delusions or hallucinations.

1. Depressed mood as indicated by either subjective report (e.g., feels sad or
empty) or observation made by others (e.g., appears tearful)
2. Markedly diminished interest or pleasure in all, or almost all, activities (as
indicated by either subjective account or observation made by others)
3. Significant weight loss when not dieting or weight gain (e.g., a change of
more than 5% of body weight in a month), or decrease or increase in
appetite
4. Insomnia or hypersomnia nearly every day
5. Psychomotor agitation or retardation (observable by others, not merely
subjective)
6. Fatigue or loss of energy
7. Feelings of worthlessness or of excessive or inappropriate guilt (not merely
self-reproach or guilt about being sick)
8. Diminished ability to think or concentrate, or indecisiveness (either by
subjective account or as observed by others)
9. Recurrent thoughts of death (not just fear of dying), recurrent suicidal
ideation without a specific plan, or a suicide attempt or a specific plan for
committing suicide

B. Symptoms do not meet criteria for a Mixed Episode (i.e., manic and depressive
symptomatology).

C. Symptoms cause clinically significant distress or impairment in social, occupational, or other important areas of functioning.

D. Symptoms are not due to the direct physiological effects of a substance
(e.g., a drug of abuse, a medication) or a general medical condition (e.g.,
hypothyroidism).

E. Symptoms are not better accounted for by Bereavement.

Note: Modified and reprinted with permission of the American Psychiatric Association.

focus on physical symptomatology. The use of the examiner's own response (i.e., feelings of increasing sadness, fatigue, and hopelessness experienced during the interview) may help to identify those patients with masked depressions. Suicidality must be assessed in every patient because it is the one lethal complication of CFS.

The major psychiatric disorders that should be considered in the differential diagnosis will now be reviewed. The theoretical and clinical implications of these disorders were discussed earlier in this volume (see Chapter 3). Although diagnoses such as mood and anxiety disorders must be evaluated in all patients, other diagnoses should be considered based on history and observations made on mental status examination. The DSM-IV diagnostic criteria for these disorders are shown in Tables 6.3 through 6.9. Self-report instruments may be helpful in the screening of patients for psychological distress and in assisting with documentation of the subjective severity of the distress. A variety of self-report psychometric instruments have been used with CFS patients—some of the most common and clinically useful are shown in Table 6.10.

TABLE 6.4. DSM-IV Diagnostic Criteria for Dysthymic Disorder

A. Depressed mood for most of the day, for more days than not, as indicated either by subjective account or observation by others, for at least 2 years.

Note: In children and adolescents, mood can be irritable and duration must be at least 1 year.

B. Presence, while depressed, of two (or more) of the following:

1. Poor appetite or overeating
2. Insomnia or hypersomnia
3. Low energy or fatigue
4. Low self-esteem
5. Poor concentration or difficulty making decisions
6. Feelings of hopelessness

C. During the 2-year period of the disturbance, the person has never been without the symptoms in criteria A and B for more than 2 months at a time.

D. No Major Depressive Episode has been present during the first 2 years of the disturbance.

E. There has never been a Manic Episode, a Mixed Episode, or a Hypomanic Episode, and criteria have never been met for Cyclothymic Disorder.

F. The disturbance does not occur exclusively during the course of a chronic Psychotic Disorder.

G. The symptoms are not due to the direct physiological effects of a substance or a general medical condition.

H. The symptoms cause clinically significant distress or impairment in social, occupational, or other important areas of functioning.

Note: Modified and reprinted with permission of the American Psychiatric Association.

TABLE 6.5. DSM-IV Diagnostic Criteria for Seasonal Pattern Specific Mood Disorder

A. There has been a regular temporal relationship between the onset of Major Depressive Episodes and a particular time of the year (e.g., regular appearance of the Major Depressive Episode in the fall or winter).

    Note: Do not include cases in which there is an obvious effect of seasonal-related psychosocial stressors (e.g., regularly being unemployed every winter).

B. Full remissions (or a change from depression to mania or hypomania) also occur at a characteristic time of the year (e.g., depression disappears in the spring).

C. In the past 2 years, two Major Depressive Episodes have occurred that demonstrate the temporal seasonal relationships defined in criteria A and B, and no nonseasonal Major Depressive Episodes have occurred during that same period.

D. Seasonal Major Depressive Episodes (as described above) substantially outnumber the nonseasonal Major Depressive Episodes that may have occurred over the individual's lifetime.

Note: Modified and reprinted with permission of the American Psychiatric Association.

TABLE 6.6. DSM-IV Diagnostic Criteria for Generalized Anxiety Disorder

A. Excessive anxiety and worry (apprehensive expectation), occurring more days than not for at least 6 months, about a number of events or activities (e.g., work or school performance).

B. The person finds it difficult to control the worry.

C. The anxiety and worry are associated with three (or more) of the following six symptoms (with at least some symptoms present for more days than not for the past 6 months).

    1. Restlessness or feeling keyed up or on edge
    2. Being easily fatigued
    3. Difficulty concentrating or mind going blank
    4. Irritability
    5. Muscle tension
    6. Sleep disturbance (e.g., difficulty falling or staying asleep, or restless unsatisfying sleep)

D. The focus of the anxiety and worry is not confined to features of an Axis 1 disorder.

E. The anxiety, worry, or physical symptoms cause clinically significant distress or impairment in social, occupational, or other important areas of functioning.

F. The disturbance is not due to the direct physiological effects of a substance (e.g., a drug of abuse or a medication) or a general medical condition (e.g., hyperthyroidism) and does not occur exclusively during a Mood Disorder, Psychotic Disorder, or Pervasive Developmental Disorder.

Note: Modified and reprinted with permission of the American Psychiatric Association.

TABLE 6.7. DSM-IV Diagnostic Criteria for Panic Disorder

Criteria for Panic Attack

A. A discrete period of intense fear or discomfort, in which four (or more) of the following symptoms developed abruptly and reached a peak within 10 minutes.

1. Palpitations, pounding heart, or accelerated heart rate
2. Sweating
3. Trembling or shaking
4. Sensations of shortness of breath or smothering
5. Feelings of choking
6. Chest pain or discomfort
7. Nausea or abdominal distress
8. Feeling dizzy, unsteady, lightheaded, or faint
9. Derealization (feelings of unreality) or depersonalization
10. Fear of losing control or going crazy
11. Fear of dying
12. Paresthesias (numbness or tingling sensations)
13. Chills or hot flushes

Diagnostic Criteria for Panic Disorder without Agoraphobia

A. Both (1) and (2):
1. Recurrent unexpected panic attacks
2. At least one of the attacks has been followed by 1 month (or more) of one (or more) of the following:
   a. Persistent concern about having additional attacks
   b. Worry about the implications of the attack or its consequences (e.g., losing control, having a heart attack, or "going crazy")
   c. A significant change in behavior related to the attacks

B. Absence of Agoraphobia

C. The Panic Attacks are not due to the direct physiological effects of a substance (e.g., a drug of abuse or a medication) or a general medical condition (e.g., hyperthyroidism)

D. The Panic Attacks are not better accounted for by another mental disorder

Diagnostic Criteria for Panic Disorder with Agoraphobia

A. Both (1) and (2):
1. Recurrent unexpected Panic Attacks
2. At least one of the attacks has been followed by 1 month (or more) of one (or more) of the following:
   a. Persistent concern about having additional attacks
   b. Worry about the implications of the attack or its consequences (e.g., losing control, having a heart attack, or "going crazy")
   c. A significant change in behavior related to the attacks

B. The presence of Agoraphobia

C. The Panic Attacks are not due to the direct physiological effects of a substance (e.g., a drug of abuse or a medication) or a general medical condition (e.g., hyperthyroidism)

D. The Panic Attacks are not better accounted for by another mental disorder

Note: Modified and reprinted with permission of the American Psychiatric Association.

TABLE 6.8. DSM-IV Diagnostic Criteria for Somatization Disorder

A. A history of many physical complaints beginning before age 30 years that occur over a period of several years and result in treatment being sought or significant impairment in social, occupational, or other important areas of functioning.

B. Each of the following criteria must have been met, with individual symptoms occurring at any time during the course of the disturbance:

   1. *Four pain symptoms:* a history of pain related to at least four different sites or functions (e.g., head, abdomen, back, joints, extremities, chest, rectum, during menstruation, during sexual intercourse, or during urination)

   2. *Two gastrointestinal symptoms:* a history of at least two gastrointestinal symptoms other than pain (e.g., nausea, bloating, vomiting other than during pregnancy, diarrhea, or intolerance of several different foods)

   3. *One sexual symptom:* a history of at least one sexual or reproductive symptom other than pain (e.g., sexual indifference, erectile or ejaculatory dysfunction, irregular menses, excessive menstrual bleeding, vomiting throughout pregnancy)

   4. *One pseudoneurological symptom:* a history of at least one symptom or deficit suggesting a neurological condition not limited to pain (conversion symptoms such as impaired coordination or balance, paralysis or localized weakness, difficulty swallowing or lump in the throat, aphonia, urinary retention, hallucinations, loss of touch or pain sensation, double vision, blindness, deafness, seizures; dissociative symptoms such as amnesia or loss of consciousness other than fainting)

C. Either (1) or (2):

   1. After appropriate investigation, each of the symptoms in criterion B cannot be fully explained by a known general medical condition or the direct effects of a substance (e.g., a drug of abuse or a medication)

   2. When there is a related general medical condition, the physical complaints or resulting social or occupational impairment are in excess of what would be expected from the history, physical examination, or laboratory findings

D. The symptoms are not intentionally produced or feigned (as in Factitious Disorder or Malingering)

Note: Modified and reprinted with permission of the American Psychiatric Association.

MAJOR DEPRESSION

A major depressive episode is the most likely comorbid diagnosis in a patient with CFS. The difficulties and controversies related to making a diagnosis of a major depressive episode in patients with CFS are reviewed in Chapter 3 (this volume). The assessment of major depression should include a review of the diagnostic criteria shown in Table 6.3. Assessment may be complicated when the patient presents primarily with somatic symptoms of depression rather than cognitive and affective symptoms. The clinician must listen carefully to the patient and observe his or her own internal

TABLE 6.9. DSM-IV Diagnostic Criteria for Conversion Disorder

A. One or more symptoms or deficits affecting voluntary motor or sensory function that suggest a neurological or other general medical condition.

B. Psychological factors are judged to be associated with the symptom or deficit because the initiation or exacerbation of the symptom or deficit is preceded by conflicts or other stressors.

C. The symptom or deficit is not intentionally produced or feigned (as in Factitious Disorder or Malingering).

D. The symptom or deficit cannot, after appropriate investigation, be fully explained by a general medical condition, or by the direct effects of a substance, or as a culturally sanctioned behavior or experience.

E. The symptom or deficit causes clinically significant distress or impairment in social, occupational, or other important areas of functioning or warrants medical evaluation.

F. The symptom or deficit is not limited to pain or sexual dysfunction, does not occur exclusively during the course of Somatization Disorder, and is not better accounted for by another mental disorder.

Note: Modified and reprinted with permission of the American Psychiatric Association.

response to the patient—if the clinician begins to feel dragged out, tired, sad, or hopeless, this is a good clue that the patient may be depressed. Similarly, it is important to look at symptoms of low mood for which the initial attribution of the patient or the physician is that the symptoms are "understandable." Many clinicians find self-report instruments useful in the assessment of depression, as shown in Table 6.10. An example of a patient with a recurrent major depressive disorder that was misdiagnosed as CFS is shown in the following case vignette.

Case Vignette: The Misdiagnosis of Recurrent Major Depressive Disorder as CFS

Mrs. C, a 37-year-old divorced mother of two, was brought to the hospital by friends because they were alarmed at her inability to care for herself. She had been increasingly unwell over a 6-month period and had been housebound for 2 months. Over the 2 weeks prior to admission, she had been sofabound, and in the 2 days prior to admission had been unable to get up and go to the bathroom on her own. She reported feelings of profound fatigue that worsened with exertion and were accompanied by a generalized feeling of malaise. Mrs. C reported a plethora of somatic symptoms, including: a profound sleep disturbance with initial insomnia of 4- to 5-hours' duration, and brief, fragmented, unrestorative sleep when she was able to fall

TABLE 6.10. Self-Report Psychometric Instruments Used in the Clinical and Research Psychiatric Assessment of Patients with CFS

Depression rating scales:

    Beck Depression Inventory (Beck et al., 1961)
    Center for Epidemiological Studies—Depression (Radloff, 1977)
    Self-Rating Depression Scale (SDS) (Zung, 1965)

Anxiety rating scales:

    Self-Rating Anxiety Scale (SAS) (Zung, 1971)
    Spielberger State–Trait Anxiety Inventory (STAI) (Spielberger et al., 1970)

Measures of personality attributes:

    Minnesota Multiphasic Personality Inventory (MMPI)—Version I (Hathaway &
        McKinley, 1940) or II (Butcher et al., 1991)
    Millon Clinical Multiaxial Inventory—II (MCMI-II) (Millon, 1987)

Measures of somatic symptoms:

    Hopkins Symptom Checklist–90 somatization subscale (Derogatis et al., 1974)
    Pennebaker Inventory of Limbic Languidness (PILL) (Pennebaker, 1982)
    Minnesota Multiphasic Personality Inventory (MMPI)—Version I (Hathaway &
        McKinley, 1940) or II (Butcher et al., 1991)

Measures of increased sympathetic activity and heightened awareness of bodily functioning:

    Modified Symptom Perception Questionnaire (MSPQ) (Main, 1983)

Measures of pain:

    McGill Pain Questionnaire (Melzack, 1975)
    West Haven–Yale Multi-Dimensional Pain Inventory (WHYMPI) (Kerns et al.,
        1985)

Measures of somatic amplification:

    Somatosensory Amplification Scale (Barsky et al., 1988)

Measures of preoccupation with health issues and illness:

    Illness Behavior Questionnaire (Pilowsky, 1967)
    Illness Attitudes Scale (Kellner, 1987)

---

asleep; a marked decrease in appetite with a 30-pound weight loss; constipation; amenorrhea; myalgias and arthralgias; recurrent headaches; and hot and cold chills. Physical examination in the emergency room revealed a cachectic woman with marked psychomotor retardation but no focal neurological or other abnormalities. Mental status examination was positive for psychomotor retardation, a flattening and constriction of affect, and impairment on tests of concentration and attention such as serial 7s, and spelling the word "world" backward. With considerable encouragement, she was able to say the months of the year backward. She knew the month and year but not the day, and she was oriented to place and person. She was very slow in copying figures and completing a drawing of a clock, but was able to do so without evidence of any constructional apraxia.

On the seventh hospital day, her sister returned from vacation and informed the resident that Mrs. C had experienced two similar episodes—the first had been five years prior to this admission, when she had severe headaches and was investigated for a brain tumor, and the second had occurred 2 years earlier, when she had presented in a very weakened and psychomotor slowed state and was convinced that she had AIDS. The sister was aware that, in both cases, the feared diagnosis was not substantiated and no other physical disorder was found that would account for her symptoms. The sister was unsure whether a diagnosis of major depression had been made but was clear that her sister seemed to improve with "tablets." Neither she nor Mrs. C could remember the name of the medication, but when her pharmacist was contacted it was determined that she had been treated in both cases with amitriptyline (Elavil) and had a complete remission of symptoms over 6 to 8 weeks. In each case, she had discontinued the medication of her own initiative after approximately 16 weeks of treatment because of the anticholinergic side effects of dry mouth and blurred vision.

Mrs. C was assessed by an infectious disease consultant who noted that her symptoms were consistent with CFS. She was treated with nortriptyline (Aventyl), which was chosen because it is a metabolite of amitriptyline and has a better side effect profile (e.g., decreased risk of anticholinergic symptoms). Mrs. C showed an improvement in her symptoms beginning 2 weeks after starting the nortriptyline. She was discharged from the hospital at that point and was followed up as an outpatient. She showed a full remission of symptoms by 8 weeks, at which point she was able to return to work and had resumed her busy social schedule and physical fitness routine. She was not seen in follow-up by the infectious disease consultant but has continued to answer a yearly follow-up questionnaire. She has had intermittent contact with psychiatry. Subsequently, she has had three recurrences of her major depressive illness—in each case, an initial physical attribution was made (fibromyalgia, chronic fatigue syndrome, AIDS) and testing was undertaken by a new internal medicine specialist. On each occasion, she called her psychiatrist of her own accord to ask for help in dealing emotionally with the "serious medical problem" that was being investigated. On each recurrence, she accepted nortriptyline with the greatest reluctance. Each episode was resolved over 6 to 8 weeks. On each occasion, she discontinued the medication on her own initiative after 12 to 20 weeks and remained well for approximately 12 to 18 months before again becoming ill. She still is not able to conceptualize these episodes as major depression and notes that coming for psychiatric help is done with the greatest reluctance because of the profound sense of shame and stigma she experiences. The shame and stigma relate to issues around an exaggerated concern with privacy in her family of origin and embarrassment about the "poor marriage" that she "made." She has strong fears of being labeled "crazy." Mrs. C is not sure whether the nortriptyline is helpful in her recovery but feels it may "boost immune function."

DYSTHYMIC DISORDER

Dysthymic disorder is a mood disorder characterized by a chronically low or depressed mood that occurs more often than not for a minimum of 2 years and is associated with significant distress or functional impairment. In addition to lowered mood, there are other symptoms as shown in Table 6.4. Because of the chronic nature of the symptoms, individuals may not report them spontaneously but only in response to direct questioning.

SEASONAL AFFECTIVE DISORDER

In DSM-IV, seasonal affective disorder has been classified as recurrent major depressive disorder with a seasonal pattern (Table 6.5). The characteristic timing of the symptoms is that they begin in the fall or early winter and remit by spring.

ANXIETY DISORDERS: GENERALIZED ANXIETY AND PANIC DISORDER

Generalized anxiety disorder is diagnosed using the criteria shown in Table 6.6. Panic disorder is characterized by a range of symptoms including very prominent physical symptoms as shown in Table 6.7. In some patients, CFS has been the mistaken diagnosis for a primary panic disorder, and the episodic physical symptoms have been attributed to variations in viral activity. An example is summarized in the following case vignette.

Case Vignette: The Misdiagnosis of Panic Disorder as CFS

Mr. N, a 34-year-old, married father of five, was extremely successful in the family law firm. While traveling to the Far East to supervise the completion of a large contract, he became ill while on the airplane. He noted the sudden onset of a feeling of unwellness and over the ensuing ten minutes developed a number of physical symptoms including: tachycardia; difficulty breathing; the sensation that his esophagus and trachea were closing off; pins and needles in his fingertips and around his mouth; muscular trembling and twitching in the large muscles of his arms and legs; a sensation of dizziness; and a feeling of terror that he was going to die on the airplane, thus abandoning his family and losing a great deal of money for the firm, which had been faltering in the recession. A doctor traveling on the flight assessed him. Although the doctor was initially concerned about a heart attack, she was relieved to watch the symptoms resolve over 35 minutes. Mr. N could not recall receiving a diagnosis from the doctor. He did not see a doctor on landing because he was feeling better, but he then had repeated episodes almost daily during the 3 weeks he was in Asia. A North American physician, recommended by the Canadian embassy, diagnosed a viral illness, and Mr. N had this diagnosis confirmed by his own physician on returning home. When his episodic symptoms continued, his three physician brothers-in-law arranged a series of evaluations for him. By the time he was seen by an infectious disease specialist, he had undergone three cardiovascular consultations, with investigations that included four negative Holter examinations; four negative stress tests; two negative thallium scans; four neurological consultations, including three negative CT scans; two negative EMG studies; four evoked potential studies, the first "equivocal" and the next three "normal"; and two MRIs.

The infectious disease specialist felt that panic disorder was the most likely diagnosis and referred him for psychiatric consultation. Mr. N was a pleasant, cooperative man who was continuing to experience episodic symptoms 2 years after their onset. He had experienced a 6-month period free of symptoms, but they had returned in the context of multiple serious negative life stressors. On consultation with the physician brothers-in-law, it became clear that Mr. N had a longstanding tendency to become bodily preoccupied and fearful of catastrophic diseases. The group was comfortable with a diagnosis of CFS and thought this explained the problem better than a diagnosis of panic disorder, but was nonetheless agreeable to a trial of an antipanic benzodiazepine. This treatment was chosen rather than an antipanic antidepressant because Mr. N was extremely debilitated occupationally and socially and because of concerns that he would not tolerate the side effects associated with a tricyclic antidepressant (this was prior to the introduction of the SSRIs). Mr. N experienced a remission of symptoms over 2 weeks and continued in cognitive therapy for 6 months to address his bodily preoccupation and hypochondriacal fears. He refused behavioral treatment for the panic attacks because of its threat to his physiological model for his symptoms. He could not understand how a "psychological treatment" could help "physical symptoms." He felt "stigmatized enough" by taking the benzodiazepine, but this was acceptable because it "altered brain biochemistry." Mr. N discontinued the benzodiazepine after 6 months and has had 2 relapses over the past 4 years that have remitted promptly with treatment.

SOMATOFORM DISORDERS

The most common somatoform disorder diagnosed in CFS patients is somatization disorder, which is defined by a history of multiple medically unexplained physical complaints beginning before the age of 30. The DSM-IV criteria are shown in Table 6.8. An example of somatization disorder misdiagnosed as CFS is shown in the following case vignette.

Case Vignette: The Misdiagnosis of Somatization Disorder as CFS

Miss V, a 48-year-old, single woman living on her own, was receiving long-term disability payments because she was unable to work as a nurse due to her fatigue and pain. She was referred as a potential participant in a group program for psychosocial rehabilitation for CFS patients. Miss V expressed some initial concern and dismay at finding that the study was being conducted by a psychiatrist, but settled when she was given ample opportunity to review her physical symptoms. She provided a detailed description of her physical symptomatology, which included all of the minor symptom criteria in the 1988 CDC case definition (Holmes et al., 1988). She noted that there was an "acute presentation" of her illness with an onset following the flu, although on the second interview she talked about an 18-month period of deteriorating occupational and social functioning, and lowered energy that preceded the flu and began in the context of her mother's terminal illness. She endorsed 28 of 35 symptoms of the DSM-III-R somatization disorder criteria. On the second interview, she reported that she had been sickly since early in her childhood, described multiple social models of chronic illness behavior in her nuclear and extended family, and noted that times of illness were the only occasions on which she experienced a sense of being nurtured or cared for by her overextended immigrant mother who held two jobs in addition to her work around the house caring for the patient and her five siblings. Prior to becoming ill with CFS, Miss V had attended special practitioners or clinics for diagnoses of endometriosis, premenstrual syndrome, temporomandibular joint dysfunction, systemic Candidiasis, "behavioral food allergies," and chronic back pain. She had also had a period of approximately a year's duration when she felt herself to be allergic to a wide variety of common environmental stimuli. Psychiatric distress was only alluded to on the second interview, and then only with great reluctance and in the context of much "normalizing" by the interviewer. On the third assessment interview, Miss V indicated that she had tried to kill herself by slashing her wrist while hospitalized for an appendectomy. The slashing occurred impulsively and she did not have any insight into why she had behaved in that way. A transfer to psychiatry had been recommended, but she had refused and was ultimately discharged, against medical advice, from the surgical floor. She acknowledged periods of low mood and instability in her mood, and she reported that she was very sensitive to any perceived criticism or rejection by colleagues or acquaintances. Social supports were extremely limited—she had "lived life around my family"—and she noted that she had a hard time relating to coworkers. Although she "enjoyed the opportunity to unload," she did not feel that psychiatry had anything to offer her. Follow-up, obtained via the yearly questionnaires sent out by her infectious disease specialist, revealed that over the next 3 years she was diagnosed with dental amalgam mercury syndrome by a naturopath, and allergy to electrical lines by a nontraditional healer.

OTHER PSYCHIATRIC DISORDERS THAT PRECLUDE A DIAGNOSIS OF CFS

Patients with conversion disorder may also present with self- or physician-diagnosed CFS. The DSM-IV diagnostic criteria for CFS are shown in Table 6.9. The case definition criteria for CFS (Fukuda et al., 1994; Holmes et al., 1988; Schleuderberg et al., 1992) define a number of psychiatric disorders as exclusionary criteria for a CFS diagnosis. Although this method has been controversial, many clinicians feel that these disorders are so severe and complex that it is not possible to reliably diagnose CFS in their presence. The most common of these disorders are psychotic disorders, eating disorders, and substance use disorders.

Psychotic Disorders and Mood Disorders Complicated by Psychosis

A wide range of psychotic disorders, including schizophrenia, bipolar mood disorder (formerly known as manic–depressive disorder), and psychotic depression have been listed as exclusionary conditions for the diagnosis of CFS. These diagnoses are usually obvious to the physician and are associated with an extensive past psychiatric history. On the rare occasion when prominent fatigue is part of the initial presentation of these disorders, other symptoms and signs of the disorder are usually easily elicited.

Eating Disorders

Anorexia nervosa is characterized by a refusal to maintain body weight at a minimally normal weight for age and height. The disorder is associated with an intense fear of gaining weight, a disturbed experience of body weight and shape, and amenorrhea (American Psychiatric Association, 1994). Bulimia nervosa is defined as recurrent episodes of binge eating and inappropriate compensatory behavior undertaken to prevent weight gain (e.g., self-induced vomiting and laxative or diuretic misuse) in an individual whose self-evaluation is excessively influenced by body weight or shape (American Psychiatric Association, 1994).

Substance Use Disorders

The most recent case definition criteria (Fukuda et al., 1994) exclude alcohol or other substance abuse within 2 years before the onset of chronic fatigue or at any time afterward. Low energy and easy fatigability may be part of the symptomatology of a range of substance use disorders in either the intoxicated or withdrawal periods. The clinician may neglect to ask about the use of caffeine, alcohol, sedative-hypnotics, marijuana, or cocaine, and thus may miss the diagnosis. The following case vignette highlights this issue.

Case Vignette: The Misdiagnosis of Substance Abuse as CFS

Mr. B was a 36-year-old self-employed house painter who was now on welfare because of his difficulties in working. He was referred for a second opinion by his psychiatrist. Mr. B had been reporting profound fatigue for the past 2 years and had received a diagnosis of CFS from his primary care practitioner. His primary care practitioner was concerned about a comorbid diagnosis of major depression and had referred him to the community psychiatrist. The psychiatrist noted that he was amotivational, reported a decreased ability to experience pleasure, and had quite significant problems with concentration. He reported severe fatigue and extremely easy fatigability. He also appeared psychomotor retarded. Mr. B reported "some problems" with his sleep, which was quite erratic, and described his appetite as erratic. He denied feelings of worthlessness or guilt, or suicidal ideation. The most concerning symptom for Mr. B was his profound fatigue; he noted that he had been unable to work consistently for a number of months. An antidepressant was prescribed and was ineffective. After a second antidepressant failed to produce a significant improvement in symptoms, Mr. B was referred for a second opinion.

Mr. B presented as a well-groomed man who appeared to be very worried about his symptomatology and the impairment associated with it in both his occupational and social life. He felt that the antidepressants had produced some improvement in his sleep and his general sense of well-being but had not "attacked the central problems—my concentration is shot and I have no energy." In interviewing Mr. B, the consulting psychiatrist noted that he did not appear to be depressed nor was there an internal response in the interviewer of low mood or fatigue. Mr. B was verbose and the assessment was running overtime. Just as the interview was about to come to an end, it was realized that substance use had not been queried. He "did not look like a drug user" but, in a drive for completeness, was asked about substance use. He then reported that he grew Dutch marijuana through hydroponic gardening in his basement and smoked twenty tokes per day. When it was commented that this might be relevant to his ongoing fatigue and problems with concentration, he looked surprised and perplexed. After a minute of silence, he laughed and noted that this made "complete sense" and stated, "You know, no one ever asked me before and I just didn't make the connection on my own."

On follow-up 6 months later, Mr. B. had decreased his marijuana consumption and was using some of the "lighter stuff." He had begun to cultivate a "lighter brand" after a discussion with a substance abuse specialist who noted that the type he was growing and the hydroponic technique were resulting in a much more potent product. On reviewing his growing records, he realized that he had changed his brand and technique in the couple of months preceding the onset of his symptoms. He was now able to work again and had resumed dating.

UNDERSTANDING AND MANAGING COUNTERTRANSFERENCE AND REACTIONS TO THE PATIENT

Mental health professionals vary in their comfort and capacity to work with different patient populations. These variations relate to their own personality styles, countertransference issues, and other reactions to patients. Managing one's countertransference and reactions to patients is a fundamental task for the clinician. Working with medical populations and populations at the interface of medicine and psychiatry, where there is often much that is not clear-cut, may be poorly tolerated by many practitioners. For others, it may be taxing and may lead to periods of burnout if appropriate care is not taken. One needs to accurately assess one's ability to work with patients who have poorly understood illnesses and protracted clinical courses, and shape one's practice accordingly. CFS patients may be particularly difficult for some clinicians to work with because of our limited knowledge about CFS and because of the distressing experiences that these patients go through (i.e., multiple losses, ongoing distress, and protracted periods of illness and rehabilitation). For other clinicians who are comfortable working with CFS patients, significant events in their own lives may adversely impact their ability to continue working with CFS patients for a period of time. For example, practitioners struggling with their own issues of personal illness, illness in a loved one, or other significant disruptions in their lives, may find it more difficult to work effectively with CFS patients. Clinicians need to evaluate their capacity to work with this population and tailor their practices based on this self-knowledge. At times, it may be necessary to transfer the care of patients to other colleagues either temporarily or permanently.

REFERENCES

Abbey, SE. Physical symptoms and somatoform disorders. In Rundell, J, Wise, M, eds., *American Psychiatric Press textbook of consultation–liaison psychiatry.* Washington, DC: American Psychiatric Press, 1996.

Abbey, SE, Garfinkel, PE. Chronic fatigue syndrome and the psychiatrist. *Can J Psychiatry* 1990; 35:625–633.

Abbey, SE, Garfinkel, PE. Chronic fatigue syndrome and depression: Cause, effect or covariate. *Rev Infect Dis* 1991; 13(Suppl 1):S73–S83.

American Psychiatric Association. *Diagnostic and statistical manual of mental disorders,* third edition, revised. Washington, DC: American Psychiatric Association, 1987.

American Psychiatric Association. *Diagnostic and statistical manual of mental disorders,* fourth edition. Washington, DC: American Psychiatric Association, 1994.

Barsky, AJ, Goodson, JD, Lane, RS, Cleary, PD. The amplification of somatic symptoms. *Psychosom Med* 1988; 50:510–519.

Beck, AT, Ward, CH, Mendelsohn, M, Mock, J, Erbaugh, J. An inventory for measuring depression. *Arch Gen Psychiatry* 1961; 4:561–571.

Burszatjn, H, Barsky, AJ. Facilitating patient acceptance of a psychiatric referral. *Arch Intern Med* 1985; 145:73–75.

Butcher, JN, Dahlstrom, WG, Graham, JR, Tellegen, A, Kaemmer, B. *Minnesota Multiphasic Personality Inventory-2: Manual for administration and scoring.* Minneapolis: University of Minnesota Press, 1991.

Butler, S, Chalder, T, Ron, M, Wessely, S. Cognitive behaviour therapy in chronic fatigue syndrome. *J Neurol Neurosurg Psychiatry* 1991; 54:153–158.

Creed, F, Guthrie, E. Techniques for interviewing the somatising patient. *Br J Psychiatry* 1993; 162:467–471.

Derogatis, LR, Lipman, RS, Rickels, K, Uhlenhuth, EH, Covi, L. The Hopkins Symptom Check List (HSCL): A self-report symptom inventory. *Behav Sci* 1974; 19:1–15.

Fisher, GC. *Chronic fatigue syndrome: A victim's guide to understanding, treating and coping with this debilitating illness.* New York: Warner Books, 1987.

Fukuda, K, Straus, SE, Hickie, I, Sharpe, MC, Dobbins, JG, Komaroff, A, the International Chronic Fatigue Syndrome Study Group. Chronic fatigue syndrome: A comprehensive approach to its definition and study. *Ann Int Med* 1994; 121:953–59.

Gabbard, K, Gabbard, GO. *Psychiatry and the cinema.* Chicago: University of Chicago Press, 1989.

Hathaway, ST, McKinley, JC. A multiphasic personality schedule (Minnesota): 1. Construction of the schedule. *J Psychol* 1940; 10:249–254.

Holmes, GP, Kaplan, JE, Gantz, NM, et al. Chronic fatigue syndrome: A working case definition. *Ann Int Med* 1988; 108:387–389.

Kellner, R. Psychological measurements in somatization and abnormal illness behavior. *Adv Psychosom Med* 1987; 17:101–118.

Kerns, RD, Turk, DC, Rudy, TE. The West Haven-Yale Multidimensional Pain Inventory (WHYMPI). *Pain* 1985; 23:345–356.

Main, CJ. The Modified Somatic Perception Questionnaire (MSPQ). *J Psychosom Res* 1983; 27:503–514.

Melzack, R. The McGill Pain Questionnaire: Major properties and scoring methods. *Pain* 1975; 1:277–299.

Millon, T. *Millon Clinical Multiaxial Inventory II: Manual for the MCMI-II.* Minneapolis, Minnesota: National Computer Systems, 1987.

Pennebaker, JW. *The psychology of physical symptoms.* New York: Springer-Verlag, 1982.

Pilowsky, I. Dimensions of hypochondriasis. *Br J Psychiatry* 1967; 113:89–93.

Radloff, LS. The CES-D scale: A self-report depression scale for research in the general population. *App Psychol Meas* 1977; 1:385–401.

Rodin, G, Craven, J, Littlefield, C. Depression in the medically ill: An integrated approach. New York: Brunner/Mazel, 1991.

Schluederberg, A, Straus, SE, Peterson, P, Blumenthal, S, Komaroff, AL, Spring, SB, Landay, A, Buchwald, D. NIH conference. Chronic fatigue syndrome research. Definition and medical outcome assessment. *Ann Intern Med* 1992; 117:325–331.

Sharpe, M, Peveler, R, Mayou, R. The psychological treatment of patients with functional somatic symptoms: A practical guide. *J Psychosom Res* 1992; 38:515–529.

Smith, GR. *Somatization disorder in medical settings.* Washington, DC: American Psychiatric Press, 1991.

Spielberger, CD, Gorsuch, RL, Luchene, RE. *Manual for the State–Trait Anxiety Inventory.* Palo Alto, California: Consulting Psychologist Press, 1970.

Stewart, D. Emotional disorders misdiagnosed as physical illness: Environmental hypersensitivity, candidiasis hypersensitivity, and chronic fatigue syndrome. *Int J Ment Health* 1990; 19:56–68.

Taylor, MA. *The neuropsychiatric guide to modern everyday psychiatry.* New York: Free Press, 1993.

Wessely, S. What your patients may be reading: ME. *Br Med J* 1989; 298:1532–1533.

Wessely, S. Old wine in new bottles: Neurasthenia and "ME." *Psychol Med* 1990; 20:35–53.

Wessely, S, Butler, S, Chalder, T, David, A. The cognitive behavioral management of the post-viral fatigue syndrome. In Jenkins, R, Mowbray, J, eds., *Post-viral fatigue syndrome.* London: John Wiley & Sons, 1991; 305–334.

Zung, WK. A self-rating depression scale. *Arch Gen Psychiatry* 1965; 12:63–70.

Zung, WK. A rating instrument for anxiety disorders. *Psychosomatics* 1971; 12:371–379.

7

Medical Assessment of Fatigue and Chronic Fatigue Syndrome

Anthony L. Komaroff, M.D.
Laura Fagioli, Ed.M.

C hronic fatigue syndrome (CFS), at least as it is currently defined, is a rare cause of the presenting complaint of chronic fatigue. Even when the patient walks in the door and says, "I think I have chronic fatigue syndrome," the clinician is obligated to first consider the broader differential diagnosis of chronic fatigue. This chapter will therefore discuss, first, the assessment of chronic fatigue, and then the assessment of CFS.

Many patients seek medical care for the problem of chronic fatigue. Chronic fatigue is among the most common problems seen by the primary care physician: along with sore throat, cough, chest pain, abdominal pain, dizziness, and headache, these problems account for 10 to 15 million office visits per year in the United States (Allan, 1944; Katerndahl, 1983; Kroenke et al., 1988; Morrison, 1980; Nelson et al., 1987; Solberg, 1984).

Chronic fatigue comes in many flavors. The nature of the fatigue may be quite different from one patient to the next. The word "fatigue" means different things to different patients: an increased need to sleep, trouble finding the energy to start new tasks, poor endurance for completing a task that has been started, difficulty concentrating on any task, or weakness or fatigability of muscles during physical effort. The differential diagnosis of each of these various types of fatigue can be quite different, and much effort in the medical assessment of fatigue can be wasted by a failure to clarify just what fatigue means to the patient.

Fatigue can also vary in its severity—or, at least, in its impact on the patient's level of function. Some patients describe a condition of marked severity that hobbles them in every activity of daily life, often being as restricted in their levels of activity as patients with well-characterized major medical disorders (Kroenke et al., 1988). Others describe a condition that is obviously causing enormous apprehension but has not really impaired their ability to function at home or in the workplace. In one British survey, 20% of adults said that during the preceding month they "always felt tired" (Cox et al., 1987). When the patient seeks care for a fatiguing condition that has not apparently interfered with the ability to function, the physician often wonders why the patient has sought medical care at all, because fatigue is a universal human experience and the patient's level of function does not seem compromised. Indeed, although community surveys indicate that many people endorse the statement that they feel "tired all the time," only a few of these people seem to perceive the fatigue as a problem requiring medical care.

Not only do the nature and severity of fatigue differ from one patient to the next, but so does the context: the patient's past medical and psychiatric history, the recent pace of the patient's life and burden of life stresses, the manner in which the fatigue began, and other symptoms besides fatigue that have become a part of the chronic, fatiguing illness.

Thus, an assessment of the nature, severity, and context of the fatigue are all important parts of the evaluation of a patient with chronic fatigue. A careful assessment of these issues can provide evidence in favor of the diagnosis of chronic fatigue syndrome, or of other medical and psychiatric illnesses that can produce chronic fatigue.

THE DIFFERENTIAL DIAGNOSIS OF CHRONIC FATIGUE

The Difficulties in Diagnosing and Treating Fatigue

The clinician's attempt to diagnose and treat a patient with chronic fatigue— and, in particular, to diagnose and treat CFS—can be difficult and frustrating. Although chronic fatigue is a very common problem in medical practice, the cause of most cases of chronic fatigue remains obscure, even after intensive medical and psychiatric evaluation. Moreover, CFS is currently a syndrome identified by a pattern of symptoms and signs, without a proven cause or pathophysiological abnormality, without a definitive diagnostic test, and without a form of proven treatment.

Fatigue can be a frustrating condition to diagnose and treat because many patients with generalized anxiety will "medicalize" symptoms and experiences that have no pathological implications. Unfortunately, many primary care physicians do not like to care for patients who, they believe, have a psychological disorder: they may feel that psychological disorders are "not real" and therefore not worth their time. Fatigue is also a frustrating complaint for physicians because we know from the moment the patient expresses the presenting complaint that there is a good chance that we will fail in our attempts to diagnose and treat the illness. Not only is the diagnosis often obscure, but attempts at treatment often are unsuccessful (Kroenke et al., 1990).

The Most Common Causes of Chronic Fatigue

In our experience, and that of most clinicians we know, the most common causes of the presenting complaint of chronic fatigue are overwork and depression. As discussed elsewhere in this volume, the diagnosis of depression is often missed, particularly when the patient presents with somatic manifestations of the depression (Barsky, 1981; Kessler et al., 1985; Hoeper et al., 1979; Nielsen et al., 1980; Reifler et al., 1979; Stoeckle et al., 1964). Chronic fatigue syndrome is a rare cause of the complaint of chronic fatigue; most patients seeking medical care for chronic fatigue probably do not have CFS (Bates et al., 1993; Kroenke et al., 1988; Manu et al., 1988).

As for overwork, the pace of life in late 20th-century America is escalating. Only 30 years ago, the workweek in America was continuing to shrink, and many social scientists studied how society would use the anticipated growth of its leisure time. Instead, over the past 30 years, far from evolving toward a "leisure society," Americans are working increasingly longer hours and have less time for relaxation (Schor, 1992). One current theory is that, as a result of this increased pace of life, many citizens of the developed nations may suffer from a chronic state of sleep deprivation (Dement, 1992).

Although overwork and depression are important causes of chronic fatigue, when they are present they are not the inevitable causes of a patient's chronic fatigue. After establishing that either or both are present, the clinician should not immediately leap to the conclusion that the patient's fatigue has been explained.

Organic Causes of Fatigue

This chapter uses the terms "organic" and "psychiatric" to describe different kinds of illnesses, because these concepts are so familiar. Nevertheless, we reject the implication that "organic" afflictions result only from tangible changes in the chemistry and structure of the body, whereas "psychiatric" afflictions result only from disordered responses to life experiences. Indeed, the suffering from most organic afflictions is very much influenced by psychological and societal factors, and neurochemical alterations probably play an important role in psychiatric illnesses.

The medical causes of fatigue are legion. Several of the more common diseases that can cause fatigue are shown in Table 7.1. Even these more common organic illnesses do not frequently explain the complaint of chronic fatigue. They may explain the complaint of fatigue in fewer than 10% of patients (Allan, 1944; Katerndahl, 1983; Kroenke et al., 1988; Morrison, 1980; Nelson et al., 1987). Many organic diseases that produce fatigue can easily be recognized by patient history, physical examination, or simple laboratory testing. This ease of diagnosis is particularly true for fatigue due to cardiac or respiratory insufficiency. These illnesses generally are accompanied by clear physical signs, the fatigue is predictably reproduced by exercise and relieved by rest, and symptoms become progressively more severe over time. Infectious, neoplastic, and hematologic diseases that are sufficiently severe to produce fatigue usually also produce weight loss, fever, pallor, lymphadenopathy, and other findings.

A description of the approach to the diagnosis of each of the organic diseases listed in Table 7.1 is beyond the scope of this chapter. However, it is important to point out that the diagnosis of these well-characterized diseases can be extremely difficult. The main reason for this difficulty is that the diseases do not always become manifest in full-blown form, with all of the symptoms, signs, and laboratory abnormalities that the textbooks describe. Indeed, in such cases, one laboratory test may indicate the disease is present and another test may not.

Multiple sclerosis (MS) and systemic lupus erythematosus are good examples of this problem, because each can be very difficult to diagnose and each shares many symptoms in common with CFS. For many patients with mild multiple sclerosis (MS) or lupus, the predominant symptom for which they seek medical care is not a focal neurological deficit, a malar rash, or other characteristic manifestation of the illness; instead, the presenting symptom is fatigue. If and when the illness becomes full-blown, the diagnosis becomes clear. But, because these diseases do not always become full-blown, different clinicians may make different diagnoses, including no diagnosis or a diagnosis of psychiatric disease.

In one study, it was found that, in a group of 60 consecutive patients who finally were diagnosed with MS, the average time that had elapsed between the first symptom of the disease and the diagnosis was 43 months (Scheinberg et al., 1984). Had these patients experienced two or more unambiguous focal neurological deficits, separated in space and time, the diagnosis of MS would have been apparent to any neurologist and probably any physician. However, their disease did not present that way.

TABLE 7.1. Some Causes of Fatigue

Physiological
  Increased physical exertion
  Inadequate rest
  Sedentary lifestyle
  Environmental stress (e.g., noise, vibration, or heat)
  New physical disability, recent illness, surgery, or trauma

Habit patterns
  Caffeine habituation
  Alcoholism
  Other substance abuse

Psychosocial
  Depression
  Dysthymia and grief
  Anxiety-related disorders
  Stress reaction

Pregnancy

Autoimmune disorders
  Systemic lupus erythematosus
  Multiple sclerosis
  Thyroiditis (with or without thyroid dysfunction)
  Rheumatoid arthritis
  Myasthenia gravis

Sleep disorders
  Sleep apnea
  Narcolepsy

Infectious diseases
  Mononucleosis
  Human immunodeficiency virus infection
  Chronic hepatitis B or C virus infection
  Lyme disease
  Fungal disease
  Chronic parasitic infection
  Tuberculosis
  Subacute bacterial endocarditis

Endocrine disorders
  Hyperparathyroidism
  Hypothyroidism
  Apathetic "hyperthyroidism"
  Adrenal insufficiency
  Cushing syndrome
  Hypopituitarism
  Diabetes mellitus

(continued)

TABLE 7.1. (Continued)

Syndromes of uncertain etiology
  Chronic fatigue syndrome
  Fibromyalgia (fibrositis)
  Sarcoidosis
  Wegener granulomatosis

Occult malignancy

Hematological problems
  Anemia
  Myeloproliferative syndromes

Hepatic disease
  Alcoholic hepatitis or cirrhosis

Cardiovascular disease
  Low output states
  "Silent" myocardial infarction
  Bradycardias
  Mitral valve dysfunction

Metabolic disorders
  Hyponatremia
  Hypokalemia
  Hypercalcemia

Renal disease
  Chronic renal failure

Respiratory disorders
  Chronic obstructive pulmonary disease

Miscellaneous
  Medications
  Autonomic overactivity
  Reactive hypoglycemia

Note: This list is not meant to be an exhaustive catalog of every illness that can cause chronic fatigue. Rather, it is intended to highlight some of the illnesses that most commonly cause chronic fatigue. Adapted from Komaroff (1994). Adapted by permission.

Schur (1989) describes the experience of some patients with lupus in obtaining a diagnosis:

> . . . Patients . . . are often labeled as hysterical. . . . They often present their symptoms in a dramatic manner; have incorporated the symptoms into their daily life; fly from doctor to doctor seeking explanations, convinced that their symptoms cannot be explained by known biologic processes; and hang on to any positive laboratory test to confirm their

suspicions. This pattern is often initiated and perpetuated by episodes of stress with which the individual cannot deal appropriately or adequately. Patients often relate . . . a long history of frustration in obtaining the proper diagnosis. Unfortunately, physicians often dislike [such] patients . . . . On the other hand, many of the symptoms turn out to be the first signs of organic disease. . . .

The parallels between this description and the description of patients with other fatiguing illnesses of obscure etiology, such as CFS, are obvious.

Fatigue That Is Neither Clearly Organic nor Psychiatric

It would be wonderful if a careful, systematic evaluation were always able to identify the organic or psychiatric cause of fatigue. Unfortunately, this is not the case. Kroenke and his colleagues performed a systematic evaluation of patients seeking medical care for chronic fatigue, including assessment of organic and psychiatric illness, on several hundred patients (Kroenke et al., 1988). Despite the extensive evaluation, a substantial number of the patients fell into a gray zone where some features of their illness suggested organic or psychiatric diseases, but they did not meet established diagnostic criteria for any organic or psychiatric disease.

CHRONIC FATIGUE SYNDROME: ISSUES AFFECTING MEDICAL ASSESSMENT

As summarized in Chapter 1 of this volume, CFS is an illness of uncertain etiology, and it lacks a clearly defined pathogenic process or diagnostic test. CFS is a syndrome, defined by its symptoms and physical examination findings. The U.S. Centers for Disease Control and Prevention (CDC) (Holmes et al., 1988), and British (Sharpe et al., 1991) and Australian (Lloyd et al., 1990) investigators have proposed case definitions. Each of the case definitions was developed through a discussion among clinicians experienced in caring for patients with CFS. A revision of the CDC case definition was recently published and is discussed in Chapter 1 of this volume (Fukuda et al., 1994). The purpose of any case definition is to make predictions about the etiology of an illness, its pathogenesis, its responsiveness to particular treatments, or its prognosis. It will not be possible to test the ability of the case definitions to predict the presence of a particular etiologic agent or pathogenetic process until such agents and processes are demonstrated. The ability of the case definitions to predict prognosis is currently a subject of active study.

CONTROVERSIES SURROUNDING THE CAUSE OF CFS, AND THEIR IMPLICATIONS FOR MEDICAL ASSESSMENT OF PATIENTS WITH SUSPECTED CFS

As with any illness without a proven cause or pathological process, controversies surround CFS. Each of the controversies also raises questions about the medical assessment of the patient with suspected CFS.

Is CFS Organic or Psychiatric?

Whether CFS is an organic or psychiatric illness is the most commonly debated question. As mentioned earlier, we find this distinction of little value. In this section, we will briefly describe our current views on this question.

Some of the symptoms of CFS are also characteristic of depression, generalized anxiety disorder, and somatization disorder (e.g., headaches, myalgias, sleep disturbance, and difficulty with concentration). However, other CFS symptoms are not (e.g., the sudden onset with an "infectious-like" syndrome, recurrent fevers, adenopathy, arthralgias, and photophobia).

The most direct way to evaluate this issue is to perform a careful psychiatric assessment of patients with CFS, with regard to their experience in the years before and since the onset of CFS. Most studies of the question have found that the majority of patients with CFS become depressed and anxious after the (usually sudden) onset of their disorder. For many patients, the depression and anxiety become the most debilitating parts of their illness, and it is imperative that they be recognized and treated. At the same time, it should be noted that these studies also indicate that a substantial fraction of patients with CFS (25% to 60%) have no evidence of any active psychiatric disorder since the onset of CFS (Gold et al., 1990; Hickie et al., 1990; Kruesi et al., 1989; Taerk et al., 1987; Wessely & Powell, 1989).

Most studies have found a relatively higher frequency of a past history of psychiatric disorders in the years before the onset of CFS, in comparison to the population at large: the average across all studies is around 30% (range, 20% to 50%) of CFS patients (Gold et al., 1990; Hickie et al., 1990; Kruesi et al., 1989; Taerk et al., 1987; Wessely & Powell, 1989). On one hand, this past history of psychiatric disorders is greater than is found in the population at large (range, 5% to 10%) (Robins et al., 1984); on the other hand, despite extensive psychiatric evaluation, no evidence of a preexisting psychiatric disorder can be found in the majority of patients with CFS.

In our own studies of over 250 patients who meet the CDC, British, or Australian criteria for CFS, we have found less psychiatric illness than was reported in other studies, except one (Hickie et al., 1990). Major depression, dysthymia, generalized anxiety disorder, somatization disorder, and panic disorder have been found in 46%, 26%, 49%, 4%, and 21%, respectively, either before or after the onset of CFS. In 41% of the patients, there is no evidence of any of these psychiatric disorders at any time in their lives.

All studies may have underestimated the real prevalence of psychiatric disorders before and after the onset of CFS, because patients have attempted to avoid being identified as having a psychiatric disorder, and because patients' responses to a psychiatric evaluation are the basis for the results of the evaluation. Making the diagnosis of depression can be difficult because the patients may find the diagnosis stigmatizing. This feeling may lead sophisticated patients to consciously or subconsciously suppress certain aspects of their condition (such as the feeling of sadness or the experience of crying).

Is CFS Caused by Infectious Agents?

As previously noted, CFS often begins suddenly, with an infectious-like syndrome characterized by fever, respiratory, and/or gastrointestinal symptoms. The symptoms suggest the possibility that a new infection, reactivation of an old infection, or both, may be responsible for CFS. At this time, however, the evidence in support of that hypothesis is limited.

If CFS were caused by a single, novel infectious agent, one to which only a small fraction of human beings had been exposed—in other words, if CFS was in this respect like acquired immunodeficiency syndrome (AIDS)—then finding such an agent in patients with this syndrome would provide strong evidence that the agent was etiologically related to CFS. Although some claims have been made that such an agent (in particular, a retrovirus like the AIDS virus) might be present in patients with CFS (DeFreitas et al., 1991), other investigators have failed to confirm this report (Gunn et al., 1992; Khan et al., 1993). It remains possible that an infectious agent is responsible for a fraction of CFS cases, but, at this time, no credible evidence for such an agent has emerged.

Some evidence suggests that several viruses that cause latent infections in many people may be reactivated in some patients with CFS. The evidence is strongest for the enteroviruses (Archard et al., 1988; Cunningham et al., 1990; Gow et al., 1991; Yousef et al., 1988), and for human herpesvirus-6 (Buchwald et al., 1992; Patnaik et al., 1995; Strayer et al., 1994). However, the reactivation of these viruses may be an epiphenomenon secondary to immune dysregulation: it may have nothing to do with the forces that initiated the illness, or with the perpetuation of the symptoms of the illness.

One of the difficulties in relating infection to CFS is that very few patients have been carefully studied for infectious agents at the time of the sudden infectious-like illness that seems to initiate the CFS symptoms in many patients. Because this initial "flu" seems like many previous self-limited infections, neither the patient nor the doctor has any reason to attempt to diagnose the infectious agent.

This unfortunate state of affairs has some exceptions, however, and we believe that such exceptions may suggest (if not prove) the rule. In some cases, CFS has followed in the wake of well-characterized primary infection with an infectious agent. Before discussing these reports, it is worth considering what they might mean. In each instance, the patients were healthy prior to the infection, and have remained ill for years after the infection; therefore, the parsimonious assumption is that these agents triggered the illness and may be playing a role in perpetuating the symptoms of the illness. Two questions immediately follow:

1. What was the nature of the illness triggered by these agents?
2. Does the triggering agent actually remain physically present, or has it simply initiated a pathological process that can continue without its presence?

Some clinicians have speculated that the illness triggered by the infectious agent is primarily the unmasking of an underlying psychiatric disorder. Support for this hypothesis is found in studies that have revealed a more frequent past history of psychiatric illness in patients who have unusual debility following influenza infection (Imboden et al., 1961; see Chapter 1, this volume). The problem with this inference is that the same studies have found a large fraction of patients with lingering postinfluenzal debility but without evidence of an underlying psychiatric disorder.

Other researchers have speculated that the illness involves a chronic immunological response to a chronic infection. This group divides into two camps. One camp believes the chronic infection cannot be eradicated and, thus, is constantly calling forth an ongoing immune response. The immune response, as described in more detail later, is what produces many of the illness symptoms.

The second camp believes that the illness is triggered by the infectious agent in a kind of "hit-and-run" fashion. The triggering infectious agent somehow perturbs immune system function, causing an immunological dysregulation that continues (for reasons that are unexplained) long after the triggering infectious agent has "left the scene." Again, the case of post-influenza infection syndrome (Imboden et al., 1961) is cited, because it is generally believed that influenza virus infections are fully eradicated within weeks of the initial infection. One problem with this hypothesis is that the infectious agents that have been strongly incriminated as triggers of CFS all have the capacity to produce long-standing, even ineradicable infection.

What about the evidence linking new infection with some infectious agents to CFS? In our judgment, there is convincing evidence that CFS, in a small number of cases, has been triggered by infection with the Epstein–Barr virus (EBV), parvovirus, and the bacterium that causes Lyme disease (*Borrelia burgdorferi*). Although several other agents have been suggested as triggers of CFS (Salit, 1985), detailed evidence has not been presented.

In a few cases (7% of the patients with CFS that we have seen), CFS has begun not with a nondescript infectious-like illness but with classic acute infectious mononucleosis, characterized by the clinical, serological (heterophil antibody), and hematological (relative lymphocytosis and atypical lymphocytosis) findings. We refer to the illness suffered by these patients as "chronic mononucleosis," although a more precise term might be "postmononucleosis CFS." Because the vast majority of mononucleosis cases are caused by primary infection with EBV, and because EBV produces a permanent, lifelong infection, the parsimonious assumption is that EBV has somehow triggered and perpetuated the pathological process that leads to the symptoms of CFS. The two problems with this assumption are: (1) in most of these cases, EBV-specific serological studies have not been performed at the time of the onset of mononucleosis—thus, primary infection with EBV has not been proven; and (2) in most of the patients we have seen, the levels of EBV antibodies in the years following the onset of the illness are unremarkable; thus, there is no strong evidence in most of these patients of an unusual immunological reaction to chronic EBV infection, or of an unusual level of active replication by EBV. However, in a few of the patients we have seen with "chronic mononucleosis," there is evidence of an unusual infection with EBV and/or an unusual immunological response to EBV infection: heterophil antibody or IgM antibody to EBV remains detectable for years after the acute mononucleosis, or there are unusually high levels of IgG antibodies to the viral capsid antigen and early antigens. In our experience, these patients are clinically indistinguishable from those chronic mononucleosis patients who have unremarkable heterophil and EBV antibody studies. In summary, there is ambiguous evidence regarding EBV's role in perpetuating the CFS that can occasionally follow primary EBV infection.

A handful of cases of fibromyalgia have been triggered by new infection with parvovirus (Leventhal et al., 1991). Fibromyalgia is a syndrome very similar to CFS (Buchwald et al., 1987; Goldenberg et al., 1990; see Chapter 1, this volume); indeed, many patients meet criteria for both syndromes. Therefore, we believe there is reasonable evidence that new infection with parvovirus can cause CFS; however, currently there is no information as to how often parvovirus might cause CFS. Because the arthritis, neutropenia, and thrombocytopenia that can be caused by parvovirus B19 infection are virtually never seen in CFS, there is little evidence to suggest that parvovirus infection is a common cause of CFS.

Recently, several groups have reported that CFS can follow in the wake of primary infection with Borrelia burgdorferi (Coyle & Krupp, 1990; Dinerman & Steere, 1992; Steere et al., 1993). Interestingly, CFS develops despite adequate antibacterial therapy that has successfully alleviated many of the primary symptoms of Lyme disease (e.g., arthritis, carditis, and mononeuritis). Because the antibacterial therapy would seem to have eliminated the bacterial infection, it is tempting to speculate that the CFS is due to a chronic immunological (or psychological) process that does not require continued infection. However, Coyle and colleagues have found evidence that there continues to be a reservoir of bacterial antigen, against which antibodies are being formed, even though living organisms may have been killed (Patricia Coyle, personal communication).

Is CFS a Primarily Immunological Disorder?

The growing belief is that CFS is characterized by a state of chronic immunological activation, although not all studies are consistent in their findings, and no study has found immunological abnormality in all patients. In this regard, it is important to note that conflicting immunological results frequently have been reported in well-defined disorders of immunity, such as HIV infection (deMartini & Parker, 1989), multiple sclerosis, and systemic lupus erythematosus. However, many studies have found clear differences in the results of immunological studies, when patients with CFS have been compared to healthy control subjects. The specificity of these findings, based on studies comparing patients with CFS to those in various disease comparison groups (e.g., major depression, multiple sclerosis, and systemic lupus erythematosus) has not been established (Buchwald et al., 1992; Buchwald & Komaroff, 1991), although such studies are under way. Perhaps the most important question is whether CFS can be distinguished from major depression. Indeed, there is growing evidence of immune activation in major depression (Maes et al., 1992).

Several groups have found circulating immune complexes (Bates et al., 1995; Straus et al., 1985), in low levels, in patients with CFS who are without evidence of immune-complex-mediated disease. In blinded studies, our group formally compared the presence of immune complexes in patients with CFS and in healthy control subjects (Bates et al., 1995). Using a sensitive radiolabeled C1q-binding assay, the relative risk of immune complexes in patients with CFS was remarkably high, after adjusting for age and gender (odds ratio 28:1, 95% CI 4–313, $p < 0.000001$). In similar blinded, controlled studies, we have found significantly higher levels of immunoglobulin G (IgG) in CFS patients than in matched healthy control subjects (odds ratio 9:1, 95% CI 2–38, $p < 0.000001$) (Bates et al., 1995). In a few of our patients with CFS, IgG levels are below the normal range; however, unlike others (DuBois et al., 1984), we have not found frequent hypogammaglobulinemia. A few of our patients have had remarkably elevated levels of IgM (two to five times above the top of the normal range, and, in all cases, polyclonal). However, IgM values for our entire group of patients are not greater than for healthy control subjects. In recently completed extensive studies of CFS patients and matched control subjects, we have not found any significant differences in the levels of any of the four IgG subsets (IgG 1–4). This finding is in contrast to a small preliminary study we previously published (Komaroff et al., 1988) and a brief report by Linde et al. (1988).

Most of the studies that have reported evidence of a state of chronic immune activation in CFS have employed expensive and/or experimental tests, performed reliably in only a few laboratories. As such, these tests are not currently indicated in the evaluation of possible CFS. However, the collective data from a growing number of well-conducted controlled studies indicate that patients with CFS are different from healthy control subjects. Indeed, the data are most consistent with the hypothesis that, in CFS, the immune system is chronically responding to a "perceived" antigenic challenge.

The most consistently reported abnormalities, across multiple-patient groups and in multiple-immunology laboratories, have been diminished NK cell function (Aoki et al. 1987; Caligiuri et al., 1987; Kibler et al., 1985; Klimas et al., 1990; Whiteside & Herberman, 1989), skin test anergy and/or impaired T-cell responses to mitogenic or antigenic stimulation (Gupta & Vayuvegula, 1991; Klimas et al., 1990; Lloyd et al., 1989; Murdoch, 1988), and activated T-cell subsets (Gupta & Vayuvegula, 1991; Klimas et al., 1990; Landay et al., 1991).

Recently, an interesting immunological abnormality has been reported. The lymphocyte 2,5-A enzymatic pathway, which is believed to have an important antiviral function, was found to be upregulated in patients with CFS (Suhadolnik et al., 1994). High levels of the two end-products of the pathway, 2,5-A and RNAse-L, were found in patients with CFS from four different American communities, but not in healthy control subjects. In what may have been a harbinger of this work, Straus et al. (1985) demonstrated a significant increase in levels of leukocyte 2′,5′-oligoadenylate synthetase (2,5-OAS) activity, the enzyme that leads to the production of 2,5-A and (ultimately) RNAse-L, although the levels of 2,5-OAS are much lower than those observed in patients with AIDS.

Is CFS an Encephalopathy?

Our group studied approximately 250 patients from one geographic area (northern California and Nevada) who had an illness much like CFS. These patients were generally unlike the typically sporadic cases of CFS that we and others have studied: most became ill within a relatively narrow window of time, and, in many cases, family members or coworkers also were affected, suggesting that many were part of an epidemic. In this group, by using magnetic resonance imaging (MRI), we found areas of abnormal signal in the white matter of the central nervous system in 79% of patients with CFS versus 20% of healthy control subjects of similar age and sex ($p < 10^{-8}$) (Buchwald et al., 1992). In a subsequent study of patients in New England, we found a lower frequency of white matter MRI abnormalities (about 40% of patients)—a frequency that still was higher than was found in healthy control subjects (Schwartz et al., 1994a).

We have also found abnormalities of the brain using single photon-emission positron tomography (SPECT). Abnormalities on SPECT reflect either diminished blood flow or dysfunction of central nervous system cells, or both. In this study, patients with CFS were compared not only to healthy control subjects but also to patients in two disease comparison groups: patients with encephalopathy from AIDS and patients with major depression. Using the objective measurement of radioactivity in a mid-cerebral plane, patients with CFS had a significantly reduced signal in comparison to patients with major depression and to healthy control subjects. The reduced signal in patients with CFS was similar to the reduced signal seen in patients with AIDS encephalopathy (Schwartz et al., 1994b).

Other technologies for evaluating the central nervous system have been used (see Chapter 4, this volume), including neuropsychological testing of cognition, electroencephalography, and evoked potentials. In our judgment, the fairest summary of currently published data is that some inflammatory process involving the central nervous system may be present in some patients with CFS.

Is CFS a Neuroendocrine Disorder?

As discussed in Chapter 4 of this volume, several abnormalities of the hypothalamic–pituitary–adrenal (HPA) axis have been demonstrated in CFS and the similar syndrome, fibromyalgia (Bennett et al., 1992; Demitrack et al., 1991). Although these findings are of great interest, HPA axis studies should also be regarded as experimental, and not for routine use in patients with suspected CFS. Also, the value of random morning cortisol levels, or of cortrosyn stimulation tests, has not been established in CFS. Moreover, these findings do not provide evidence that CFS should be treated with low-dose steroid replacement. Such treatment is currently under study.

DIAGNOSING CFS: OBTAINING CLINICAL INFORMATION

Medical History

Illness Onset

In our experience, one of the most important questions to ask a patient with chronic fatigue is how the fatigue started. The chronic fatigue that stems from depression or overwork usually begins insidiously. In contrast, in nearly 90% of the patients we have seen with CFS, the fatigue began suddenly, most often with a flu-like illness characterized by fever, respiratory tract, and/or gastrointestinal symptoms. Less frequently, the fatigue is described as beginning suddenly following physical trauma (such as an accident or surgery). Rarely, the fatigue is described as beginning suddenly with an emotionally traumatic event. We are currently studying whether the prognosis or psychiatric profile of patients whose fatigue starts suddenly (particularly with a flu-like illness) is different from that of patients whose fatigue begins gradually.

We must emphasize that the description of the sudden onset of the fatigue was elicited without prompting. The patients stated that they had been feeling well and functioning very well in meeting their responsibilities at work and at home until "one day" they became acutely ill, never regaining full health or function thereafter: they stated that "it all started with that flu." This history was given just as often by patients seen in our practice before 1987, when media coverage of CFS became extensive; thus, it does not appear that this history offered by the patients is likely to reflect either outright malingering or the power of suggestion, after being educated about CFS by the media.

Principal Symptoms

Table 7.2 shows the current tabulation of the symptoms experienced by 260 patients who met the CDC case definition for CFS, followed in our practice over the past 7 years. In general, our experience is representative of that of others. The 260 patients summarized in Table 7.2 were selected for study from a group of about 2,000 subjects who have sought care in our practice. Participants were selected largely because they indicated that their condition was significantly interfering with their lives; thus, these patients are a highly

TABLE 7.2. Frequency of Symptoms and Signs in Chronic
Fatigue Syndrome

Symptom/Sign	Frequency
Fatigue	100%
Intermittently bedridden or shut-in	55
Regularly bedridden or shut-in	28
Systemic symptoms	
Night sweats, frequent and recurrent	52
Unintentional weight loss (median, 10 pounds)	54
Unintentional weight gain (median, 15 pounds)	57
Low-grade fever (by self-report), frequent and recurrent	50
Temperature > 99.3°F (by examination)[a]	20
Temperature < 97.0°F (by examination)[a]	22
Respiratory tract symptoms	
Sudden onset with flu-like illness	85
Swollen lymph glands in neck, frequent and recurrent	64
Sore throat, frequent and recurrent	47
Cough, frequent and recurrent	29
Palpable posterior cervical nodes[a]	48
Musculoskeletal symptoms	
Muscles hurt, frequent and recurrent	88
Postexertional malaise, frequent and recurrent	89
Joints painful but not red or swollen, frequent and recurrent	78
Generalized muscle weakness, frequent and recurrent	73
Morning stiffness, frequent and recurrent	60
Gelling, after sitting for hours, frequent and recurrent	60
Digits turn blue/white with cold, then red when warm	22
Neuropsychological symptoms	
Awaken most mornings unrested	91
Difficulty concentrating, frequent and recurrent	86
Headaches, new or different in character, frequent and recurrent	77
Unusually forgetful, frequent and recurrent	74
Depression (by self-report)	
Following onset of CFS	4
Before onset of CFS	68
Anxiety (by self-report)	
Following onset of CFS	67
Before onset of CFS	11
Alcohol regularly makes symptoms worse	46
Tingling/numbness in extremities, frequent and recurrent	57
Bright lights hurt eyes, frequent and recurrent	61
Dizzy when moving head suddenly, frequent and recurrent	51
Visual blurring, frequent and recurrent	53
Impaired tandem gait (by examination)[a]	23
Abnormal Romberg test (by examination)[a]	22
Impaired serial 7's test (by examination)[a]	43

(continued)

TABLE 7.2. (Continued)

Symptom/Sign	Frequency
Miscellaneous symptoms	
Premenstrual exacerbation of fatigue, frequent and recurrent	67
Nocturia, frequent and recurrent	47
Nausea, frequent and recurrent	61
Sudden rapid heartbeat, frequent and recurrent	45

Note: Summarized from formal studies of 260 patients who meet the CDC criteria for CFS, as of September 1993 (A. L. Komaroff, unpublished data).

[a] As detected on at least one physical examination.

selected, unusually sick group and may not be representative of the universe of patients with this syndrome.

The mean and median ages at onset of the illness are 32.5 years and 31 years, respectively. Although we have not studied children with this illness, others have done so (Bell et al., 1991; Jones, et al., 1985). Of our patients, 7% were older than age 50 when their illness began; these patients were just as likely to note an acute onset of the illness with a flu-like syndrome. Women constituted 76% of the sample, and 58% of the patients were college graduates. The mean and median durations of illness, as of August 1993, were 7.8 years and 7.4 years, respectively.

Each patient completed the same detailed questionnaire regarding symptoms. The data in Table 7.2 indicate how frequently patients stated that the symptoms were recurrently and frequently present. Symptoms that were experienced occasionally, for brief periods, were not counted. Also, all patients were asked to indicate whether the symptoms had been experienced chronically before versus after the onset of their chronic fatigue. Only the data on symptoms experienced regularly after the onset of the illness are included in Table 7.2; the frequency of each symptom in the years before the onset of illness was much lower, typically being reported by fewer than 5% of the patients (data not shown).

Patients who regularly experienced a symptom after the onset of the illness were also asked if they would describe the symptom as severe.

The symptom of fatigue was quite severe in this selected group of patients: 55% are periodically bedridden or shut-in, 18% are unable to work at all, and 52% are unable to work full-time. Of those able to work, 46% state that their work performance has suffered; 91% report having to cut down social or recreational activities, and 72% state that they are less able to fulfill their responsibilities to their families. Although their friends, coworkers, and families were initially sympathetic about their illness, the patients perceived these people as often becoming unsympathetic or even hostile after the patients' debility continued without a clear diagnosis.

A striking aspect of the illness has been the number of patients who describe postexertional malaise (89%). Even modest physical exertion (e.g., walking half a mile or raking leaves for 15–30 minutes) typically produces a worsening of their illness. The worsening fatigue does not usually occur during the exercise or immediately after, but 1 to 2 days afterward. The fatigue is not just in the muscles used in the exercise (which could simply reflect deconditioning). In addition, exercise also regularly provokes new or worse fevers (26% of patients), new or worse swelling of lymph nodes in thee neck (35%), new or worse sore throat (38%), and increased difficulty with concentration(57%). The great majority of the patients explicitly deny any such postexertional symptoms in the years before they became ill.

Interestingly, prior to the onset of their illness, the patients stated that they were unusually physically vigorous: 61% stated that they were more "full of energy than most people" they knew, and 91% stated that they had regularly engaged in moderate or vigorous exercise.

Also striking is how often the patients we have seen describe regular night sweats. After the onset of the illness, 52% of patients report experiencing recurrent night sweats; before the onset of the illness, only 1.5% of the patients reported experiencing recurrent night sweats. These sweats are not merely the dew of nocturnal anxiety, but drenching night sweats, requiring changes of bedclothes or sheets. In some patients, this occurs several times a week; in others, less frequently. Night sweats can be a nightly phenomenon for some patients when other symptoms are more severe, but then remit when the other symptoms improve. Whatever the pattern, it is a new experience since the onset of the illness.

A few patients with CFS have had transient acute neurological events, typically in the first 6 months of the illness: primary seizures; acute, profound ataxia; focal weakness; transient blindness; and unilateral paresthesias (not in a dermatomal distribution). The seizures have been witnessed by reliable observers; the ataxia, focal weakness, and unilateral sensory deficits (which sometimes accompany the paresthesias) have been documented by physicians and neurologists; but the blindness has never been documented. Similar acute and transient neurological events have been reported occasionally in outbreaks of myalgic encephalomyelitis. Other investigators (Stephen Straus, James Jones, personal communications), who have studied many contemporary sporadic cases of CFS, have told us that they have not seen patients with such acute neurological events, so our experience may not be generalizable.

Among the patients we have seen, a worsening of their symptoms is not only regularly provoked by physical exertion and the premenstrual period (as mentioned above) but also by humid weather (61% of patients), hot weather

(41% of patients), changes in weather (36% of patients), drinking alcoholic beverages (46% of patients), and stress (85% of patients).

Past Medical History

Several investigators have reported that, in patients with CFS, there is a high frequency of atopic or allergic illness: 60% to 80% of patients with CFS have long-standing atopic disorders, versus a point prevalence of approximately 20% in the general U.S. population (Olson et al., 1986a, 1986b; Salvaggio, 1992; Straus et al., 1988). In general, this has been our experience as well.

Physical Examination

Although several physical examination findings are included in the CDC case definition, only one controlled study has demonstrated that any physical examination abnormalities distinguish patients with CFS from healthy subjects or from disease controls (Buchwald et al., 1995). Having begun with this caveat, it is my impression that the following abnormal physical findings may be seen more often in patients with CFS than in healthy subjects: fevers; unusually low basal body temperature (below 97°F); posterior cervical adenopathy; the tender points described in patients with a similar illness, fibromyalgia (Goldenberg et al., 1990); and abnormal tests of balance (Romberg and tandem gait) (Table 7.2).

Psychological Assessment

Given the importance of psychiatric illness in many patients with the complaint of fatigue, it is crucial for the clinician to assess each patient for the presence of an underlying primary psychiatric disorder. Most clinicians do this, with greater or lesser success, during the course of taking an open-ended history. The use of formal instruments—first, a brief screening instrument, and then, if psychiatric illness is suggested, a more extensive instrument—is unusual in most primary care practices. The value of brief screening instruments in patients with possible CFS has not been studied. We routinely administer the Diagnostic Interview Schedule (DIS) to patients with chronic fatigue, but our practice is heavily engaged in research.

The process of making the psychiatric diagnosis can make the patient aware of how his or her feelings relate to the symptoms, an essential first step in management. Thus, the patient's emotional status is explored while the medical history is being obtained. A simple interviewing technique can be based on the biopsychosocial approach developed by Engel (1977) and the medical interviewing techniques developed by Bird et al. (1983) and Cohen-Cole et al. (1984). Occult alcohol abuse (and other forms of substance abuse) often produces chronic fatigue, either directly, as a result of chronic intoxication, or indirectly, through its disruptive effects on sleep or its production of inflammatory disease of the liver. A psychiatric assessment should always evaluate the possibility of substance abuse in the patient with chronic fatigue.

In sum, the clinician should be vigilant in looking for evidence of psychological disorders, and should have a low threshold for having patients formally evaluated for such disorders. The same principles apply even when the patient fully meets criteria for CFS, given that psychological disorders can often be present in CFS and can be the most disabling part of the illness.

Standard Laboratory Testing in Patients with Chronic Fatigue

In patients with fatigue of modest severity and relatively short duration (e.g., 1 to 3 months)—who probably are most typical of patients seeking medical care for fatigue—no laboratory testing may be warranted. This approach is particularly true when a patient has many lifestyle features that are likely to explain fatigue, when a psychological disorder is deemed likely, and when no other symptoms suggest an organic abnormality.

In patients with fatigue of greater duration (6 months or more) or severity (significantly interfering with their ability to work or maintain their responsibilities at home), a modest screening evaluation, to look for evidence of an underlying organic disorder, is warranted. A panel of tests recently recommended by a 1991 National Institutes of Health conference (Schluederberg et al., 1992; see Chapter 1, this volume) is shown in Table 7.3. Although not all of these tests are highly sensitive for organic disease, nor highly specific for any particular disease, they serve as a useful screen for organic illness. As stated earlier, the various immunological, neurological, and virological tests mentioned in the discussion of chronic fatigue syndrome should be considered experimental and not appropriate for general use at this time.

The history obtained for a patient with severe chronic fatigue should include questions that screen for the large number of conditions that can cause chronic fatigue, some of which are summarized in Table 7.1. Extensive testing for all of these conditions is definitely not to be routinely performed in patients with chronic fatigue. Rather, such testing should be reserved for cases in which any of these conditions is suggested by the history, according to the clinical judgment of the examining physician.

TABLE 7.3. Case-Finding Laboratory Tests

- Complete blood count
- Manual differential white blood cell count (unless automated counts accurately determine atypical lymphocytes)
- Erythrocyte sedimentation rate (Westergren technique)
- Chemistry panel including assessment of renal and hepatic function, glucose, electrolytes, calcium, phosphate, total cholesterol, albumin, and globulin
- Thyroid function tests (highly sensitive TSH is sufficient)
- Antinuclear antibodies and rheumatoid factor, if there are prominent arthralgias and myalgias
- Urinalysis

Note: Adapted from National Institutes of Health conference, March 1991 (Schluderberg et al., 1992).

Standard Laboratory Testing in Suspected CFS

Standard laboratory testing is generally unremarkable in CFS (Buchwald & Komaroff, 1991). Controlled studies by our group have found that a few abnormalities may occur more frequently in CFS than in healthy control subjects of similar age and sex: atypical lymphocytosis, elevated alkaline phosphatase, and elevated total cholesterol (Bates et al., 1995). None of these abnormalities is seen in more than 50% of patients with CFS, however; thus, none constitutes a sufficiently sensitive diagnostic test. Because each can be seen in other disorders, none is a sufficiently specific test.

Immunological Testing

As mentioned earlier, we have found increased levels of circulating immune complexes and IgG much more often in patients with CFS than in healthy control subjects. Tests to determine immune complexes and immunoglobulin levels are readily available to the clinician, relatively inexpensive, and reliably performed. Our studies suggest that these tests have some value in patients with CFS, but this remains to be confirmed by others.

Neurological Studies

As previously suggested, MRI and SPECT are relatively insensitive, nonspecific, and expensive diagnostic tests. For these reasons, we do not believe that routine use of MRI or SPECT is indicated in patients with suspected CFS. When the history or physical examination suggests the possibility of MS (as is the case in some patients with CFS), MRI may be useful.

Infectious Disease Studies

At this time, there is no reason to routinely test patients with suspected CFS for the various infectious agents previously mentioned, because their etiological relationship to CFS remains unestablished. In our practice, we obtain an antibody profile to EBV (IgG and IgM to the viral capsid antigens, IgG to the early antigens, and IgG to the Epstein–Barr nuclear antigen) in those patients whose chronic illness has begun with what was a classic case of acute infectious mononucleosis. We obtain serological tests for Lyme disease when there is a likelihood of exposure and a history of symptoms suggesting Lyme disease (not simple fatigue), because this is the one treatable infectious agent that has been suggested as a trigger for some cases of CFS.

Sleep Laboratory Testing

Sleep laboratory testing is indicated when the patient has a history of prominent snoring (particularly if snoring was not frequent or prominent before the chronic fatigue) or witnessed apneic periods during sleep, frequent jerking movements of the legs during sleep, or an overwhelming urge to sleep during the day.

Recent studies have suggested that important sleep disorders—including, but not limited to, the alpha intrusion pattern that has been reported in fibromyalgia (Moldofsky, 1989; Moldofsky et al., 1975; Moldofsky & Scarisbrick, 1976) and CFS (Moldofsky, 1993)—may be reasonably common in patients with severe chronic fatigue and CFS even though these patients may not experience these symptoms (Buchwald et al., 1994; Morriss et al., 1993). However, because it is not clear that these conditions respond to treatment in patients with CFS, and because sleep laboratory testing is expensive, the role of such testing remains uncertain at this time.

Medical Follow-Up in Patients with Fatigue

No longitudinal studies of patients with chronic fatigue, including CFS, have been reported. Therefore, there are no empiric data on which to base recommendations regarding the medical follow-up of patients with fatigue. In our view, when a patient continues to have a debilitating chronic fatigue that significantly interferes with his or her life, and no organic or psychological cause of the fatigue has been uncovered, it is appropriate to obtain an interval history and to repeat, every 6 to 12 months, the physical examination and the panel of tests shown in Table 7.3.

REFERENCES

Allan,FN. The differential diagnosis of weakness and fatigue. *N Engl J Med* 1944; 231:414–418.

Aoki, T, Usuda, Y, Miyakoshi, H, Tamura, K, Herberman, RB. Low natural killer syndrome: Clinical and immunologic features. *Nat Immun Cell Growth Regul* 1987; 6:116–128.

Archard, LC, Bowles, NE, Behan, PO, Bell, EJ, Doyle, D. Postviral fatigue syndrome: Persistence of enterovirus RNA in muscle and elevated creatine kinase. *J Roy Soc Med* 1988; 81:326–329.

Barsky, AJI. Hidden reasons some patients visit doctors. *Ann Intern Med* 1981; 94:492–498.

Bates, DW, Buchwald, D, Lee, J, Kith, P, Doolittle, T, Rutherford, C, Churchill, WH, Schur, P, Wener, M, Wybenga, D, Winkelman, J, Komaroff, AL. Clinical laboratory test findings in patients with the chronic fatigue syndrome. *Arch Int Med* 1995; 155:97–103.

Bates, DW, Schmitt, W, Ware, NC, Lee, J, Thoyer, E, Kornish, RJ, Komaroff, AL. Prevalence of fatigue and chronic fatigue syndrome in a primary care practice. *Arch Int Med* 1993; 153:2759–2765.

Bell, KM, Cookfair, D, Bell, DS, Reese, P, Cooper, L. Risk factors associated with chronic fatigue syndrome in a cluster of pediatric cases. *Rev Infect Dis* 1991; 13(suppl 1):S32–S38.

Bennett, RM, Clark, SR, Campbell, SM, Burckhardt, CS. Low levels of somatomedin C in patients with the fibromyalgia syndrome: A possible link between sleep and muscle pain. *Arthritis Rheum* 1992; 35:1113–1116.

Bird, J, Cohen-Cole, SA, Boker, J, Freeman, A. Teaching psychiatry to non-psychiatrists: I. The application of educational methodology. *Gen Hosp Psychiatry* 1983; 5:247–253.

Buchwald, D, Cheney, PR, Peterson, DL, Henry, B, Wormsley, SB, Geiger, A, Ablashi, DV, Salahuddin, SZ, Saxinger, C, Biddle, R, Kikinis, R, Jolesz, FA, Folks, T, Balachandran, N, Peter, JB, Gallo, RC, Komaroff, AL. A chronic illness characterized by fatigue, neurologic and immunologic disorders, and active human herpesvirus type-6 infection. *Ann Intern Med* 1992; 116:103–113.

Buchwald, D, Goldenberg, DL, Sullivan, JL, Komaroff, AL. The "chronic, active Epstein–Barr virus infection" syndrome and primary fibromyalgia. *Arthritis Rheum* 1987; 30:1132–1136.

Buchwald, D, Komaroff, AL. Review of laboratory findings for patients with chronic fatigue syndrome. *Rev Infect Dis* 1991; 13(Suppl 1):S12–S18.

Buchwald, DS, Pascualy, R, Bombardier, C, Kith, P. Sleep disorders in patients with chronic fatigue. *Clin Infect Dis* 1994; 18:S68–72.

Buchwald, DS, Umali, P, Umali, J, Kith, P, Pearlman, T, Komaroff, AL. Chronic fatigue and the chronic fatigue syndrome: Prevalence in a Pacific Northwest health care system. *Ann Int Med* 1995; 123:81–88.

Caligiuri, M, Murray, C, Buchwald, D, Levine, H, Cheney, P, Peterson, D, Komaroff, AL, Ritz, J. Phenotypic and functional deficiency of natural killer cells in patients with chronic fatigue syndrome. *J Immunol* 1987; 139: 3306–3313.

Cohen-Cole, SA, Bird, J. Teaching psychiatry to nonpsychiatrists: II. A model curriculum. *Gen Hosp Psychiatry* 1984; 6:1–11.

Cox, B, Blaxter, M, Buckle, A, Fenner, NP, Golding, JF, Gore, M, Huppert, FA, Nickson, J, Roth, M, Stark, J, Wadsworth, MEJ, Whichelow, M. *The health and lifestyle survey*, 61–62. London: Health Promotion Research Trust, 1987.

Coyle, PK, Krupp, L. Borrelia burgdorferi infection in the chronic fatigue syndrome. *Ann Neurol* 1990; 28:243–244.

Cunningham, L, Bowles, NE, Lane, RJM, Dubowitz, V, Archard, LC. Persistence of enteroviral RNA in chronic fatigue syndrome is associated with the abnormal production of equal amounts of positive and negative strands of enteroviral RNA. *J Gen Virol* 1990; 71:1399–1402.

DeFreitas, E, Hilliard, B, Cheney, PR, Bell, D, Kiggundu, E, Sankey, D, Wroblewska, Z, Palladino, M, Woodward, JP, Koprowski, H. Retroviral sequences related to human T-lymphotropic virus type II in patients with chronic fatigue immune dysfunction syndrome. *Proc Natl Acad Sci USA* 1991; 88:2922–2926.

deMartini, RM, Parker, JW. Immunologic alterations in human immunodeficiency virus infection: A review. *J Clin Lab Anal* 1989; 3:56–70.

Dement, W. *The sleepwatchers.* Stanford, CA: Stanford University Press, 1992.

Demitrack, MA, Dale, JK, Straus, SE, Laue, L, Listwak, SJ, Kruesi, MJP, Chrousos, GP, Gold, PW. Evidence for impaired activation of the hypothalamic–pituitary–adrenal axis in patients with chronic fatigue syndrome. *J Clin Endocrinol Metab* 1991; 73:1224–1234.

Dinerman, H, Steere, AC. Lyme disease associated with fibromyalgia. *Ann Int Med* 1992; 117:281–285.

DuBois, RE, Seeley, JK, Brus, I, Sakamoto, K, Ballow, M, Harada, S, Bechtold, TA, Pearson, G, Purtilo, DT. Chronic mononucleosis syndrome. *South Med J* 1984; 77:1376–1382.

Engel, GL. The need for a new medical model: A challenge for biomedicine. *Science* 1977; 196:129–136.

Fukuda, K, Straus, SE, Hickie, I, Sharpe, MC, Dobbins, JG, Komaroff, A, and the International Chronic Fatigue Syndrome Study Group. The chronic fatigue syndrome: A comprehensive approach to its definition and study. *Ann Int Med* 1994; 121(12):953–959.

Gold, D, Bowden, R, Sixbey, J, Riggs, R, Katon, WJ, Ashley, R, Obrigewitch, R, Corey, L. Chronic fatigue: A prospective clinical and virologic study. *JAMA* 1990; 264:48–53.

Goldenberg, DL, Simms, RW, Geiger, A, Komaroff, AL. High frequency of fibromyalgia in patients with chronic fatigue seen in a primary care practice. *Arthritis Rheum* 1990; 33:381–387.

Gow, JW, Behan, WMH, Clements, GB, Woodall, C, Riding, M, Behan, PO. Enteroviral RNA sequences detected by polymerase chain reaction in muscle of patients with postviral fatigue syndrome. *Br Med J* 1991; 302:692–696.

Gunn, WJ, Komaroff, AL, Levine, SM, Connell, DB, Bell, DS, Cheney, PR. Inability of retroviral tests to identify persons with chronic fatigue syndrome. *MMWR* 1993; 42:183–190.

Gupta, S, Vayuvegula, B. A comprehensive immunological study in chronic fatigue syndrome. *Scand J Immunol* 1991; 33:319–327.

Hickie, I, Lloyd, A, Wakefield, D, Parker, G. The psychiatric status of patients with the chronic fatigue syndrome. *Br J Psychiatry* 1990; 156:534–540.

Hoeper, EW, Nycz, GR, Cleary, PD, Regier, DA, Goldberg, ID. Estimated prevalence of RDC mental disorder in primary medical care. *Int J Ment Health* 1979; 8:6–15.

Holmes, GP, Kaplan, JE, Gantz, NM, Komaroff, AL, Schonberger, LB, Straus, SE, Jones, JF, DuBois, RE, Cunningham-Rundles, C, Pahwa, S, Tosato, G, Zegans, LS, Purtilo, DT, Brown, N, Schooley, RT, Brus, I. Chronic fatigue syndrome: A working case definition. *Ann Int Med* 1988; 108:387–389.

Imboden, JB, Canter, A, Cluff, LE. Convalescence from influenza. *Arch Intern Med* 1961; 108:393–399.

Jones, JF, Ray, CG, Minnich, LL, Hicks, MJ, Kibler, R, Lucas, DO. Evidence for active Epstein–Barr virus infection in patients with persistent, unexplained illnesses: Elevated anti-early antigen antibodies. *Ann Int Med* 1985; 102:1–7.

Katerndahl, DA. Fatigue of uncertain etiology. *Fam Med Rev* 1983; 1:26–38.

Kessler, LG, Cleary, PD, Burke, JD. Psychiatric disorders in primary care. *Arch Gen Psychiatry* 1985; 42:583–587.

Khan, AS, Heneine, WM, Chapman, LE, Gary, Jr, H.E., Woods, TC, Folks, TM, Schonberger, LB. Assessment of a retrovirus sequence and other possible risk factors for the chronic fatigue syndrome in adults. *Ann Int Med* 1993; 118:241–245.

Kibler, R, Lucas, DO, Hicks, MJ, Poulos, BT, Jones, JF. Immune function in chronic active Epstein–Barr virus infection. *J Clin Immunol* 1985; 5:46–54.

Klimas, NG, Salvato, FR, Morgan, R, Fletcher, M. Immunologic abnormalities in chronic fatigue syndrome. *J Clin Microbiol* 1990; 28:1403–1410.

Komaroff, AL. Chronic fatigue. In Branch, WT, Jr, ed., *Office practice of medicine,* third edition. Philadelphia: W.B. Saunders Co., 1994; 810–820.

Komaroff, AL, Geiger, AM, Wormsley, S. IgG subclass deficiencies in chronic fatigue syndrome. *Lancet* 1988; 1:1288–1289.

Kroenke, K, Arrington, ME, Mangelsdorff, AD. The prevalence of symptoms in medical outpatients and the adequacy of therapy. *Arch Int Med* 1990; 150:1685–1689.

Kroenke, K, Wood, DR, Mangelsdorff, AD, Meier, NJ, Powell, JB. Chronic fatigue in primary care. Prevalence, patient characteristics, and outcome. *JAMA* 1988; 260:929–934.

Kruesi, MJP, Dale, J, Straus, SE. Psychiatric diagnoses in patients who have chronic fatigue syndrome. *J Clin Psychiatry* 1989; 50:53–56.

Landay, AL, Jessop, C, Lennette, ET, Levy, JA. Chronic fatigue syndrome: Clinical condition associated with immune activation. *Lancet* 1991; 338:707–712.

Leventhal, LJ, Naides, SJ, Freundlich, B. Fibromyalgia and parvovirus infection. *Arthritis Rheum* 1991; 34:1319–1324.

Linde, A, Hammarstrom, L, Smith, CIE. IgG subclass deficiency and chronic fatigue syndrome. *Lancet* 1988; 1:885–886.

Lloyd, AR, Hickie, I, Boughton, CR, Spencer, O, Wakefield, D. Prevalence of chronic fatigue syndrome in an Australian population. *Med J Aust* 1990; 153:522–528.

Lloyd, AR, Wakefield, D, Boughton, CR, Dwyer, JM. Immunological abnormalities in the chronic fatigue syndrome. *Med J Aust* 1989; 151:122–124.

Maes, M, Lambrechts, J, Bosmans, E, Jacobs, J, Suy, E, Vandervorst, D, DeJonckheere, C, Minner, B, Raus, J. Evidence for a systemic immune activation during depression: Results of leukocyte enumeration by flow cytometry in conjunction with monoclonal antibody staining. *Psychol Med* 1992; 22:45–53.

Manu, P, Lane, TJ, Matthews, DA. The frequency of the chronic fatigue syndrome in patients with symptoms of persistent fatigue. *Ann Int Med* 1988; 109:554–556.

Moldofsky, H. Fibromyalgia, sleep disorder and chronic fatigue syndrome. In Bock, GR, Whelan, J, eds., *Chronic fatigue syndrome,* 262–279. New York: John Wiley & Sons, 1993.

Moldofsky, H. Sleep-wake mechanisms in fibrositis. *J Rheumatol Suppl* 1989; 19:47–48.

Moldofsky, H, Scarisbrick, P. Induction of neurasthenic musculoskeletal pain syndrome by selective sleep stage deprivation. *Psychosom Med* 1976; 38:35–44.

Moldofsky, H, Scarisbrick, P, England, R, Smythe, H. Musculoskeletal symptoms and non-REM sleep disturbance in patients with "fibrositis syndrome" and healthy subjects. *Psychosom Med* 1975; 37:341–351.

Morriss, R, Sharpe, M, Sharpley, AL, Cowen, PJ, Hawton, K, Morris, J. Abnormalities of sleep in patients with chronic fatigue syndrome. *Br Med J* 1993; 306:1161–1164.

Morrison, JD. Fatigue as a presenting complaint in family practice. *J Fam Pract* 1980; 10:795–801.

Murdoch, JC. Cell-mediated immunity in patients with myalgic encephalomyelitis syndrome. *N Zealand Med J* 1988; 101:511–512.

Nelson, E, Kirk, J, McHugo, G, Douglass, R, Ohler, J, Wasson, J, Zubkoff, M. Chief complaint fatigue: A longitudinal study from the patient's perspective. *Fam Pract Res J* 1987; 6:175–188.

Nielsen, ACI, Williams, TA. Depression in ambulatory medical patients. *Arch Gen Psychiatry* 1980; 37:999–1004.

Olson, GB, Kanaan, MN, Gersuk, GM, Kelley, LM, Jones, JF. Correlation between allergy and persistent Epstein–Barr virus infections in chronic-active Epstein–Barr virus-infected patients. *J Allergy Clin Immunol* 1986a; 78:308–314.

Olson, GB, Kanaan, MN, Kelley, LM, Jones, JF. Specific allergen-induced Epstein–Barr nuclear antigen-positive B cells from patients with chronic-active Epstein–Barr virus infections. *J Allergy Clin Immunol* 1986b; 78:315–320.

Patnaik, M, Komaroff, AL, Conley, E, Ojo-Amaise, EA, Peter, JB. Prevalence of IgM antibodies to human herpesvirus-6 early antigen (p41/38) in chronic fatigue syndrome. *J Infect Dis* 1995; 172:1364–1367.

Reifler, BV, Okimoto, JT, Heidrich, FE, Inui, TS. Recognition of depression in a university-based family medicine residency program. *J Fam Pract* 1979; 9:623–628.

Robins, LN, Helzer, JE, Weissman, MM, Orvaschel, H, Gruenberg, E, Burke, JD, Regier, DA. Lifetime prevalence of specific psychiatric disorders in three sites. *Arch Gen Psychiatry* 1984; 41:949–958.

Salit, IE. Sporadic postinfectious neuromyasthenia. *Can Med Assoc J* 1985; 133:659–663.

Salvaggio, JE. Allergic rhinitis. In Wyngaarden, JB, Smith, LH, Jr, Bennett, JC, eds., *Cecil textbook of medicine*. Philadelphia: W.B. Saunders Co., 1992; 1457–1462.

Scheinberg, LC, Kalb, RC, Larocca, NG, Giesser, BS, Slater, RJ, Poser, CM. The doctor-patient relationship in multiple sclerosis. In Poser, CM, Paty, DW, Scheinberg, LC, McDonald, WI, Ebers, GC, eds., *The diagnosis of multiple sclerosis*. New York: Thieme-Stratton, 1984; 205–215.

Schluederberg, A, Straus, SE, Peterson, P, Blumenthal, S, Komaroff, AL, Spring, SB, Landay, A, Buchwald, D. Chronic fatigue syndrome research: Definition and medical outcome assessment. *Ann Int Med* 1992; 117:325–331.

Schor, JB. *The overworked American. The unexpected decline of leisure*. New York: Basic Books, 1992.

Schur, PH. Clinical features of SLE. In Kelley, WN, Harris, ED, Ruddy, S, Sledge, CB, eds., *Textbook of rheumatology*. Philadelphia: W.B. Saunders Co., 1989; 1101–1129.

Schwartz, RB, Komaroff, AL, Garada, BM, Gleit, M, Doolittle, TH, Bates, DW, Vasile, RG, Holman, BL. SPECT imaging of the brain: comparison of findings in patients with chronic fatigue syndrome, AIDS dementia complex, and major unipolar depression. *AJR Am J Roentgenol* 1994a; 162:943–951.

Schwartz, RB, Garada, BM, Komaroff, AL, Tice, HM, Gleit, M, Jolesz, FA, Holman, BL. Detection of intracranial abnormalities in patients with chronic fatigue syndrome: comparison of MR imaging and SPECT. *AJR Am J Roentgenol* 1994b; 162:935–941.

Sharpe, MC, Archard, LC, Banatvala, JE, Borysiewicz, LK, Clare, AW, David, A, Edwards, RHT, Hawton, KEH, Lambert, HP, Lane, RJM, McDonald, EM, Mowbray, JF, Pearson, DJ, Peto, TEA, Preedy, VR, Smith, AP, Smith, DG, Taylor, DJ, Tyrrell, DA, Wessely, S, White, PD. A report—chronic fatigue syndrome: Guidelines in research. *J Roy Soc Med* 1991; 84:118–121.

Solberg, LI. Lassitude. A primary care evaluation. *JAMA* 1984; 251:3272–3276.

Steere, AC, Taylor, E, McHugh, GL, Logigian, EL. The overdiagnosis of Lyme disease. *JAMA* 1993; 269:1812–1816.

Stoeckle, JD, Zola, IK, Davidson, GE. The quantity and significance of psychological distress in medical patients. *J Chronic Dis* 1964; 17:959–970.

Straus, SE, Dale, JK, Wright, R, Metcalfe, DD. Allergy and the chronic fatigue syndrome. *J Allergy Clin Immunol* 1988; 81:791–795.

Straus, SE, Tosato, G, Armstrong, G, Lawley, T, Preble, OT, Henle, W, Davey, R, Pearson, G, Epstein, J, Brus, I, Blaese, RM. Persisting illness and fatigue in adults with evidence of Epstein–Barr virus infection. *Ann Int Med* 1985; 102:7–16.

Strayer, DR, Carter, WA, Brodsky, I, Cheney, P, Peterson, DL, Salvato, P, Thompson, C, Loveless, M, Suhadolnik, RJ, Reichenbach, N, Hitzges, P, Walters, D, Breaux, EJ, Einck, L, Shapiro, DE, Elsasser, W, Gillespie, DH. A controlled clinical trial with a specifically configured RNA drug, poly(I):poly (C12U) in chronic fatigue syndrome. *Clin Infect Dis* 1994; 18:S88–95.

Suhadolnik, RJ, Reichenbach, NL, Hitzges, P, Sobel, W, Peterson, DL, Henry, B, Ablashi, DV, Carter, WA, Strayer, DR. Upregulation of the 2-5A synthetase/RNase L antiviral defense pathway associated with chronic fatigue syndrome (CFS). *Clin Infect Dis* 1994; 18:S96–104.

Taerk, GS, Toner, BB, Salit, IE, Garfinkel, PE, Ozersky, S. Depression in patients with neuromyasthenia (benign myalgic encephalomyelitis). *Int J Psychiatry Med* 1987; 17:49–56.

Wessely, S, Powell, R. Fatigue syndromes: A comparison of chronic "postviral" fatigue with neuromuscular and affective disorders. *J Neurol Neurosurg Psychiatry* 1989; 52:940–948.

Whiteside, TL, Herberman, RB. The role of natural killer cells in human disease. *Clin Immunol Immunopathol* 1989; 53:1–23.

Yousef, GE, Bell, EJ, Mann, GF, Murugesan, V, Smith, DG, McCartney, RA, Mowbray, JF. Chronic enterovirus infection in patients with postviral fatigue syndrome. *Lancet* 1988; 1:146–150.

III
TREATMENT

8

Psychotherapeutic Perspectives on Chronic Fatigue Syndrome

Susan E. Abbey, M.D.

Psychotherapeutic techniques may offer important benefits to individuals with chronic fatigue syndrome. Recently, there has been an explosion of interest in the use of psychotherapy in individuals with acute and chronic medical illnesses. This literature may guide us in the development of appropriate psychotherapies for individuals with chronic fatigue syndrome. This chapter reviews the psychology of medical illness and the psychological aspects of fatigue. It also presents an overview of psychotherapy in medical illness in general, specific techniques that may be of use in the management of individuals with chronic fatigue syndrome, and a discussion of important issues involved in combining psychotherapy with pharmacotherapy.

THE PSYCHOLOGY OF MEDICAL ILLNESS

All patients with medical illness experience an emotional impact associated with their illness; in fact, it has been described as "an integral part of the disease process" (Green, 1993, p. 16). The psychological response to a given illness can be quite variable and is dependent on multiple factors, including the type of medical illness, the life stage at which the illness presents, the individual's personality and psychology (including emotional conflicts and vulnerabilities), and the individual's social and cultural milieu (Rodin, 1995). Successful adaptation to a chronic medical illness varies among individuals, but, in general, it is characterized by intact self-esteem, compliance with the medical regimen, and active participation in as many facets of life as is possible, given the illness (Rodin, 1995). Individuals who have achieved a satisfactory adaptation are able to contain and tolerate the emotional reactions evoked by illness.

A variety of components affect an individual's response to illness, including the total experience of illness, perceptual–cognitive responses to illness, and the personal meanings of illness that are related to the individual's psychodynamics, based on prior subjective experiences (Lipowski, 1985). Five basic categories of the personal meaning of illness have been described (Lipowski, 1985). They are:

1. Threat
2. Loss (both concrete and symbolic)
3. Source of gain or relief
4. Challenge
5. Insignificance

Each of these categories impacts on perceptual–cognitive processes. For example, threat may elicit psychophysiological responses that, in turn, alter a variety of body systems and may produce or accentuate bodily symptoms. The patient's attributions of illness etiology interact with these categories of personal meaning. For example, belief that the cause of illness is a personal failure, moral weakness, or punishment for real or imaginary misdeeds increases the likelihood that the individuals will experience the illness as a loss that they have brought on themselves and that there will be a concomitant loss of self-esteem.

Illness dynamics is a term used to refer to the diverse biological, psychological, and social factors that affect an individual's response to a specific disease at a specific point in the life cycle (Green, 1985, 1993). Green argued that "illness dynamics derive from the interplay between the singular components of one's biologic, psychologic, and social existence, transforming an episode of ill health into a highly subjective experience. By shaping its meaning in this fashion, they can convert the same disease process into seemingly different illnesses in two individuals requiring identical diagnostic workup, acute treatment, and ongoing care. Because illness dynamics span an enormous and complex range . . . combinations of these many biologic, psychologic, and social issues cause patients to define their particular ailments in highly idiosyncratic terms . . ." (Green, 1993).

Although psychiatry has conventionally focused on the intrapsychic world of the ill person, medical anthropology and sociology have reminded us that illness is, at its most basic, a social event (Kleinman, 1980, 1986, 1988; Ware, 1992; Ware & Kleinman, 1992). Illness occurs within the context of the individual's social world and both impacts on and is impacted by social relationships. An understanding of the social course of illness, including the ways in which the severity of symptomatology is influenced by aspects of the social environment and the way in which the illness impacts on the sufferer's environment and life is important. The social course of chronic fatigue syndrome is now being delineated (Ware, 1992; Ware & Kleinman, 1992) as will be discussed in the following themes, which are commonly brought to therapy.

PSYCHOLOGICAL ASPECTS OF FATIGUE

Although fatigue is an extremely common sensation, it has received remarkably little attention in the psychodynamic literature. A discussion of fatigue and the closely aligned concept of neurasthenia is not found in most psychoanalytic treatises on psychosomatic medicine. A search of psychoanalytic databases revealed several papers on fatigue in psychoanalysts, related to their countertransference to patients. Remarkably few papers were found related to fatigue in the analysand or to a psychodynamic understanding of fatigue.

Neurasthenia was a popular diagnosis in the 19th century, and a variety of primarily physical etiologies were proposed (Abbey & Garfinkel, 1991). An offshoot of neurasthenia was "psychasthenia," which emphasized psychological etiologies for neurasthenic symptoms. The development of the concept of psychasthenia has been seen as a theoretical reaction against the "organicity" of neurasthenia (Berrios, 1990). In 1920, Cobb commented that it was not surprising that a theoretical school would arise in opposition to the view of neurasthenia as organic, but he emphasized that "neurasthenia was caused by abnormal mental process, which produced the disorder by means of mental mechanisms. . . ." (cited in Berrios, 1990). Psychasthenia and neurasthenia "were themselves disaggregated" (Berrios, 1990).

Freud, writing about neurasthenia in 1895, argued that there were grounds for detaching from it a particular syndrome that he called "anxiety neurosis" (Freud, 1962). He separated anxiety neurosis as an example of the psychoneuroses (including transference neuroses) that were felt to originate in earlier life circumstances. Freud felt that the anxiety neuroses had their etiology in "noxae and influences from sexual life." In contrast, neurasthenia was an example of an actual neurosis. Actual neuroses had causes that were "purely contemporary and do not, as in the case of the psychoneuroses, have their origin in the patient's past life" (Freud Lecture 24, "The Common Neurotic State" 1916–1917, p. 433, as cited in Freud, 1973). The actual neuroses had physical symptoms with "no 'sense,' no psychical meaning" (Freud, 1973, p. 435). Freud thus concluded that the psychoanalytic techniques he had discovered would be of no use in the treatment of neurasthenia.

More recent developments in psychoanalytic theory have focused on understanding the dynamic meaning of medical disorders and symptoms to patients. Self-psychology, an important theoretical perspective, has been recently applied to the understanding of the mind–body interaction in illness. Self-psychology notes that illness produces disruptions in the sense of self because illness is a threat to the integrity of the self (Mohl & Burstein, 1982; Rodin, 1984, 1991; Taylor, 1987, 1992). Some researchers have suggested that there is an increased susceptibility to disease in individuals with deficits in their capacity to regulate their internal states, both physiological and psychological (Taylor, 1987, 1992). These deficits include problems in identifying and regulating affects, a decreased capacity for symbolization, and a tendency to express distress in physical rather than psychological symptoms (Taerk & Gnam, 1994). The theoretical paradigm of self-psychology has recently been applied to the understanding and treatment of chronic fatigue syndrome (Berger, 1993; Taerk & Gnam, 1994), although some controversy has surrounded the role of self-pathology in regard to vulnerability to or genesis of the syndrome. Taerk and Gnam have used self-psychology and object relations theory to develop the integrated model of chronic fatigue syndrome shown in Figure 8.1. They propose that a psychological vulnerability in chronic fatigue syndrome patients contributes to the clinical expression of the syndrome. One of the most important advantages of their model is that it validates the use of psychological therapies while avoiding the useless mind–body dichotomy that alienates patients. In contrast to more traditional models that, as McDougall (1989) notes, have dismissed the importance of

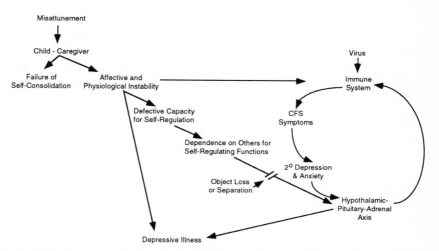

FIGURE 8.1. An explanatory model for disease susceptibility applied to chronic fatigue syndrome. From Taerk and Gnam (1994). Copyright 1994 by Elsevier Science, Inc., New York. Reprinted by permission.

somatic symptoms, a self-psychological model allows the therapist to "listen to the patient's symptoms empathically without trying to convince the patient that his disease is strictly psychological."

The particular importance of the therapist as a self object cannot be underestimated. A self object has been defined as an important figure who is perceived as part of the self and performs vital functions in a relationship that "evoke, maintain, or positively affect the sense of self" such as attunement to and containment of affective states, tension regulation, soothing, validation of subjective experience, and recognition of uniqueness and creative potential (Bacall & Newman, 1990; Taerk & Gnam, 1994). In the two cases reported by Taerk and Gnam (1994), it was noted that there was an "intimate relationship over time of fatigue symptoms to disturbances in object relationships, particularly within the transference" and that "improvement in symptoms" occurred when the relationship was "seen and understood by the patient."

PSYCHOTHERAPY IN MEDICAL ILLNESSES

Psychotherapy is often an important part of the psychosocial care of patients with acute and chronic medical illnesses. Psychotherapy may be the sole treatment modality or it may be part of an integrated program with pharmacotherapy, social therapies, and practical supports. Psychotherapy may be directed to the development or enhancement of adaptive coping strategies, or to the understanding and management of feelings evoked by the illness experience (Rodin, 1995).

Psychotherapy is a diverse field with a range of treatment approaches that vary in terms of the theoretical underpinning of the treatment, the focus and goals of treatment, and whether it is provided in individual or group settings. All forms of psychotherapy share as a foundation the therapist–patient relationship, which should be consistent, reliable, and empathic, and should maintain the patient's morale and hope (Rodin, 1995).

Psychotherapies used with the medically ill can be broadly categorized into two major therapeutic approaches: (1) supportive therapies that are anxiety-suppressing, and (2) introspective or analytical therapies that are anxiety-provoking (Green, 1993). The clinician's fundamental decision in delineating therapeutic goals is whether to support the patient's usual style of emotional functioning or to encourage a more introspective, psychodynamically informed process (Green, 1993). This decision is based on an assessment of the presence of major Axis I disorders, the patient's level of ego functioning (as assessed by occupational and educational achievements, psychosexual adjustment, degree of autonomy, and ability to assume responsibility), the quality and maturity of object relationships, the capacity for self-introspection, intelligence, and psychological-mindedness (Green, 1993). Supportive and introspective or analytical approaches to therapy may be delivered in individual, group, couple, or family formats.

The two broad sets of psychological tasks that may form appropriate targets for intervention or treatment goals for psychotherapeutic work with the medically ill are: (1) illness-specific tasks such as symptom management, and dealing with health care providers and the hospital environment; and (2) general psychological issues such as the maintenance of self-esteem, emotional equilibrium, and interpersonal relationships (Moos & Schaefer, 1984).

The effectiveness of psychotherapy in the medically ill can be assessed in a number of different ways. Outcomes of potential interest include improved psychological well-being, amelioration or prevention of physical symptoms, improved medical management, and reduction in health care utilization (Levenson & Hales, 1993).

COMMON THEMES IN PSYCHOTHERAPY WITH CHRONIC FATIGUE SYNDROME PATIENTS

Chronic fatigue syndrome patients bring a wide range of concerns to therapy. These concerns vary with their experience of illness and with their life history. Duff (1993) describes her personal experience with chronic fatigue syndrome and the multiplicity of meanings associated with her symptomatology and experiences. The major themes commonly seen in chronic fatigue syndrome patients are briefly described below.

The Search for Legitimacy and Problems of Stigmatization

The dichotomization of mind and body remains central to our culture (Kirmayer, 1988; Kirmayer & Robbins, 1991; Ware, 1992). In the medical realm, it is paralleled by the dichotomization of illnesses into "organic" or "physical" illnesses, and "functional" or "psychological" illnesses. Associated with this distinction is the commonly held belief that organic or physical illnesses are "real," but functional or psychological illnesses are "not real." The latter quality can be extended to include pejorative concepts such as "imaginary," "all in the head," "faked," or "malingered." Organic or physical illnesses are seen as externally caused, and the individual is absolved of blame for them, but functional or psychological illnesses are seen as blameworthy and under the control of the individual (Kirmayer & Robbins, 1991). Chronic fatigue syndrome is vulnerable to being seen as a not-real illness because of the lack of laboratory markers defining the diagnosis. This possibility parallels the experience of chronic pain patients (Jackson, 1992). Thus, the search for legitimacy of their illness becomes integral to the lives of chronic fatigue syndrome patients (Abbey & Garfinkel, 1991; Ware 1992, 1994; Ware & Kleinman, 1992). The prominence of the delegitimation of illness experience in the lives of patients with chronic fatigue syndrome has been described by Ware (1992). Forms of delegitimation include the trivialization of chronic fatigue syndrome symptoms that are seen as "common" or "part of normal life" (e.g., "You're tired? We're all tired!") and the definition of the illness as "psychosomatic" by some health care providers, which is construed as meaning it is "all in your head." Ware notes that the disconfirmation of the patient's subjective experience by significant others and the health care system leads to increased suffering. This suffering arises from the still widespread stigma associated with psychological disorder, the alienation that results from the decision by many chronic fatigue syndrome patients to keep the illness secret, and the shame in being labeled as "wrong," by physicians, family, or friends, with regard to one's sense of reality. Thus, the search for legitimacy is important for most patients. Unfortunately, the search is often complicated by self-doubt about one's own experiences and symptoms, arising from repeated disconfirmation of reality by significant others. Ware (1992) describes the two major strategies used by patients to dispute the definition of chronic fatigue syndrome as psychosomatic: (1) the argument that the illness is physical with the redefinition of it as somatopsychic, and (2) the presentation of evidence that one is not psychologically disturbed. "[W]hat is at issue in the struggle over the proper definition of reality in chronic fatigue syndrome— physical or psychosomatic condition, real or unreal illness—is whether patients will be accorded the status of sane persons who are genuinely sick. If so, much of their psychic, if not their physical, suffering will be alleviated" (Ware, 1992).

Overextended, Overcommitted Lifestyle Preceding Chronic Fatigue Syndrome

An overextended lifestyle was anecdotally described early in the history of the study of chronic fatigue syndrome (Salit, 1985). Recently, Ware and Kleinman (1992) have documented the "lives of intense activity and involvement" reported by chronic fatigue syndrome patients prior to the onset of their illness. They note that "a desire for accomplishment and success, underwritten by exacting standards for personal performance, impelled these individuals always to try harder, go further, in an attempt to meet the expectation they had set for themselves at work, at home, and at school. The result was an overextended, overcommitted lifestyle that left them feeling breathless—fragmented by competing demands, straining toward achievement and 'perfection,' constantly pressed for time" (Ware & Kleinman, 1992, p. 551). A tendency to place the interests of others ahead of their own interests was also documented. As a result of the illness, a "gradual dismantling of established ways of living" in patients with chronic fatigue syndrome occurs. For 44% of the 50 patients studied, this was ultimately seen to be part of a positive lifestyle transformation with changes in lifestyle leading to a sense of "contentment and relief." For these patients, "the authorization of sickness mediated life changes in the direction of greater personal efficacy . . ." (Ware & Kleinman, 1992, p. 557) However, this experience is not uniform. A profound sense of loss was reported by 32% of their sample, and ongoing negatively valued limitations were described by 12%.

Perfectionism and Other Maladaptive Beliefs

The clinician working with chronic fatigue syndrome patients often notes that rehabilitation is impeded by unhelpful or inaccurate beliefs. These beliefs are also relevant to the previously discussed pattern of an overextended, overcommitted lifestyle prior to the onset of chronic fatigue syndrome. High standards for work performance, responsibility in personal conduct, and perfectionism were noted by the Oxford group in their discussion of cognitive behavioral therapy ($n = 50$) and psychological assessment ($n = 100$) (Surawy et al., 1995). Perfectionism and other maladaptive or dysfunctional beliefs may impede rehabilitation through a variety of mechanisms, including perpetuating the use of ineffective coping strategies, and inducing or maintaining negative mood states that may be associated with adverse psychophysiological states (e.g., depression or anxiety) (Sharpe et al., 1996; Surawy et al., 1995). Similar relationships are reported for chronic pain (Ciccone & Grzesiak, 1990; Skinner et al., 1990) and major depression (Beck et al., 1979; Burns, 1980). The self-help literature labels such beliefs as cognitive distortions (Burns, 1980) or mind traps (Borysenko, 1987). An example of one such cognitive distortion or mind trap is all-or-nothing thinking. In all-or-nothing thinking, one is either well or sick. This stance precludes a return to activity. The recognition that one is functioning at 30% of normal allows for the specification of those activities that are possible at 30% and the hope of moving forward to a 40% level of functioning and beyond. The cognitive distortion or mind trap of catastrophization is a common cognitive error in patients with chronic fatigue syndrome. An example of catastrophization is an excessive reaction to a setback in the rehabilitation process. Our clearest example of catastrophization was the response of a patient in a chronic fatigue syndrome rehabilitation group to experiencing the flu that had been widespread in the community. The patient started the group discussion by noting that he still had symptoms from the flu that had prevented his attendance at the prior week's session. He then talked about his conviction that he was never going to get better, that he would lose his family, job, and home, and would end up dying of hypothermia in front of the Salvation Army hostel to which he had not been admitted because he arrived too late to obtain a bed. This statement was the first time that group members spontaneously recognized the concept of cognitive distortions or mind traps, and they challenged their copatient with respect to the statement. The patient was slowly convinced that his current situation had been "blown way out of proportion." The group now understood the concept of catastrophization, and other group members proceeded to relate their own episodes of catastrophization related to chronic fatigue syndrome. Cognitive therapy directed toward these beliefs has been shown to be helpful in an open trial that included cognitive therapy but relied more heavily on behavioral therapy (Butler et al., 1991), in a group format combining cognitive therapy and mindfulness meditation (P. Kelly, personal communication), and in the randomized controlled trial of cognitive therapy (Sharpe et al., 1996).

Illness as the Sole Problem

Many patients with chronic fatigue syndrome identify the illness as their sole problem and the focus for intervention when, in fact, a number of other important issues may impact on their level of functioning and their psychosocial distress, and may be amenable to intervention. This focus on chronic fatigue syndrome as the sole or principal problem is at variance with the experience of most clinicians, who note the multiple psychosocial problems troubling many chronic fatigue syndrome patients. Although many of these troubles may be subsequent to the illness, others may have antedated it. These troubles may not be an etiological factor in the illness, but they nevertheless contribute to the distress of the patient and their amelioration may be associated with a significant improvement in quality of life. The prevalence of other psychosocial troubles has been corroborated by a study using detailed research interviews in which many patients report both acute negative life events and chronic psychosocial difficulties prior to the onset of illness (Ware & Kleinman, 1992). Life history data obtained from a sample of 50 individuals with chronic fatigue syndrome revealed that 42% reported negative life events (e.g., serious injury, divorce, job loss, or death of a close friend or family member), 40% reported chronic life difficulties (e.g., serious illness in immediate family, serious marital problems, or persistent work problems), and 42% reported histories of physical or sexual abuse, low self-esteem, or serious family dysfunction in childhood (Ware & Kleinman, 1992). Among these chronic fatigue syndrome patients, almost half implicated stress as having some role in their illness.

The preferential attribution of all problems to illness may be a useful strategy in decreasing stigma (Watts, 1982) and preserving self-esteem (Powell et al., 1990), but it limits the patient's ability to address potentially reversible or solvable problems (Wessely et al., 1991).

Coping with Chronic Fatigue Syndrome

Coping with illness has been defined as the "cognitive and motor activities which a sick person employs to preserve his bodily and psychic integrity, to recover reversibly impaired function and compensate to the limit for any irreversible impairment" (Lipowski, 1970, p. 93). The coping strategies used to deal with chronic fatigue syndrome have been identified as: (1) maintaining activity despite unwellness; (2) accommodating to the illness (e.g., organizing one's life to avoid overexertion and control stress); (3) focusing on symptoms (e.g., a preoccupation with symptoms was linked with an appraisal of helplessness and of one's life as dominated by illness); and (4) information seeking (e.g., seeking information and readiness to try remedies) (Ray et al., 1993). In a preliminary cross-sectional study of coping with chronic fatigue syndrome, it was found that maintaining activity protects everyday functioning but is associated with increased anxiety. Accommodating to the illness is associated with better emotional adjustment but greater functional impairment. Focusing on symptoms had negative implications for both functional and emotional status. The researchers cautioned that the directionality of the relationships between coping and functional and emotional status have not been determined (Ray et al., 1993).

Cognitive Impairment

Reports of cognitive impairment are commonly described by patients with chronic fatigue syndrome and are reported by them to be an important cause of social and occupational dysfunction. The basis for these complaints is discussed in Chapter 5 of this volume. Despite the prominence of these complaints and their impact on daily life, most therapists treating chronic fatigue syndrome patients have not experienced these symptoms as precluding psychotherapeutic treatment.

TYPES OF PSYCHOTHERAPY APPLICABLE TO CHRONIC FATIGUE SYNDROME

The past ten years have witnessed an explosion in the development of psychotherapeutic techniques that are potentially helpful to patients with medical illnesses. The major categories of psychotherapeutic techniques with relevance to the treatment of the chronic fatigue syndrome patient are discussed here. Although the techniques vary with regard to the degree to which the patient's psychodynamics are the focus for treatment, the choice of treatment should be dynamically informed so that the proposed treatment is consistent with an assessment of the patient's functioning and needs (Blacher, 1984; Gabbard, 1990; Levenson & Hales, 1993). In addition to current difficulties associated with illness, patients often find that their illness evokes memories, distress, and conflicts associated with earlier periods in their life. The comprehensive psychiatric assessment of individuals with chronic fatigue syndrome was discussed in Chapter 6 of this volume and is summarized in Table 8.1.

As in other medical illnesses, the therapist may be perplexed as to the directionality of the relationships between psychologically meaningful factors and physical functioning (Burke, 1992). At the present time, it seems appropriate to treat what can be treated and to not become stalemated by questions of the directionality of these relationships.

Cognitive-Behavioral Therapy and Cognitive Therapy

Cognitive-behavioral therapy (CBT) and cognitive therapy (CT) have been advocated for CFS patients based on prior work with CBT as an adjuvant treatment in a variety of medical illnesses, including cancer (Moorey & Greer, 1989) and rheumatoid arthritis (O'Leary et al., 1988), and in medically unexplained syndromes such as irritable bowel syndrome (Blanchard et al., 1992; Greene & Blanchard, 1994), fibromyalgia (Goldenberg et al., 1994), chronic pain (Ciccone & Grzesiak, 1990; Skinner et al., 1990), temporomandibular disorders (Dworkin et al., 1994), and noncardiac chest pain (Mayou, 1992). CBT originated as a treatment for depression (Beck et al., 1979; Fennell, 1989) and has subsequently been adapted for the treatment

---

TABLE 8.1. Comprehensive Psychiatric Assessment of the Individual with Chronic Fatigue Syndrome

• Axis I Psychiatric Diagnoses
  Depression and dysthymia
  Anxiety disorders
  Current and past traumatic events
  Somatoform disorders
  Substance use disorders
  Factitious disorders
	• Axis II Personality Disorders
	
	• Psychosocial stressors
	  Current and past traumatic events
	  Interpersonal difficulties
	  Work-related stressors
	
	• Illness behavior and the sick role

of panic disorder (Clarke, 1986, 1989; Craske, 1988), hypochondriasis (Salkovskis, 1989; Salkovskis & Warwick, 1986), phobias (Beck et al., 1985; Butler, 1989), and bulimia nervosa (Fairburn, 1985; Wilfley et al., 1993). The expanding use of CBT in a variety of different disorders results from the fact that it allows for a flexible, individualized approach, it has documented efficacy in randomized controlled trials, and it is attractive to many patients as an alternative to pharmacotherapy. Table 8.2 describes CBT. Components of CT may be integrated into other forms of psychotherapy to address the patient's attributional style, maladaptive cognitions, and dysfunctional attitudes (Rodin et al., 1991). Attention to these factors may change the significance or meaning of the illness and the current situation for the patient. CBT and CT are among the most commonly used interventions for chronic fatigue syndrome, and have received the most research attention. CBT and CT are discussed in detail in Chapter 10 of this volume.

TABLE 8.2. Cognitive-Behavioral Therapy

Indications	Difficulties coping with illness associated with behavioral avoidance, demoralization, anxiety, or depression and maladaptive or unhelpful beliefs and attitudes
Goals	1. Identify thoughts, attitudes, assumptions, and behaviors that are associated with distress and ineffective coping 2. Develop specific strategies leading to more adaptive appraisal and coping methods
Techniques	Negotiation of therapy content—patient as collaborator and scientist General techniques 　Self-monitoring and recording of thoughts and activities 　Homework assignments and behavioral experiments 　Scheduling activities Specific techniques 　Recognizing maladaptive cognitions 　Examining available evidence 　Testing beliefs prospectively 　Searching for alternative explanations 　Assessing adaptive value of beliefs 　Planning alternative behaviors 　Skills training 　Evaluating social context
Frequency	Weekly sessions
Duration	8–20 weeks
Format	Individual or group sessions

Supportive Psychotherapy

Supportive psychotherapy is one of the most common forms of therapy. Unfortunately, it has traditionally been seen as inferior to analytic forms of therapy and thus has not received the attention that it deserves (Green, 1993; Rockland, 1993). Interest in the theoretical and technical foundations of supportive psychotherapy has recently increased (Rockland, 1993). Two recent reviews have been published on the use of supportive psychotherapy with medical patients (Green, 1993; Rockland, 1993). The major goals of supportive psychotherapy in the medically ill are: (1) eliciting and maintaining a positive therapeutic relationship; (2) supporting the patient's defensive structure and mobilizing healthier ego functioning; and (3) dealing with diminished self-esteem and demoralization (Green, 1993). See Table 8.3 for a description of supportive psychotherapy.

Clinical experience suggests that supportive therapy may be critical in sustaining patients with chronic fatigue syndrome and that it may be the most appropriate form of therapy for a subgroup of these patients. Over time, the relationship with the therapist may serve as an anchor for the individual whose social world has been significantly disrupted by illness. Supportive psychotherapy may also be helpful for those patients who do not demonstrate specific psychological conflicts or deficits, but who are in need of support and assistance with maintaining self-esteem and a sense of hopefulness in the context of a disabling illness.

TABLE 8.3. Supportive Psychotherapy

Indications	1. Healthy individuals faced with crises
	2. Individuals who are unable or not motivated to make use of insight-oriented therapies
Goals	1. Bolster adaptive coping mechanisms
	2. Minimize maladaptive coping mechanisms
	3. Decrease adverse psychological reactions such as fear, shame, and self-disparagement
Techniques	Structured approach
	Education
	Appropriate reassurance and advice
	Reality testing
Frequency	Variable—once a week to once every 4 to 6 weeks
Duration	Variable
Format	Individual or group sessions

Psychodynamically Informed Psychotherapy

Traditional psychodynamically informed psychotherapy has focused on the recovery and expression of unconscious mental contents. More recent approaches have emphasized the creation of meaning (Rodin et al., 1991). In medically ill patients, the meaningful incorporation of the present illness into the life narrative and an increase in the capacity to tolerate and organize subjective experience may be very useful.

Recently, attention has turned to the development of the brief psychotherapies (MacKenzie, 1988; Ursano & Hales, 1986). Levenson and Hales (1993) have reviewed the literature on brief psychodynamically informed therapy for medically ill patients and have described the application of specific models of brief psychotherapy to medically ill patients. A variety of dynamically informed brief psychotherapies have been used with the medically ill. These brief psychotherapies share certain fundamental characteristics, including a persistent pursuit of unconscious material, the therapist's taking an active and confronting stance, and a central focus of attention on the patient's emotional reaction to physical illness (Green, 1993). Although brief psychotherapies may be helpful for many patients, there is a caveat: patients with a chronic medical illness may require a longer or more open-ended approach to psychotherapy because of the ongoing difficulties in adjustment, and the uncertainty and unpredictability associated with the illness (Rodin et al., 1991).

Several case reports of the role of insight-oriented or expressive psychotherapeutic treatment in the management of patients with chronic fatigue syndrome have been published. (See Table 8.4 for a description of this type of psychotherapy.) Burke (1992) has described the long-term insight-oriented psychotherapy of a woman with chronic fatigue syndrome whose illness occurred against a backdrop of preexisting emotional problems. Burke hypothesized that working through earlier stressful life events and relationships and alleviating long-standing depression led to more energy being available for the patient's current life and relationships. The therapy provided the opportunity to observe the longitudinal course of the illness. At times, chronic fatigue syndrome symptoms were reported to coincide with emotional issues, but, at other times, it was unclear whether there was any connection between the work of therapy and her physical symptoms. This variable relationship led to uncertainty and frustration on the part of the therapist with regard to the type of intervention that was indicated at different points in the course of therapy.

Taerk and Gnam (1994) have reported on two cases of long-term intensive psychoanalytic psychotherapy of chronic fatigue syndrome patients. They noted that the intensity of their treatment provided a unique vantage point from which to view the nature of chronic fatigue syndrome and the

TABLE 8.4. Insight-Oriented/Expressive Psychotherapy

Indications	1. Identifiable and significant psychological or interpersonal problems impeding rehabilitation 2. Motivation and capacity to understand feelings 3. Supportive relationships available in present and past
Goals	1. Resolve psychological conflicts interfering with rehabilitation or medical care 2. Provide stabilization for individuals who have a defective sense of self 3. Promote self-understanding and psychological growth
Techniques	Uncover unconscious mental processes through free association Reconstruct intrafamilial and intrapersonal experiences from childhood, and understand their role in present distress Implement clarification, suggestion, and learning through experience Interpret defense and transference
Frequency	Weekly sessions
Duration	Brief therapies—8–20 weeks; longer therapies—variable
Format	Individual or group sessions

intimate relationship, over time, of fatigue symptoms to stressful life events and to the vicissitudes of the transference. Taerk and Gnam reported an improvement in symptoms when these relationships were recognized and understood by the patient. The importance of the patient–therapist bond in facilitating clinical improvement was also noted. They described the important self-object function of the therapist and how disruptions in the therapeutic relationship were associated with heightened symptomatology. The importance of naming affective states was described, and it was noted that the two chronic fatigue syndrome patients they treated had difficulty identifying and labeling internal states. They posit that an internalization of the tension-regulating components of the therapeutic relationship had a positive impact on the course of the illness.

For most therapists and patients, the question of the relationship between symptomatology and the work of therapy is a vexing one. The most commonly cited example is the question of how to deal with a patient's experience of fatigue or other somatic symptoms during the course of a session. In the patient without chronic fatigue syndrome, the onset of prominent fatigue during a session would be seen as resistance and would lead to an attempt to link the fatigue with suppressed or repressed material. For the chronic fatigue syndrome patient, such a relationship may not hold. Over time, most therapists and patients develop an awareness of the characteristics and patterning of fatigue, which appears to be related to illness, versus factors that appear to be related to resistance.

Interpersonal Psychotherapy

Interpersonal psychotherapy (IPT) was devised by Klerman and colleagues (1984a, 1984b) as a psychotherapeutic treatment for major depression. (See Table 8.5 for an outline.) IPT focuses on "reassurance, clarification of feeling states, improvement in interpersonal communication, testing of perception, and interpersonal skills" (Ursano & Hales, 1986). IPT involves a delineation of psychological symptomatology related to problems in grief, role transitions, interpersonal disputes, and interpersonal deficits that impact the individual's interpersonal network. These issues are particularly salient in the treatment of patients with chronic medical illness, where role transitions and loss, disappointment, and demoralization are prominent (MacKenzie, 1988). Interpersonal disputes or interpersonal deficits may interfere with the patients' receiving the social support they need. Interpersonal therapy has recently been modified for use in patients with HIV, AIDS (Markowitz et al., 1993), and breast cancer (L. Gillies, personal communication).

TABLE 8.5. Interpersonal Therapy

Indications	Mild to moderate depression
Goals	Address issues relevant to the genesis and maintenance of depression, including difficulties in interpersonal relationships, role transitions, and grief
Techniques	Vary with focus of therapy (e.g., role transition—mourn loss of old role and achieve mastery of new role)
	Focus on current psychosocial functioning (e.g., recent life events, stresses in family, home, workplace, and friendship patterns)
	Use exploratory techniques
	Encourage affect
	Analyze communication
Frequency	Weekly sessions
Duration	6–20 sessions (with follow-up maintenance)
Format	Individual or group sessions

Group Psychotherapy

Group psychotherapy offers patients the opportunity to interact with other individuals and share experiences related to illness and its impact. Although the literature with respect to the use of group psychotherapy in the medically ill is developing, there is an increasing interest in both therapist-led and leaderless groups for the medically ill (Spira & Spiegel, 1993). In addition to the theoretical benefits associated with group treatment, it has become an increasingly popular form of therapy because of its relatively low cost. Spira and Spiegel (1993) reviewed the literature on the use of group psychotherapy in the medically ill and delineated the various approaches that have been used in this population, including interpersonal–existential, interpersonal–psychodynamic, interpersonal–systems, cognitive restructuring, behavioral medicine, and supportive–expressive modes of therapy. Group psychotherapy may be conducted in disease homogeneous groups (e.g., all chronic fatigue syndrome patients) or in disease heterogeneous groups (e.g., chronic fatigue syndrome patients in groups consisting of patients with various other medical illnesses). A variety of theoretical reasons are offered to explain why a patient might do better in a heterogeneous versus a homogeneous group (Green, 1993). As a result of illness, individuals may become aware of concerns about aspects of their interpersonal relationships that are independent of the illness and may seek out group treatment related to interpersonal relationships rather than to coping with illness.

The curative factors in group psychotherapy have been described as including: installation of hope, universality (i.e., discovery of the similarity of one's concerns to those of others), imparting of information, altruism, the corrective recapitulation of the primary family group, development of socializing techniques, imitative behavior, interpersonal learning, catharsis, existential factors, and group cohesiveness (Yalom, 1975). A variety of theoretical schools of therapy may be delivered in a group format, including psychodyamically oriented therapies, interpersonal therapy, supportive psychotherapy, and cognitive-behavioral and cognitive therapies. Groups may be time-limited with a predetermined group membership, or may be open-ended in terms of both the time an individual spends in the group and when new members may join the group. Typical indications for group psychotherapy include: longer-term difficulties in personal or professional relationships, interpersonal communication, work, or family roles. Some patients will find that prior patterns of interaction that were adaptive for them when healthy are no longer helpful when they are ill. Some groups may be focused solely on difficulties in coping with medical illness. The goals of group psychotherapy with medically ill patients vary with the specific theoretical stance of each group. In general, these goals include: enhancing coping skills related to the symptoms and management of medical illness; receiving social support; exploring and understanding the meaning of illness and its impact on individual roles and activities, communication styles, and relationship patterns; and the development of more effective interpersonal relationships. Group psychotherapy may be particularly useful for individuals who are socially isolated and for those with personality styles that would be difficult to address in individual psychotherapy.

Relaxation- and Meditation-Based Therapies

In recent years, we have seen an explosion of interest in relaxation therapies, meditation, self-hypnosis, and guided imagery. A wide variety of educational materials are available, including books and tapes that may be useful for patients. However, most people find it easier to learn these techniques with some guidance or assistance, either in an individual or a group setting. Courses specifically directed to the medically ill are offered in many health care settings, and more generic courses are available through adult education programs and private practitioners (see Table 8.6 for an outline of these therapies).

In addition to the use of these techniques as single modalities of treatment, the additive benefit of the integration of concentration meditation or mindfulness meditation with psychotherapy has been described (Kutz et al., 1985). Although both forms of meditation involve the regulation of attention, they vary in how attention is regulated. In concentration meditation (e.g., Benson's "relaxation response," transcendental meditation), attention is restricted to a single repetitive stimulus (e.g., a mantra). In mindfulness meditation, only a portion of attention is directed to a focal stimulus (e.g., aware-

TABLE 8.6. Relaxation- and Meditation-Based Therapies

Indications	Chronic physiological arousal
Goals	1. Induction of relaxation response 2. Decreased sympathetic nervous system activity
Techniques	Meditation—concentration- or mindfulness-based techniques Relaxation response Self-hypnosis and guided imagery Yoga
Frequency	Weekly sessions
Duration	8–16 sessions
Format	Individual or group sessions

ness of breathing) and the remainder of attention is allowed to observe the mental contents with a detached quality (Kabat-Zinn, 1982; Kutz et al., 1985). The physiological changes induced by either form of meditation have been documented by numerous authors and are similar (Benson, 1975; Benson et al., 1974; Kutz et al., 1985). These physiological changes have been labeled the "relaxation response" by Benson (Benson, 1975; Benson et al., 1974).

The use of mindfulness meditation in chronic illness has been popularized by Kabat-Zinn (1990). The practice of mindfulness meditation encourages a "witnessing" stance in which the individual learns to observe his or her ever-changing mental contents and physical symptoms without being carried away by them. Over time, there is increasing awareness of the interplay of mind and body. Studies have noted that mindfulness meditation combines the benefits of physiological changes with aspects of cognitive therapy, including acknowledging automatic thoughts but achieving some distance in viewing them (Kaplan et al., 1993). Kabat-Zinn (1982) has argued that mindfulness meditation, in many medical patients, disengages the cognitive–affective and sensory aspects of pain or other physical symptoms.

There is evidence of the efficacy of mindfulness meditation in improving physical condition and psychosocial functioning in patients with chronic pain (Kabat-Zinn, 1982; Kabat-Zinn et al., 1987) and fibromyalgia (Kaplan et al., 1993). "Our group has begun to use mindfulness meditation with chronic fatigue syndrome patients and have found it efficacious in terms of a decreasing of the distress associated with somatic symptoms, a decreasing of symptoms of muscular tension, and improving mood. We have also observed that as a result of their experiences with mindfulness meditation, some patients have identified emotional issues contributing to their fatigue that have then been treated using other forms of psychotherapy" (P. Kelly, personal communication).

Marital and Family Therapy

Unfortunately, partners and families of the medically ill have traditionally been neglected by the health care system, and their suffering, which is often equal to or greater than the patients', is not attended to. Their importance is often conceptualized as a "background factor" influencing the patient's well-being (McDaniel et al., 1992). Partners and families have been traditionally either marginalized or involved as a "cotherapist" or adjunctive aid in treating the patient (Doherty & Campbell, 1988), and "not as a group of people who need help in their own right" (McDaniel et al., 1992). The impact of chronic fatigue syndrome on marital and family functioning is strikingly absent in the scientific literature. The only attention paid to family members has been as potential cotherapists for cognitive-behavioral treatment (Wessely et al., 1989, 1991; Sharpe, 1990, 1993).

Clinical work suggests that chronic fatigue syndrome can have a significant impact on the marital dyad and the family system as life begins to revolve increasingly around the limitations of the chronic fatigue syndrome patient. This change in focus can produce a wide range of pragmatic problems in the present and may reactivate conflicts and psychological distress from earlier stages in the individual's or family member's personal history. These problems can then serve to further interfere with the functioning of the chronic fatigue syndrome patient, impede rehabilitation, and cause significant personal and interpersonal distress and problems for family members, including derailment from their own personal developmental lines.

Jacobs (1993) traces the development of theoretical models of families and medical illness from early formulations that placed the family in a pathogenic role to more recent biopsychosocial formulations that conceptualize illness as an external stressor for the family. As with other forms of therapy, a wide variety of theoretical models, with assorted goals and techniques of treatment, can be delivered in a marital or family format. These models range from psychoeducational treatments focusing attention on the illness to forms of therapy with broader goals and more intensive techniques aimed at fundamental family problems. McDaniel et al. (1992) described the importance of medical family therapy that consciously attends to the medical illness and its role in the interpersonal life of the family. They noted that the goals of therapy may include better coping with chronic illness or disability, feeling less conflicted about handling the medical regimen, improving communication with medical professionals, and making lifestyle adjustments required by the illness or disability (McDaniel et al., 1992). In the process, patients and their families develop increased capacity for active involvement in decision making related to the illness and its impact on the patient and family, enhanced communication patterns, and experience in healing the disruptions in family functioning and interpersonal relationships within the family that are related to illness. The importance of grounding family therapy in the medical context offers significant benefits in contrast to more traditional forms of family therapy that have minimized the medical context and the impact of illness.

The importance of understanding the context of an illness for a given family has been emphasized, "one striking element of family stress in the context of medical illness is that the severity of the illness alone does not seem to be a strong predictor of caregiver functioning. Rather, one must understand what type of challenge a particular illness constitutes in the context of a particular family environment" (Jacobs, 1993, p. 19). Certain areas of family life are particularly vulnerable to disruption from chronic illness, including dimensions of functioning within the family (e.g., boundary regulation, role allocation, problem solving, communication, and family beliefs),

TABLE 8.7. Marital and Family Therapy

Indications	Marital or family problems that are a source of distress to patient or interfere with rehabilitation
Goals	1. Identify the problems 2. Develop strategies to deal with the problems 3. Enhance intimacy within the couple relationship or functioning within the family
Techniques	Enlist different types of therapy Vary the techniques according to theoretical orientation
Frequency	Weekly or biweekly sessions
Duration	Variable
Format	Individual or group sessions

and between the family and the external world (e.g., problems between the family and the medical care team, and financial problems) (Jacobs, 1993). The significant components of assessing a family with a member who has a chronic illness include an assessment of the illness characteristics, the phase of the illness, the specific features of the illness (e.g., degree of unpredictability, uncertain prognosis, degree of disability, need for monitoring, stigma, and disfigurement), and the family's response to illness (e.g., the fit between the family style and the demands of the illness, reallocation of family roles, and the effect on preillness activities and traditions), the developmental phase of family members and the relationship of illness management to long-standing family problems (Jacobs, 1993). Techniques that are important components of medical family therapy include clarifying issues, externalizing the illness (i.e., separating the illness from the person who is ill), removing blame, normalizing negative feelings, maintaining and enhancing communication within the family and with medical providers, and recognizing the impact of the illness on the developmental phase of the family unit and of its individual members. (See Table 8.7 for a summary of the therapeutic approach.)

Chronic fatigue syndrome is a particularly difficult illness for families to deal with because of the lack of information about the illness, its unpredictability, the degree of disability associated with it, and the ongoing debate as to its legitimacy.

COMBINING PSYCHOTHERAPY AND PHARMACOTHERAPY

Traditionally, there was opposition to the use of pharmacotherapy in patients undergoing psychotherapy unless it was absolutely necessary to ensure the safety of the patient. This view was based on concerns that medication would decrease the level of symptomatic distress (thus, weakening the motivation for or investment in psychotherapy) or that insights derived during periods of pharmacotherapy would dissipate when the medication was discontinued (Green, 1993). More recently, theoretical and empirical work supports the combined use of psychotherapy and pharmacotherapy. Many theorists and clinicians have noted the beneficial effects of pharmacologically containing state-related neurobiological symptoms associated with depression, panic disorder, and generalized anxiety disorder, to allow the patient to better participate in psychotherapy. The particular compatibility of supportive psychotherapy and pharmacotherapy has been emphasized (Rockland, 1993). An illness such as chronic fatigue syndrome, for which psychopharmacological treatments may confer substantial benefits in terms of symptom relief, particularly highlights the importance of successfully integrating psychotherapy and pharmacotherapy.

REFERENCES

Abbey, SE, Garfinkel, PE. Chronic fatigue syndrome and the psychiatrist. *Can J Psychiatry* 1990; 35:625–633.

Abbey, SE, Garfinkel, PE. Neurasthenia and chronic fatigue syndrome: The role of culture in the making of a diagnosis. *Am J Psychiatry* 1991; 148:1638–1646.

Bacall, HA, Newman, MK. *Theories of object relations: Bridges to self-psychology.* New York: Columbia University Press, 1990.

Beck, AT, Emery, G, Greenberg, R. *Anxiety disorders and phobias: A cognitive perspective.* New York: Basic Books, 1985.

Beck, AT, Rush, AJ, Shaw, BF, Emery, G. *Cognitive therapy of depression.* New York: Guilford Press, 1979.

Benson, H. *The relaxation response.* New York: Morrow, 1975.

Benson, H, Beary, JF, Carol, MP. The relaxation response. *Psychiatry* 1974; 37:37–46.

Berger, S. Chronic fatigue syndrome: A self-psychological perspective. *Clin Soc Work J* 1993; 21:71–84.

Berrios, GE. Feeling of fatigue and psychopathology: A conceptual history. *Compr Psychiatry* 1990; 31:140–151.

Blacher, RS. The briefest encounter: Psychotherapy for medical and surgical patients. *Gen Hosp Psychiatry* 1984; 6:226–232.

Blanchard, EB, Scharff, L, Payne, A, Schwartz, SP, Suls, JM, Malamood, H. Prediction of outcome from cognitive-behavioral treatment of irritable bowel syndrome. *Behav Res Ther* 1992; 30:647–650.

Borysenko, J. *Minding the body, mending the mind.* New York: Bantam Books, 1987.

Burke, SG. Chronic fatigue syndrome and women: Can therapy help? *Soc Work* 1992; 37:35–39.

Burns, DD. *Feeling good: The new mood therapy.* New York: Avon Books, 1980.

Butler, G. Phobic disorders. In Hawton, K, Salkovskis, PM, Kirk, J, Clark, DM, eds., *Cognitive behaviour therapy for psychiatric problems: A practical guide.* Oxford: Oxford University Press, 1989; 97–128.

Butler, S, Chalder, T, Ron, M, Wessely, S. Cognitive behaviour therapy in chronic fatigue syndrome. *J Neurol Neurosurg Psychiatry* 1991; 54:153–158.

Ciccone, DS, Grzesiak, RC. Chronic musculoskeletal pain: A cognitive approach to psychophysiologic assessment and intervention. *Adv Clin Rehab* 1990; 3:197–214.

Clarke, DM. A cognitive approach to panic. *Behav Res Ther* 1986; 24:461–470.

Clarke, DM. Anxiety states: Panic and generalized anxiety. In Hawton, K, Salkovskis, PM, Kirk, J, Clark, DM, eds., *Cognitive behaviour therapy for psychiatric problems: A practical guide.* Oxford: Oxford University Press, 1989; 52–96.

Craske, MG. Cognitive behavioral treatment of panic. In Frances, A, Hale, R, eds., *Annual review of psychiatry,* Volume 7. Washington, DC: American Psychiatric Press, 1988; 121–137.

Doherty, WJ, Campbell, T. *Families and health.* Newbury, CA: Sage, 1988.

Duff, K. *The alchemy of illness.* New York: Pantheon Books, 1993.

Dworkin, SF, Turner, JA, Wilson, L, Massoth, D, Whitney, C, Huggins, KH, Burgess, J, Sommers, E, Truelove, E. Brief group cognitive-behavioral intervention for temporomandibular disorders. *Pain* 1994; 59:175–187.

Fairburn, CG. Cognitive-behavioral treatment for bulimia. In Garner, DM, Garfinkel, PE, eds., *Handbook of psychotherapy for anorexia nervosa and bulimia.* New York: Guilford Press, 1985; 160–192.

Fennell, MJV. Depression. In Hawton, K, Salkovskis, PM, Kirk, J, Clark, DM, eds., *Cognitive behaviour therapy for psychiatric problems: A practical guide.* Oxford: Oxford University Press, 1989; 169–234.

Freud, S. On the grounds for detaching a particular syndrome from neurasthenia under the description "anxiety neurosis" (1895 [1894]). In Strachey, J, Freud, A, Strachey, A, Tyson, A, trans., *The standard edition of the complete psychological works of Sigmund Freud,* Volume III (1893–1899). Early Psychoanalytic Publications. Toronto: Clarke, Irwin and Co. Ltd., 1962; 90–117.

Freud, S. *Introductory lectures on psychoanalysis, Vol. 1, The Pelican Freud Library.* Strachey, J, trans., Strachey, J, Richards, A, eds. New York: Penguin Books, 1973.

Gabbard, GO. *Psychodynamic psychiatry in clinical practice.* Washington, DC: American Psychiatric Press, 1990.

Goldenberg, DL, Kaplan, KH, Nadeau, MG, Brodeur, C, Smith, S, Schmid, CH. A controlled study of a stress-reduction, cognitive-behavioral treatment program in fibromyalgia. *J Musculoskeletal Pain* 1994; 2:53–66.

Green, S. *Mind and body: The psychology of physical illness.* Washington, DC: American Psychiatric Press, 1985.

Green, S. Principles of medical psychotherapy. In Stoudemire, A, Fogel, BS, eds., *Psychiatric care of the medical patient.* Oxford: Oxford University Press, 1993; 3–18.

Greene, B, Blanchard, EB. Cognitive therapy for irritable bowel syndrome. *J Consult Clin Psychol* 1994; 62:576–582.

Hickie, I, Lloyd, A, Wakefield, D, Parker, G. The psychiatric status of patients with chronic fatigue syndrome. *Br J Psychiatry* 1990; 156:534–540.

Jackson, JE. After a while no one believes you: Real and unreal pain. In DelVecchio Good, MJ, Brodwin, PE, Good, BJ, Kleinman, A, eds., *Pain as human experience: An anthropological perspective.* Berkeley: University of California Press, 1992; 138–168.

Jacobs, J. Family therapy in the context of chronic medical illness. In Stoudemire, A, Fogel, BS, eds., *Psychiatric care of the medical patient.* Oxford: Oxford University Press, 1993; 19–30.

Kabat-Zinn, J. An outpatient program in behavioral medicine for chronic pain patients based on the practice of mindfulness meditation: Theoretical considerations, and preliminary results. *Gen Hosp Psychiaty* 1982; 4:37–47.

Kabat-Zinn, J. *Full catastrophe living: Using the wisdom of your body and mind to face stress, pain, and illness.* New York: Delacorte Press, 1990.

Kabat-Zinn, J, Lipworth, L, Burney, R, Sellers, W. Four-year follow-up of a meditation-based program for the self-regulation of chronic pain: Treatment outcomes and compliance. *Clin J Pain* 1987; 2:159–173.

Kaplan, KH, Goldenberg, DL, Galvin-Nadeau, M. The impact of a meditation-based stress reduction program on fibromyalgia. *Gen Hosp Psychiatry* 1993; 15:284–289.

Kirmayer, LJ. Mind and body as metaphors: Hidden values in biomedicine. In Lock, M, Gordon, D, eds., *Biomedicine examined.* Dordrecht: Kluwer Academic Publishers, 1988; 57–93.

Kirmayer, LJ, Robbins, JM. Conclusion: Prospects for research and clinical practice. In Kirmayer, LJ, Robbins, JM, eds., *Current concepts of somatization: Research and clinical perspectives.* Washington, DC: American Psychiatric Press, 1991; 201–225.

Kleinman, A. *Patients and healers in the context of culture: An exploration of the borderland between anthropology, medicine and psychiatry.* Berkeley: University of California Press, 1980.

Kleinman, A. *Origins of distress and disease: Depression, neurasthenia, and pain in modern China.* New Haven: Yale University Press, 1986.

Kleinman, A. *The illness narratives: Suffering, healing and the human condition.* New York: Basic Books, 1988.

Klerman, GL, Weissman, MM, Rounsaville, BJ, Chevron, ES. *Interpersonal psychotherapy of depression.* New York: Basic Books, 1984a.

Klerman, GL, Weissman, MM, Rounsaville, BJ, Chevron, ES. Interpersonal psychotherapy for depression. In Grinspoon, L, ed., *Psychiatry update: The American Psychiatric Association annual review,* Vol. III. Washington, DC: American Psychiatric Press, 1984b; 56–66.

Kutz, I, Borysenko, JZ, Benson, H. Meditation and psychotherapy: A rationale for the integration of dynamic psychotherapy, the relaxation response and mindfulness meditation. *Am J Psychiatry* 1985; 142:1–8.

Levenson, H, Hales, RE. Brief psychodynamically informed therapy for medically ill patients. In Stoudemire, A, Fogel, BS, eds., *Medical–psychiatric practice,* Vol. 2. Washington, DC: American Psychiatric Press, 1993; 3–37.

Lipowski, ZJ. Physical illness, the individual and the coping process. *Psychiatric Med* 1970; 1:91–102.

Lipowski, ZJ. Psychosocial reactions to physical illness. In Lipowski, ZJ, ed., *Psychosomatic medicine and liaison psychiatry: Selected papers.* New York: Plenum Medical Book Co., 1985; 141–175.

MacKenzie, KR. Recent developments in brief psychotherapy. *Hosp Comm Psychiatry* 1988; 39:742–752.

Markowitz, JC, Klerman, GL, Perry, SW, Clougherty, KF, Josephs, LS. Interpersonal psychotherapy for depressed HIV-seropositive patients. In Klerman, GL, Weissamn, MM, eds., *New applications of interpersonal psychotherapy.* Washington, DC: American Psychiatric Press, 1993; 199–224.

Mayou, R. Patients' fears of illness: Chest pain and palpitations. In Creed, F, Mayou, R, Hopkins, A, eds., *Medical symptoms not explained by organic disease.* London: The Royal College of Psychiatrists and The Royal College of Physicians of London, 1992; 25–32.

McDaniel, SH, Hepworth, J, Doherty, WJ. *Medical family therapy: A biopsychosocial approach to families with health problems.* New York: Basic Books, 1992.

McDougall, J. *Theaters of the body: A psychoanalytic approach to psychosomatic illness.* New York: W. W. Norton & Co., 1989.

Mohl, PC, Burstein, AG. The application of Kohutian self psychology to consultation–liaison psychiatry. *Gen Hosp Psychiatry* 1982; 4:113–119.

Moorey, S, Greer, S. *A psychological therapy for patients with cancer: A new approach.* Washington, DC: American Psychiatric Press, 1989.

Moos, R, Schaefer, J. The crisis of physical illness: An overview and conceptual approach. In Moos, R, ed., *Coping with physical illness: 2. New perspectives.* New York: Plenum, 1984; 3–26.

O'Leary, A, Shoor, S, Lorig, K, Holman, HR. A cognitive-behavioral treatment for rheumatoid arthritis. *Health Psychology* 1988; 7:527–544.

Powell, R, Dolan, R, Wessely, S. Attributions and self-esteem in depression and chronic fatigue syndromes. *J Psychosom Res* 1990; 34:665–673.

Ray, C, Weir, W, Stewart, D, Miller, P, Hyde, G. Ways of coping with chronic fatigue syndrome: Development of an illness management questionnaire. *Soc Sci Med* 1993; 37:385–391.

Rockland, LH. A review of supportive psychotherapy, 1986–1992. *Hosp Comm Psychiatry* 1993; 44:1053–1060.

Rodin, G. Somatization and the self: Psychotherapeutic issues. *Am J Psychother* 1984; 38:257–263.

Rodin, G. Somatization: A perspective from self psychology. *J Am Acad Psychoanalysis* 1991; 19:367–384.

Rodin, G. Psychiatric care for the chronically ill and dying patient. In Goldman, H, ed., *Review of general psychiatry,* fourth edition. Norwalk, CT: Appleton & Lange, 1995; 476–482.

Rodin, G, Craven, J, Littlefield, C. *Depression in the medically ill: An integrated approach.* New York: Brunner\Mazel, 1991.

Salit, IE. Sporadic postinfectious neuromyasthenia. *Can Med Assoc J* 1985;
133:659–663.

Salkovskis, PM. Somatic problems. In Hawton, K, Salkovskis, PM, Kirk, J, Clark,
DM, eds., *Cognitive behaviour therapy for psychiatric problems: A practical guide.*
Oxford: Oxford University Press, 1989; 235–276.

Salkovskis, PM, Warwick, HMC. Morbid preoccupations, health anxiety, and reassurance: A cognitive behavioural approach to hypochondriasis. *Behav Res Ther*
1986; 24:597–602.

Schweitzer, R, Robertson, DL, Kelly, B, Whiting, J. Illness behaviour of patients
with chronic fatigue syndrome. *J Psychosom Res* 1994; 38:41–49.

Sharpe, M. Chronic fatigue syndrome: can the psychiatrist help? In Hawton, K,
Cowen, P, eds., *Dilemmas and difficulties in the management of psychiatric patients.*
Oxford: Oxford University Press, 1990.

Sharpe, M. Non-pharmacological approaches to treatment. In Brock, GR, Whelan,
J, eds., *Chronic fatigue syndrome,* CIBA Foundation Symposium 173, Toronto:
John Wiley & Sons, 1993; 298–317.

Sharpe, M, Hawton, K, Simkin, S, Surawy, C, Klimes, I, Peto, TEA, Warrell, D,
Seagroatt, V. Cognitive therapy for chronic fatigue syndrome: A randomized
controlled clinical trial. *Br Med J* 1996; 312:22–26.

Skinner, JB, Erskine, A, Pearce, S, Rubenstein, I, Taylor, M, Foster, C. The evaluation of a cognitive behavioural treatment programme in outpatients with
chronic pain. *J Psychosom Res* 1990; 34:13–19.

Spira, JL, Spiegel, D. Group psychotherapy of the medically ill. In Stoudemire, A,
Fogel, BS, eds., *Psychiatric care of the medical patient.* Oxford: Oxford University
Press, 1993; 31–50.

Surawy, C, Hackman, A, Hawton, K, Sharpe, M. Chronic fatigue syndrome: A
cognitive approach. *Behav Res Ther* 1995; 33:535–544.

Taerk, F, Gnam, W. The chronic fatigue syndrome and psychoanalytic therapy: A
model for mind–body integration. *Gen Hosp Psychiatry* 1994; 16:319–325.

Taylor, GJ. *Psychosomatic medicine and contemporary analysis.* Madison: International
Universities Press, 1987.

Taylor, GJ. Psychoanalysis and psychosomatics: A new synthesis. *J Amer Acad of Psychoanalysis* 1992; 20:251–275.

Ursano, RJ, Hales, RE. A review of brief individual psychotherapies. *Am J Psychiatry* 1986; 143:1507–1517.

Ware, NC. Suffering and the social construction of illness: The delegitimation of
illness experience in chronic fatigue syndrome. *Med Anthro Quar* 1992; 6(4):
347–461.

Ware, NC. An anthropological approach to understanding chronic fatigue syndrome. In Straus, S, ed., *Chronic fatigue syndrome.* New York: Marcel Dekker,
1994; 85–97.

Ware, NC, Kleinman, A. Culture and somatic experience: The social course of illness in neurasthenia and chronic fatigue syndrome. *Psychosom Med* 1992;
54:546–560.

Watts, FN. Attributional aspects of medicine. In Antaki, C, Brewin, C, eds., *Attributions and psychological change.* London: Academic Press, 1982; 135–155.

Wessely, S, Butler, S, Chalder, T, David, A. The cognitive behavioural management of the post-viral fatigue syndrome. In Jenkins, R, Mowbray, J, eds., *Post-viral fatigue syndrome.* Chichester: John Wiley & Sons, 1991; 305–334.

Wessely, S, David, A, Butler, S, Chalder, T. Management of chronic (post-viral) fatigue syndrome. *J Roy Coll Gen Pract* 1989; 39:26–29.

Wessely, S, Powell, R. Fatigue syndromes: A comparison of chronic "postviral" fatigue with neuromuscular and affective disorders. *J Neurol Neurosurg Psychiatry* 1989; 52:940–948.

Wilfley, DE, Agras, WS, Telch, CF, Rossiter, EM, Schneider, JA, Cole, AG, Siffor, L, Raeburn, SD. Group cognitive-behavioral therapy and group interpersonal psychotherapy for the nonpurging bulimic individual: A controlled comparison. *J Consult Clin Psychology* 1993; 61:296–305.

Yalom, ID. *The theory and practice of group psychotherapy,* second edition. New York: Basic Books, 1975.

9

Cognitive-Behavioral Therapy for Patients with Chronic Fatigue Syndrome: Why?

Simon C. Wessely, M.D.

Previous chapters in this volume have considered the role of both physical and psychological factors in the etiology of chronic fatigue syndrome (CFS). This contribution discusses the influence of social, physical, and psychological factors in the perpetuation of CFS, and hence describes the rationale for the particular treatment approach that I, and others, espouse. Practical issues will be addressed in the subsequent chapter. In other words, this chapter makes the case for the cognitive-behavioral approach (the why), and the next chapter describes the principles of treatment (the how).

Earlier chapters have already described the role of psychiatric disorder in CFS. The fact that patients with severe chronic fatigue are at a high risk for psychosocial morbidity is now beyond dispute. However, each generation of physicians seems to find it necessary to discover this fact afresh, and their observations continue to inspire the same futile "organic versus psychological" polemics (Shorter, 1992; Wessely, 1991). Once again, an increasing number of studies confirms that perhaps the majority of patients seen in specialist centers, with a chief complaint of chronic fatigue, fulfill operational criteria for psychiatric disorder (see Chapter 3, this volume). The diagnoses vary, but depression is the most common, followed by anxiety disorders and somatization disorders. The link among chronic fatigue, CFS, and psychiatric disorder is complex, but the greater the number of symptoms required for the diagnosis of CFS, the stronger the link with psychiatric disorder (Katon & Russo, 1992).

212

These findings have no single explanation (see Chapters 6 and 7, this volume). In some cases, psychological disorder is a consequence of physical disorder, although this cannot explain the illness of the majority, because the rates of psychiatric disorder in CFS cases are in excess of those seen in other chronic medical conditions (Katon et al., 1991; Wessely & Powell, 1989; Wood et al., 1991). In other cases, psychological disorder has been misdiagnosed as CFS. The possibility that both CFS and psychiatric disorder have a common origin in disturbances of cerebral function attracts considerable attention (Bearn & Wessely, 1993; see also Chapter 5, this volume), but has, as yet, few treatment implications.

However, psychiatric diagnoses per se can be misleading in the context of CFS. For example, if I receive a referral from a physician stating that he or she wishes me to see a depressed patient in my clinic, this would not give me much useful information if the patient was suffering from CFS. On the other hand, I find little clinical difference between a CFS patient who fulfills criteria for depressive illness, and one who does not, perhaps because he or she lacks one additional symptom. Finally, the old truism that the management of a patient presenting with unexplained symptoms is to "manage the underlying disease" is far from true in regard to CFS. This chapter will argue that the management of a patient with CFS and depression does not differ substantially from a subject with CFS and panic disorder, or CFS and no psychiatric disorder. However, the management of a depressed CFS patient does differ from the management of depression in normal psychiatric practice. Psychiatric diagnoses in the context of CFS are helpful, but in themselves are not sufficient to suggest a treatment course.

I argue here that cognitive (conscious thoughts), attributional (beliefs about illness), and behavioral factors play a crucial role in determining outcome and mediating disability. Crucial to this argument is the basic scheme that what starts an illness is not always the same as what determines prognosis. In some illnesses, a simple model is sufficient—a nonimmune person infected with the rabies virus will develop rabies, or a worker exposed to radiation will develop marrow failure in a dose response fashion—but CFS cannot be explained in such a simple manner. The element that triggers CFS may not be what perpetuates it; hence, treatment may not be determined by the nature of the initial insult.

THE PATHOPHYSIOLOGY OF FATIGUE IN CFS

Treatment for any disease must be based on an informed knowledge of the nature of the observed disability. In CFS, this disability is principally related to fatigue and fatigability, which remains the central feature according to all current definitions of the condition. What is the nature of this symptom?

Fatigue in CFS has frequently been assumed to be of neuromuscular origin, particularly in the United Kingdom. In what must be one of the most cited single-case studies in the literature, evidence has been presented suggesting a metabolic abnormality in the muscles of a single medical sufferer (Arnold et al., 1984). Others have found evidence of enteroviral genome in the muscles of sufferers (Gow et al., 1991). Researchers have confidently stated that CFS is a viral myopathy (Hyde & Bergmann, 1988), a "muscle membrane disorder" (Jamal & Hansen, 1989), and a postviral mitochondrial disorder (Behan et al., 1991).

However, the evidence for a neuromuscular origin of the symptoms of CFS is far from convincing. First, most clinicians agree that physical and mental fatigue and fatigability are at the heart of CFS and cannot be accounted for by any known mechanism of muscular function (Wessely & Powell, 1989). The neuropsychiatric symptoms of CFS, such as poor concentration and short-term memory impairment, are not peripheral neuromuscular disorders (Wessely & Powell, 1989; Wood et al., 1991).

A second line of argument comes from the results of studies of actual neuromuscular function (as opposed to structure). There is a surprising degree of unanimity, especially for a subject as diverse as CFS. Meticulously conducted studies of dynamic muscle function have failed to show any evidence of peripheral neuromuscular dysfunction. These studies included subjects with CFS as defined in the United Kingdom (Riley et al., 1990; Stokes et al., 1988), subjects with immune dysfunction as seen in Australia (Lloyd et al., 1988, 1991), subjects with CDC-defined CFS (Kent-Braun et al., 1993), and subjects with post Epstein–Barr virus (EBV) fatigue syndrome (Rutherford & White, 1991). The research has shown no objective evidence of a delayed appearance of abnormal postexertional muscle fatigability, as is claimed by some (Gibson et al., 1993; Lloyd et al., 1988).

Some differences have emerged. Although all researchers agree that the fatigue in CFS is centrally mediated, Lloyd et al. (1988, 1991) and Rutherford and White (1991) have found totally normal recruitment, activation, and function; and Stokes et al. (1988) and Kent-Braun et al. (1993) have found that central activation is impaired. A number of explanations, including impaired motivation and the effect of pain, are possible. Whether the symptoms are similar to those encountered in multiple sclerosis, as has been claimed (DeLuca et al., 1993), also remains to be seen. The important message regarding treatment is that "on physiological and pathological grounds it is clear that CFS is not a myopathy" (Edwards et al., 1993).

Many observers also comment on the "extreme and sudden variability of energy levels both within and between episodes of illness" (Dowsett & Welsby, 1992). Such variations cannot be explained on a neuromuscular, immune, or immunological basis, but instead fit a cognitive behavioral model, as will be shown later in this chapter.

REST AND THE TREATMENT OF CFS

At present, the mainstay of management in CFS is rest. A nurse with CFS advises others to "always remember, until an exciting medical announcement is made, that there is no one drug to cure myalgic encephalomyelitis (ME). The only cure is rest and keeping the affected parts of the body rigid so as to improve the body's defences" (Dainty, 1988) . Similar sentiments have been expressed in a popular magazine: "The only hope is that one day some substance will be isolated that has the power to zap the ME virus," and until then "the most doctors can do is to advise patients to rest, and wait for the ME to go away" (Hodgkinson, 1988). The Victorian metaphor of the supply and demand of energy reappears frequently. A sufferer must "pace myself carefully, nurturing my fragile energy like a delicate plant" (Roeber, 1989) and "use energy at a slower rate than you make it" (Holford, 1989). Another Victorian source of metaphor was the world of electricity; hence, in neurasthenia, "the storage battery has been discharged rapidly or for too long a time" (Pershing, 1904). Similarly, ME sufferers must "recharge our batteries" (Millenson, 1992)—"a person with ME is like a battery that cannot hold its charge" (MacIntyre, 1989).

The treatment always comes back to the mainstay of the Victorian approach to neurasthenia, the rest cure. An American self-help book (Feiden, 1990) heads a section with the title "Rest, Rest and More Rest," and discusses "Aggressive rest therapy," as does an English self-help title (Franklin & Sullivan, 1989). A more orthodox U.K. book has 13 entries in the index under "rest, importance of" (Shepherd, 1989). The original fact sheets produced by one of the self-help groups for CFS sufferers stated, in bold type, "For the majority of ME sufferers, physical and mental exertion is to be avoided, and adequate rest essential. Important: if you have muscle fatigue do not exercise, this could cause a severe relapse" (ME Action Campaign, 1989). A self-help book tells sufferers that they must only do "seventy five percent of what you are capable of . . . unless you want to plummet down with another relapse soon, you really must follow the rule of doing less than you think you can" (Dawes & Downing, 1989).

Although there is no doubting the good faith behind such advice, its long-term wisdom is open to question. One general practitioner who is a sufferer and author of a popular self-help guide has written that "prolonged bed rest . . . should be advised with great care in the long-term cases, who may then become trapped in a vicious circle of immobility and weakness, and become almost bedridden" (Shepherd, 1989); another popular self-help book tells readers to "gradually increase the duration and type of exercise" (Crook, 1992), but such sentiments are unusual, particularly in the United Kingdom.

The advice given to CFS sufferers, especially in the United Kingdom, is remarkably consistent, yet the advice is at odds with most medical teaching.

Rest has little place in the management of most, if not all, chronic diseases, and many acute conditions as well. Exercise is part of the standard management of a wide range of neuromuscular, orthopedic, and rheumatological conditions. Graded activity forms the basis of the standard rheumatological management of fibromyalgia, a condition that has more than a passing similarity to CFS. Even if CFS is thought to have a neuromuscular origin—in this author's opinion, it does not—it is worth noting that exercise remains a useful part of the treatment of neuromuscular disorders until muscle function is below 10% of normal (Milner-Brown & Miller, 1988; Vignos, 1981). The use of rest, even in the management of such conditions as heart failure and low back pain, is now increasingly being questioned (Coats et al., 1990). In acute low back pain, a graded activity results in an earlier return to work (Lindstrom et al., 1992), and activity in all forms is the basis of treatment for chronic back pain because it is being recognized that rest is not just ineffective, but counterproductive (Frank, 1993).

Why is rest so popular? One reason is that it appears to work. Rest is an effective short-term strategy for dealing with acute fatigue, as all of us know. In particular, rest is the usual strategy we adopt when coping with acute infections. The majority of patients with CFS who are seen in tertiary care centers can trace their disability to the aftermath of a "viral" infection. Factors such as chance (the average adult in the United Kingdom experiences three or four symptomatic viral infections annually), search after meaning and recall bias will inflate these figures, but it would be folly to discount such evidence entirely. How might a viral infection contribute to chronic fatigue? Although a great deal of attention has been given to the immunological and serological consequences of viral infection (Behan & Behan, 1988; Denman, 1990), and to the direct effects of viral agents on mood (Webb & Parsons, 1992), little attention has been paid to the behavioral consequences. During an acute viral infection, the symptoms of pain, myalgia, fatigue, and so on, force most people to rest. This need to rest may be adaptive, because there is evidence of short-term subtle abnormalities in skeletal muscle (Astrom et al., 1976), cardiac muscle (Montague et al., 1988), and neuromuscular transmission (Friman et al., 1977) during acute viral infection, although their relevance is unclear (Friman et al., 1985). The immediate behavioral consequence of these abnormalities is rest.

For most subjects, rest is used only as a short-term coping strategy, and the vast majority are able to resume normal activity. However, recovery from viral infection is almost certainly normally distributed, and some may experience a prolonged and inexplicable period of ill health. Attempts to resume previous levels of activity may continue to be difficult during this period, and may result in a resurgence of symptoms. CFS sufferers appear more likely to adopt such strategies, for a variety of reasons.

Researchers have noted that many chronic fatigue sufferers initially adopted a vigorous program of exercise. Numerous anecdotal reports have indicated chronic sufferers with a previous history of an abrupt return to dramatic physical activity (Ho-Yen, 1990; Peel, 1988). One reason for this phenomenon is that CFS, as seen in the clinic, seems to be overrepresented among the fit and athletic (Eichner, 1989; Riley et al., 1990; Wessely et al., 1989). Previously athletic patients would be at risk of rapid physical deconditioning after a period of enforced rest. Furthermore, personality and lifestyle factors may suggest that the same people are likely to adopt overaggressive early attempts at exercise following illness. Athletic sufferers are particularly prone to be overactive, unlikely to take things easy, and "the last types to take time [off from] work for no good reason" (Shepherd, 1989). Common statements are: "it seemed like a bad bout of flu from which (as usual) I did not allow myself proper time to recover" or "I refused to admit something was wrong." Athletic sufferers "work until they drop, whilst everyone else creeps to bed with the slightest headache or sniffle. . . . Lazy people don't get ME" (Bragg, 1989). A popular explanation of the fact that the Royal Free epidemic in 1955 (the paradigmatic example of ME in Britain) involved staff, and not patients, is that the former were vulnerable because of the amount of exercise involved in their jobs, unlike the patients, rendered immune by resting in bed (Shepherd, 1987).

This concept leads to the area of personality and vulnerability to CFS, recently reviewed by Abbey (1993). Few systematic studies have been undertaken in this area. The typical case history of sufferers frequently fulfills the image of the conscientious, successful, and dedicated person with high standards and responsibilities. Advocates of CFS/ME frequently attribute the illness to the pressure of life, the stresses under which people labor, and the pressure of deadlines, which affects people who refuse to rest. CFS sufferers are "do-ers" (Maros, 1991); all of them are "active, energetic, capable, competent" (Eland, 1988).

Such accounts inevitably reinforce the stereotype of "Yuppie flu," so disliked by sufferers and the self-help organizations. The step from adjectives such as successful, dedicated, and conscientious to terms such as overachiever, lifestyle-dominated, and overactive is a short one. One sufferer denied the tag "Yuppie flu," but later described herself as "an aggressive Eighties career woman" (Fleh, 1990). Articles frequently describe the label as "inaccurate and unjust" (Stacey, 1990), but then use case histories that reinforce the unwelcome image. ME patients are "active, successful people" leading "vigorously successful lives" (Hodgkinson, 1987). One article began by stating that ME was "wrongly labelled as yuppie flu," but went on to say that "career women who push themselves to attain goals, working long hours and not eating properly, are most at risk" (Willsher, 1990). The *Sunday Telegraph*

Magazine (1989) used a case history of a "26-year-old successful hard-working stock broker . . . healthy, cheerful, social and energetic, often working 12 or more hours a day but none the less enthusiastically filling her remaining hours with plenty of sport or parties." An almost identical description appeared in a self-help book (Steincamp, 1989). *The Observer* magazine (Bryan & Melville, 1989) noted, without irony, that "patients have difficulty convincing their doctors that they are not malingering, even though a significant proportion were previously high achievers (hence the nickname 'yuppie flu')." Even children must be "enthusiastic, energetic, positive-minded people who try too hard when they are ill," or "bright, bubbly, energetic . . . competitive, sports loving."

These accounts have a purpose. The current president of the ME Association, herself a doctor, stated that one of the distinctive differences between ME sufferers and depressives is that those with ME are highly motivated achievers—"they almost have too much will power, whereas depressives have virtually none" (Stacey, 1990). If depression and hysteria occur in malingerers, shirkers, and those with low moral fiber, then establishing that the CFS sufferer has none of these characteristics is a necessary part of legitimization, but, ironically, it also fuels the image of the "yuppie flu." Some CFS advocates are aware of this contradiction—one noted that it has been necessary to steer doctors away from the stereotype of the neurotic woman, in order to "convince the medical community that the disease is legitimate," but to do so portrays patients as "successful super achievers" (Jessop, cited in Feiden, 1990).

How true are these stereotypes? When Ware and Kleinman studied 50 CFS patients attending the practice of Anthony Komaroff, they found that "a desire for accomplishment and success, underwritten by exacting standards for personal performance, impelled these individuals always to try harder, go further, in an attempt to meet the expectations they had set for themselves at work, home and school." The recorded interviews were full of such phrases as "hyper," "always on the go," and "workaholic" (Ware, 1993; Ware & Kleinman, 1992).

The role of personality and achievement is confusing. Along with the alleged excess of medical personnel among CFS sufferers, one must not neglect the role of selection bias. Relevant factors may be illness behavior and access to medical care. Furthermore, assessments of personality are usually retrospective. Sufferers, recognizing the possibility of receiving a psychiatric diagnosis, might emphasize those aspects of personality and behavior that appear to provide evidence against psychiatric disorder. Sufferers are more likely to "have a good premorbid personality and work record" (Dowsett & Welsby, 1992)—indeed, "the fact that they were all known to have good premorbid personalities made us consider an organic cause for their illness" (Fegan et al., 1983). Good premorbid personality does not prevent psychiatric disorder, but many clinicians believe it does.

The publicity accorded to famous, athletic, or medical sufferers has a symbolic purpose—to dispel any suggestion that CFS sufferers are anything other than exceptional and active members of society. However, like all stereotypes, these images have a basis in the reality of the populations seen in CFS clinics. It is my opinion that these personality variables can play a significant role in prognosis and can provide another rationale for a cognitive approach to treatment.

CFS, MYALGIA, AND ACTIVITY

The evidence suggesting that the core features of CFS are centrally, and not peripherally, mediated was discussed earlier in this chapter. However, this still leaves several clinical aspects of CFS unexplored. Patients have little doubt that their symptoms are related to muscular activity—they complain bitterly of pain experienced all too clearly in muscles, and related all too clearly to activity. Why?

One possible explanation relates to the behavioral consequences of the inactivity that is the sine qua non of CFS. Are CFS patients unfit? Almost certainly, yes. Studies of subjects with fibromyalgia confirm the clinical impression of deconditioning (Klug et al., 1989), as do studies of CFS (Riley et al., 1990). The various changes in muscle metabolism and mitochondrial activity that have been reported might all be explained on the basis of physical deconditioning (Wagenmakers et al., 1988; Wong et al., 1992). However, are such changes primary or secondary? The answer is unclear. Case control designs, which at present make up almost all CFS studies, cannot answer this question. Findings similar to those in CFS can be caused by lack of activity. CFS patients are certainly characterized by inactivity—a substantial degree of functional impairment is necessary for the diagnosis in all of the current operational criteria. Only one prospective study sheds any light on the matter. In White's (1991) important cohort study of recovery from EBV, (White et al., 1995), simple measures of unfitness taken within a few weeks of the onset of definite EBV infection were significantly associated with fatigue syndrome at 4 months. There is also controlled evidence suggesting that increased activity assists recovery from fibromyalgia (McCain et al., 1988), and uncontrolled evidence from a study of CFS recovery (Butler et al., 1991) makes the same suggestion. However, whether the benefits are due to increased self-esteem and self-efficacy consequent upon achieving targets, or to increased physical fitness, is unclear.

Does being unfit matter? One of the consequences of neuromuscular deconditioning is delayed-onset postexertional muscle pain (Klug et al., 1989), resulting particularly from eccentric contractions, where the muscle lengthens while doing work (Newham, 1988), especially in the untrained person (Editorial, 1987). Postexercise muscle pain should not necessarily be regarded as pathological—it is common to all subjects who engage in movement that requires muscular activity not normally performed in their everyday life (Klug et al., 1989). The consequences of lack of physical activity, and the changes in the neuromuscular system that result, have been known to clinicians for many years. In normal individuals, bed rest causes a decline in muscle strength of around 3% per day, particularly if daily maximal achieved tension is less than 20% of the maximal strength of the muscle (Kottke, 1966). A decrease of 25% in muscle protein turnover has been observed after prolonged quadriceps immobilization (Gibson et al., 1987), but is detectable within 6 hours (Booth, 1987). In an immobilized limb, not only muscle bulk, but muscle histology, is rapidly altered (Jaffe et al., 1978). As Richard Asher (1947) warned "We should think twice about ordering a patient to bed and realize that beneath the comfort of the blanket there lurks a host of formidable dangers."

Inactivity also increases the sense of effort on exertion, both physical and mental. Normal volunteers who remained immobile for a week, but were exposed to normal environmental stimulation, showed impaired neuropsychological performance together with EEG changes (Zuber & Wilgosh, 1963).

A different but equally elegant explanation of myalgia in CFS has been proposed by Bennett and colleagues working in the related area of fibromyalgia (Bennett et al., 1992). They hypothesized that the sleep disturbance integral to both CFS and fibromyalgia caused a disruption of stage 4 sleep. Growth hormone plays a critical role in muscle homeostasis and repair. Impairment of growth hormone production might explain the features of muscle microtrauma that Bennett and others have noted in biopsy studies. Bennett et al. (1992) provided evidence in support of this theory by demonstrating lowered levels of somatomedin-C in random samples taken from fibromyalgia patients compared to normal controls. However, we have been unable to replicate this finding in a smaller series, using fasting morning samples.

The presence of eccentric contractions, and, perhaps, sleep-induced changes in muscle homeostasis, can explain at least some of the experiences of delayed muscle pain. However, along with the other consequences of disuse, these conditions cannot be regarded as the primary cause of CFS pain. Furthermore, nonpathological delayed-onset muscle pain is usually localized to the muscles used, whereas CFS patients tend to complain of more widespread and diffuse pain. Nevertheless, whether myalgia results from physiological or pathological processes, there can be no doubt as to the authenticity of the experience and the resulting distress. The neuromuscular abnormalities that are found in CFS may correspond to those observed in fibromyalgia, about which it has been written that "it is highly likely that it is not a disease *per se,* but rather an altered physiological state" (Reilly & Littlejohn, 1990).

COGNITIONS, ATTRIBUTIONS, AND CHRONIC FATIGUE

Psychiatrists and psychologists now pay considerable attention to the thoughts and beliefs ("cognitions") experienced in a wide variety of situations, especially by those with chronic illnesses that are both physical and psychological (Sensky, 1990). Two areas of particular interest are: attributional style and cognitive errors.

Most patients presenting to a specialist with chronic fatigue believe their illness is due to an external agent, usually infective in origin (Hickie et al., 1990; Wessely & Powell, 1989). This belief is the opposite of the situation in primary care (David et al., 1990), or in the community (Pawlikowska et al., 1994), where most chronically fatigued patients ascribe their condition to psychosocial adversities. Many reasons are given for such attributions. As already mentioned, many CFS sufferers trace their symptoms to an infective episode. The symptoms arising after nonspecific infection are similar to those occurring during episodes of mood disorder (Imboden et al., 1959). Although one publication on ME is subtitled "You don't get a temperature with a nervous breakdown" (Stone, 1991), both chills and fevers are not uncommon presentations of psychiatric disorder (Harding et al., 1980; Wilson et al., 1983).

The external nature of the attribution made by the chronically fatigued patient seen in hospital practice has certain consequences, irrespective of its accuracy. Some of these consequences are advantageous—"Symptoms attributed to an external cause are less disabling than symptoms attributed to a personal cause" (Watts, 1982). External attribution also protects the patient from the stigma of being labeled psychiatrically disordered—"the victim of a germ infection is therefore blameless" (Helman, 1978). In the context of CFS, "to attribute the continuing symptoms to persistence of a 'physical' disease is a mechanism that carries the least threat to a person's self-esteem" (Katz & Andiman, 1988), but "patients who suffer from unrelenting fatigue fear they have a serious, occult medical problem and worry that people will think they had a mental problem or a blameworthy characterological weakness of will" (Greenberg, 1990). The absence of guilt and the preservation of self-esteem, even in the context of mood disorder, have been noted in the postinfectious fatigue syndrome (Imboden et al., 1959; Powell et al., 1990; Webb & Parsons, 1992). Abbey, among others, has drawn attention to the important role that avoiding stigma and blame plays in the genesis of CFS (Abbey, 1993).

This concept has been captured in the media writing on CFS. A newspaper headline expressed this view in its clearest form: "Virus research doctors finally prove shirkers really are sick" (Hodgkinson, 1987). A *London Times* (1988) piece was titled "Fatigue blamed on virus: Malingering disease proved genuine." The reviewer of one self-help book for a British newspaper wrote that "an infection is respectable. It has none of the stigma of a psychologically induced illness, which implies weakness or lack of moral fibre" (Seagrove, 1989).

However, there are detrimental aspects to such an attributional style. It is common knowledge that viruses cannot be treated (Helman, 1978); thus, the attribution implicit in the label of "postviral fatigue" carries no information about how the sufferer can recover (Wessely et al., 1991). The patient feels in the grip of something that he or she is powerless to influence, be it chronic virus or chronic allergy. Furthermore, attributing chronic fatigue to "postviral fatigue" or "ME" conveys more than a simple statement of etiology. It also suggests certain beliefs about prognosis and treatment, and, in particular, emphasizes the importance of limiting activity. The nurse with CFS, previously quoted as advising sufferers to rest, also describes the effects of viruses: "These living viruses are erratic and unpredictable. The prickly-edged ones pierce their way into the body cells. If disturbed by the patient's activity they become as aggressive as a disturbed wasps' nest, and can be felt giving needle-like jabs (or stimulating the nerves to do so" (Dainty, 1988). Such opinions may reinforce the despair and helplessness so frequently reported by chronic fatigue sufferers. At present, the attribution of CFS or ME is usually associated with a belief that the condition is incurable, and that the symptoms should be managed by rest. The consequences can be helplessness, increased fatigue, lack of self-efficacy, and diminished responsibility for one's own health (Powell et al., 1990). In the context of anxiety, external attributions increase the severity of fatigue (Hoehn-Saric & McLeod, 1985). In the context of CFS, belief in a viral cause for illness was independently associated with poor prognosis in the systematic follow-up study of Sharpe et al. (1992), as was continued membership in a self-help organization.

Cognitive factors such as fear and anxiety may be implicated in the perpetuation of disability. Systematic studies have suggested a role for clinically manifest anxiety in subjects with chronic fatigue and chronic fatigue syndrome (Kroenke et al., 1988; Manu et al., 1991). The hierarchical nature of psychiatric diagnosis suggests that the true prevalence of clinical anxiety is higher than even systematic studies suggest. Less studied is the role of fear. Fear of illness is an important part of CFS, but this is not the exaggerated fear of illness found in hypochondriasis. This theory has been confirmed by Robbins, Kirmayer, and Kapusta (1990), who compared fibromyalgia patients with rheumatoid arthritis controls. Robbins et al. found no differences in fear of illness and illness worry between the two groups—the opposite of what would be predicted in hypochondriasis. Nevertheless, worry about illness did play a role in the fibromyalgia patients, and correlated highly with overall functional disability. Robbins et al. suggest that a "feeling of vulnerability and apprehension about having an illness of unknown origin may contribute to sufferers' activity limitations, inability to sustain a work effort and varied somatic distress."

There are many sources of fear in chronic fatigue sufferers. Some of the literature available to sufferers in Great Britain has anxiogenic properties. For example, a newsletter published for young sufferers tells them: "Up to 30% of patients may suffer from cardiac complications, depending upon the strain of infecting virus. There is therefore a danger of pushing a child too far physically" (Colby, 1992). The same publication goes on to state that only 25% of sufferers (i.e., children) make a complete recovery. Much of the literature details various agents, ranging from immunizations and pollution to a variety of foods (and even sunlight) that may affect the illness. Some persons with CFS merge into the realm of multiple chemical sensitivity or total allergy syndrome (Buchwald et al., 1992; Stewart, 1990a, 1990b), and their lives are ruined by fearful anticipation and avoidance of most forms of environmental stimulation.

What are adult sufferers told about outcome? The first president of the ME Association and its first medical advisor use the same words—the disease has "an alarming tendency to chronicity" (Ramsay, 1989; Smith, 1989). The president of the ME Association states that an essential clinical feature of the disease is a "prolonged relapsing course lasting years or decades" (Dowsett & Welsby, 1992). Sufferers must make "very significant changes in their lifestyle" (Shepherd, 1989). Behan and Behan (1988), who have perhaps the most extensive experience with CFS in the United Kingdom, describe the outcome of patients referred to a neurology service as follows: "Most cases do not improve, give up their work and become permanent invalids, incapacitated by excessive fatigue and myalgia."

There is evidence to support this gloomy outlook. Hellinger et al. (1988) and Gold et al. (1990) reported that half of the patients referred had significantly improved after 1 year, but the other half had not, and only 6% were symptom-free. In Canadian primary care, over one-half of fatigued patients remained fatigued 1 year later (Cathebras et al., 1992). Hinds and McCluskey (1993) found that only 18% of those referred to a immunology clinic improved, and the prognosis of fibromyalgia is similarly disheartening (Norregaard et al., 1993). Finally, in a systematic follow-up of 177 cases of postviral fatigue referred to a single infectious disease clinic in Oxford, Sharpe et al. (1992) found that short-term prognosis was poor, but two-thirds had shown some improvement by 4 years. However, only 13% considered themselves fully recovered; a similar figure was reported by Wheeler et al. (1950).

Does this mean that patients are untreatable—or do these views actually influence outcome? Can the perception of ME and related illnesses as incurable become a self-fulfilling prophecy? Because it is now accepted that self-efficacy, the judgment of how successfully the subject believes he or she can execute any course of action, is a crucial determinant of whether an activity will be engaged (Bandura, 1977; Klug et al., 1989), such beliefs could have a deleterious effect on performance.

Fear may result not only from the provision of negative information, but from the absence of any information. This problem is related to the status ambiguity that surrounds CFS and to the absence of guidance about, and information on, the nature of the illness and its symptoms. Jerome Frank wrote: "Patients suffering from unfamiliar diseases tend to develop emotional reactions which impede recovery, such as anxiety, resentment and confusion. To keep disability at a minimum, therapeutic efforts must be directed not only to overcoming the pathogenic agent but to maintaining the patient's confidence in the physician, and encouraging his expectation of return to useful activity" (Frank, 1946). CFS patients have a double jeopardy—not solely the absence of meaningful information concerning the nature of their illness, its management and its outcome, but, all too frequently, the provision of information that may be both misleading and deleterious.

The most important aspect of fear of symptoms is that it provokes and fuels avoidance behavior (Lethem et al., 1983; Philips, 1987). As the patient's expectation that symptoms will follow activity increases, so do the precautions taken to avoid such symptoms. If these precautions prove unsuccessful, fear increases. Rachman (1978) has shown that stimuli that are anticipated, but unpredictable and uncontrollable, are particularly likely to lead to the final stage, when fear becomes fixed by the development of phobic anxiety. Avoidance of situations, including work, social activity, and travel, may result in the development of a phobic response on reexposure. This response is signaled by anxiety that in turn exacerbates fatigue (Folgering & Snik, 1988; Winokur & Holeman, 1963), creating a vicious circle.

Phobic attributions and cognitions influence not only mood, but disability. Negative cognitions (e.g., belief that activities causing an increase in symptoms must be damaging, belief that any activities are impossible in the presence of symptoms, and belief that recovery is not under personal control but is at the whim of a virus) lead to a loss of self-control, and an allied tendency to symptom monitoring and increased symptom perception. The chronic pain literature suggests that patients who cope with symptoms by avoidance suffer more disability and more pain (Philips, 1987). The situation may be analogous in chronic fatigue, where strategies such as rest, although effective in the short term, may be maladaptive in the long term. A brief abstract from the research team at the University of Miami lends empirical support to a link among distorted cognitive appraisals, avoidance, and functional disability in CFS (Antoni et al., 1992).

COGNITIONS, BEHAVIOR, AND DISABILITY

We can now see the role cognition and behavior play in the otherwise mysterious progression from short-term adaptive avoidance of activity to maladaptive chronic avoidance. Prolonged convalescence causes physical deconditioning: of the four groups studied by Benjamin and Hoyt (1945), namely athletes, "normal adults," adults with effort syndromes, and adults with prolonged recovery from infectious hepatitis, the last mentioned were the most physically unfit. Efforts to resume activity at normal levels will be particularly likely to lead to failure and continuing symptoms in this group. This persistence of symptoms will be particularly demoralizing to persons who have been told that all viral infections are short-lived and recovery is always rapid.

The personality variables discussed above make a further contribution to disability. I believe, along with most clinicians, that the cornerstone of treatment is a cautious, graded resumption of activity, using clearly defined, modest, and predictable goals. However, many patients have difficulty keeping to such a program. If it is true that chronic fatigue sufferers have tried to "exercise away" their fatigue, and hence carried out activity that may be excessive in the light of their current (but not previous) fitness, or in other ways failed to adopt the cautious, slow approach suggested, then delayed myalgia is inevitable. Symptoms of fatigue and myalgia can be both severe and frightening. Using the concepts of "learned helplessness" (Abramson, Seligman, & Teasdale, 1978), it is easy to see how such potent, aversive, uncontrollable, and mysterious symptoms can give rise to both demoralization and high rates of mood disorder, especially if attributed to either an external agent (such as a virus) or an internal, primary neuromuscular cause. Mood disorder is strongly associated with fatigue and myalgia (Wessely, 1989); thus, it sets up another of the many vicious circles that contribute to chronic fatigue.

Furthermore, many patients have personalities characterized by high internal standards, devotion to duty, and perfectionism, making it hard for them to accept anything less than 100%. These expectations are frequently impossible to achieve in the setting of CFS and in the early stages of treatment, and are experienced by many patients as failure. The cognition that "if I can't do it properly, it's not worth doing at all" is a frequent one. Another cognitive factor in CFS is that many patients, in an understandable effort to control and reduce symptoms by varying activity levels, become hypervigilant and oversensitized to physical sensations. Our knowledge of attention and awareness suggests that symptom focusing may serve to further exacerbate unpleasant sensations. For example, increasing the attention paid to one's heart rate may lead to the detection of nonpathological ectopic beats that in turn gives rise to anxiety, and, hence, more palpitations.

Cognitive factors (e.g., beliefs about health and illness) and behavioral factors (the use of avoidance as a coping strategy) are important determinants

of outcome in CFS. All of these factors contribute to the vicious circle postulated in CFS (Wessely et al., 1989, 1991). However, as usual, even vicious
circles are nothing new in the pathogenesis of chronic fatigue syndrome
(Hurry, 1914, 1915).

EFFORT SYNDROME

The reference to Hurry (1914, 1915) introduces a historical dimension to the
discussion of CFS. CFS is far from new, and at least part of its origin lies in
the disease known to Victorian society as neurasthenia (Wessely, 1990,
1991), a view shared by others (Abbey & Garfinkel, 1991; Greenberg et al.,
1990; Shorter, 1992; Ware & Kleinman, 1992; White, 1989). The resem-
blances between CFS and neurasthenia, in terms of symptoms, etiology, social class, and management, are striking and beyond the scope of this chapter.
However, it is useful to consider the neglected topic of effort syndrome, also
known as neurocirculatory asthenia, Soldier's Heart, and Da Costa's syndrome (Paul, 1987). The clinical characteristics of effort syndrome are strikingly reminiscent of CFS, even down to the frequent role of an infective
trigger (MacKenzie, 1916).

   One particular set of studies, now rarely cited, is relevant to the current
discussion. These studies were carried out by Maxwell Jones at the Mill Hill
Army Hospital, where 2,324 soldiers with effort syndrome were seen during
World War II (Jones & Mellersh, 1946; Jones & Scarisbrick, 1946). Jones was
influenced by cardiologist Paul Wood, whose views on the etiology of effort
syndrome had undergone a radical transformation during his career; his final
view of the syndrome was synonymous with anxiety disorder. Jones began
studying the exercise tolerance and lactate response to activity in sufferers,
anticipating the later detailed classic work by Mandel Cohen. Jones concluded that the key difference between anxiety and effort syndrome was not
impaired exercise tolerance nor early production of lactic acid, which were
present in both. Instead, he wrote that effort syndrome patients were "conscious of their poor exercise response and tend to associate their symptoms
with physical effort (in fact develop an effort phobia); but in the anxiety
group no such awareness is present and the somatic symptoms of anxiety are
not correlated with exercise" (Jones & Scarisbrick, 1946).

   Maxwell Jones is known as the founder of psychoanalytically based
group therapy, but what he was describing was the manner in which cognitive and attributional factors played a role in mediating disability. Despite his
orientation toward psychogenic perpetuating mechanisms, he drew attention
to the role of infection in triggering effort syndromes.

   The exact nature of the hemodynamic disturbances induced by exercise
in effort syndromes and anxiety disorders remains a matter of continuing,

albeit little publicized research. Modern researchers are now describing central mechanisms that bear some resemblance to those being postulated in CFS (Mantysaari et al., 1988). However, the work of Maxwell Jones reminds us of the leitmotiv of this chapter. An organically determined central mechanism may underlie the symptoms of CFS, but the link between such dysfunction and the profound disability of CFS may lie in the cognitions of those afflicted and the strategies that result.

THE SOCIOLOGY OF CFS

Cognitive and behavioral factors such as those already discussed can influence many conditions, both physical and psychological, and not solely CFS. However, CFS has social and political implications that distinguish it from many other conditions and give an added dimension to the nature, disability, and treatment of the illness. A recent letter to a journal talked about the "highly charged, medical, social and political atmosphere" surrounding the subject of CFS (Reeves et al., 1992). Controversy seems inseparable from chronic fatigue. One journalist wrote that "there is no middle ground when it comes to CFS" (Lechky, 1990). Paul Cheney (1989), one of the most prominent doctors on the CFS scene, has written that "we who believe that this is a real disease are almost in a death grip with those forces who would stifle debate, trivialize this problem, and banish patients who suffer from it beyond the edges of traditional medicine" (which, in this context, includes psychiatry). Many people will have had similar experiences to one medical journalist, who wrote that "at any dinner party you will find the friends of sufferers, who will either support or hotly dispute this view, usually with ferocity" (Collee, 1991). CFS "falls into the category of illnesses that cannot be debated dispassionately" (Brodsky, 1991).

CFS is associated with a flourishing network of consumerism and political action. A recent American article on CFS drew attention to the "proliferation of support groups, research foundations dominated by patients with the syndrome, and fund raising and lobbying groups" (Charatan, 1990). Recently, patient organizations have started advertising campaigns in the cinema and the popular press. CFS is accompanied by a rhetoric of struggle and injustice—a typical headline is: "Justice for the neglected and maligned sufferers of ME" (*Guardian,* 1990) ME sufferers in the United Kingdom "looked to the House of Commons for justice" (Hood, 1988). Passions are high—as indicated by the perhaps infelicitous words one activist chose to describe her involvement in the cause: "This issue chose me . . . if you were in Germany during the war, you didn't get to pick your issue, yet there was no greater test of leadership" (Montgomery, cited in Feiden, 1990). Regrettably, this social and cultural atmosphere is not just of dinner-party interest. These same forces intrude into the nature of the disability in CFS and add unique problems in its management.

For many doctors, CFS and its syndromes are not considered legitimate illnesses and are certainly not in the same category as heart attacks or cancer. Many aspects of fatigue contribute to this nonmedical categorization. The principal drawback is the absence of any confirmation by physical examination or laboratory testing. The patient often does not look sick. Sufferer after sufferer notes how outsiders make comments such as "Well, you don't look sick—you look great" (cited in Ware, 1993). "My skin is clear and tanned. I don't have a plaster cast on a broken leg . . . people say, 'You look so well.'" Sue Finlay (1986) identified "looking healthy and strong" as a principal difficulty in dealings with doctors. Blakely et al. (1991), in a questionnaire study, found links between chronic fatigue and chronic pain in regard to personality and symptoms—these links may extend to social factors as well. Chronic fatigue, like chronic pain, is a private experience to which no one else has access. Baszanger (1992) argues that, in chronic pain, the absence of objective evidence is a fundamental barrier to the normal organization of relationships between sufferer and doctor—a similar situation to that of chronic fatigue.

The regrettable truth seems to be that the poor treatment and frank rudeness, described by CFS patients in the self-help literature, have both a firm basis in reality and a long tradition. Among the many similarities between neurasthenia and CFS is the ability to cause disputes between patient and doctor, and between doctor and doctor. Perhaps as a result, past patients with neurasthenia and present CFS patients frequently receive little comfort from doctors. Sir Andrew Clark (1886) called neurasthenics "always ailing, seldom ill" and stated that the "wealthy neurasthenic will be a useless, frivolous, noxious element of society" (Urquhart, 1889). Such views were echoed in the popular press: "The majority of sufferers have better reason to complain of the weakening of their moral fibres than of either their mental or physical ones" (Anon, 1894). In the United States, Jelliffe, a New York neurologist who later became a psychoanalyst and editor of the *Journal of Nervous and Mental Diseases,* described CFS sufferers as "purely mental cases. Laziness, indifference, weakness of mind and supersensitiveness characterise them all." They are "ill because of lack of moral courage" (Jelliffe, 1905). Even those sympathetic to neurasthenics could not avoid a note of irritation and condescension. Patients were "the terror of the busy physician" (Rankin, 1903). They were "occupied by their symptoms beyond reason" (Blocq, 1894), went from physician to physician (even Beard called them "rounders") where they "write down their sensations in long memoranda which they hasten to read and to explain " (Blocq, 1894). Chronic fatigue, like chronic pain, is one of those "symptoms that depress the doctor" (Merskey, 1984).

A contemporary pediatrician who received publicity for an anti-ME stance also admitted that "his views were a lot more moderate than many of his colleagues who believed that ME was nonsense" (*Sheffield Telegraph,* 1990). Journalists frequent comment on similar reactions from doctors whom they approach for their stories about CFS, although the doctors usually prefer to remain anonymous. Occasionally such views surface. One article in a medical magazine calls ME an "escape route for the middle classes" (Dalrymple, 1992), and states that those affected "suffer triumphantly, and their claim that the disease has ruined their lives is not to be believed." The writer believed CFS to be a "sickness not of the body, but of the spirit," and by his levity demonstrated that such afflictions are deserving not of sympathy but of blame.

The problem of dismissal and discourtesy from doctors is such that each generation of doctors interested in fatigue has seen fit to warn their colleagues against levity in their treatment of fatigue patients. Charles Beevor (1898), at the National Hospital for Nervous Disease, reminded his colleagues that "on no account should the patient's symptoms be laughed at," and John Mitchell (1908), at the John Hopkins Hospital, complained that his medical colleagues treated the neurasthenic patient "with ridicule or a contemptuous summing up of his case in the phrase 'there is nothing the matter, he is only nervous.'" Paul Cheney told a journalist that "there are doctors who leave the room after speaking to one of these [CFS] patients and can't stop laughing" (Johnson, 1987).

Does all this matter in regard to treatment and recovery? The answer is an unequivocal yes. The climate of opinion and controversy surrounding CFS means that the sufferer is frequently caught in a trap. The treatments suggested by a model of CFS as a unitary condition, the sole consequence of a single physical agent, are straightforward, simple to explain, and free of stigma and moral implications. Sadly, none of them appears to work. On the other hand, strategies based on a more complex model, frequently involving either psychological or behavioral interventions, are far from value-free. All of these implications are magnified in the light of the controversy surrounding CFS. Those clinicians who support CFS, and those who oppose it, frequently share the same views concerning the legitimacy (or, in this case, the nonlegitimacy) of psychological distress. Both sides believe that anything other than the narrowly organic is equated with low moral fiber and malingering. The only dispute is the status to be awarded CFS. One doctor is quoted in a self-help book as telling a medical conference that "ME is an imaginary disease . . . for which the best treatment is psychiatric" (Steincamp, 1989) (like most of the doctors who express opinions on psychiatry and CFS, he was not psychiatrically qualified). The existence, in many minds, of a link between malingering and seeing a psychiatrist may be both surprising and offensive to many psychiatrists. Many sufferers recall that the outcome of visiting their doctor was to be "accused of malingering or given a psychiatric referral" (Ho-Yen, 1987). In this climate, accepting any treatment other than those based on the single disease or external agent model is fraught with difficulty. For many, it is better to have an incurable disease such as CFS than a psychological disease even if it might be treatable. "The day Nomi Antelman learned she had an incurable disease, she rejoiced" (Ames, 1985).

The hostility toward psychological distress, perceived as synonymous with low moral fiber and blame, permeates treatment and outcome. CFS patients may be characterized by a denial of psychological distress (Blakely et al., 1991). Psychiatrists are seen as having little or no role in the management of CFS. The stigma of psychiatry, as reflected in the mirror of CFS, is too vast a subject to be addressed here, but it is all too often true that, in the CFS literature, the only good psychiatrist is the one who finds nothing wrong and declares the sufferer psychologically normal. A character who surfaced in a popular television series, "Golden Girls," addressed the subject of CFS in September 1989. In the TV script, we first saw the image of the "bad" doctor, who is rude to the patient, keeps her waiting, finds all her tests normal, and tells her to pull herself together, before finally diagnosing her condition as one of loneliness—a functional or mental problem. Another neurologist pronounces her well, and recommends that she see a psychiatrist. However, she has already done so, and produces two letters saying her problems are physical, not psychological.

A nonfictional sufferer told a popular newspaper that he had seen a neurologist who failed to find anything physically wrong, became "beside himself with wrath, and suggested that I see a psychiatrist. . . . The psychiatrist told me that I was no madder than the rest of the population and sent me back to the by-now quivering and speechless neurologist" (Monckton, 1988). Pleas are often made for a multidisciplinary approach to CFS (David et al., 1988). One distinguished epidemiologist appeared to answer these pleas when he told a journalist that "there is need for multidisciplinary approaches. We are talking about a disease, the investigation of which requires epidemiologists, virologists, psychologists." However, "Why the psychologist? To prove you're not all crazy" (Grufferman, cited in Feiden, 1990).

The consequences of these views are not in doubt. "Sufferers often reject psychiatric treatment for fear of being told it is all the mind" (*Daily Mail,* 1990), so that accepting any form of psychiatric treatment is seen as stigmatizing CFS. "I don't know anyone who has been for psychiatric treatment, because CFS is a physical illness. I'm not crazy, I'm sick" (Cherreson, 1991). Being referred to a psychiatrist is "being blackballed" (Conant, 1990). The image of being on trial is common: "For me, being a psychiatric patient was a little like being imprisoned for a crime I didn't do" (Gardner, 1988). Such views do little for the self-esteem of the average psychiatrist, but have more serious consequences. Many CFS patients are denied what may be simple but effective treatments. For others, the rejection of any social, psychological, or behavioral intervention may set in motion the maladaptive patterns that form the basis of this chapter.

Evidence from other areas attests to the malignant effect of polarization, dispute, and controversy on the outcome of diseases. When a person with an illness in which the only evidence comes from subjective experience, without any of the traditional evidence of disease, enters the public arena, the consequences in terms of recovery are dire. The outcome of many chronic pain syndromes is determined not by the nature of the injury, but by the social and political context in which it occurred. For example, the outcome for acute back pain is influenced by the presence of litigation (Rohling, Binder, & Langhinrichsen-Rohling, 1995). The Australian epidemic of regional pain syndromes (the so-called repetitive strain injury or RSI) was related to social pressures such as an adversarial legal system, ill-informed and unsympathetic employers and doctors, "sensationalist media attention and scaremongering; misguided but vocal self help groups; faulty belief about the relation between pain and injury; and socio-economic pressures in a country heading towards recession" (Reilly, 1993). With the possible exception of socioeconomic pressures, all of these problems can be clearly identified in the context of CFS. The moving personal accounts of RSI sufferers show how such macro pressures can be translated into an individual experience with malign effects (Reid et al., 1991).

The cognitive-behavioral model outlined in this chapter has many theoretical and practical advantages—not the least being that it leads to a plan of treatment, as opposed to the therapeutic nihilism that can result from other illness models. However, it is not without hazards. One sufferer touched on these hazards in a letter to a Sunday newspaper (Merrigan, 1991): "Why do some doctors still insist on telling us that the illness is caused by depression rather than depression being caused by the illness?," and continued that sufferers "do not need to be told that they are somehow the cause of their own condition: this just places an extra burden on them." Many CFS sufferers and their doctors might misinterpret the explanations advanced in this paper as implying that sufferers are responsible for their illness. Any such imputation would indeed contribute to psychological distress. The models outlined above have no connection with simulated or malingered illness. In the context of fibromyalgia, Yunus (1988) has pointed out that "operant conditioning is not the same as malingering, and any hint that the patient is consciously avoiding duties should be avoided"—because it is not true.

Contrary to some ill-formed medical opinions, CFS patients are not responsible for their illness and do not wish to be ill, but frequently feel powerless to effect recovery. Treatment aims to combat this feeling of helplessness in the face of a mysterious assailant, to restore a sense of responsibility for recovery without engendering any stigma of guilt for being ill, and to suggest strategies for how this recovery might take place. Carrying out this treatment in practice is the subject of Chapter 10.

REFERENCES

Abbey, S. Somatization, illness attribution and the sociocultural psychiatry of chronic fatigue syndrome. In Kleinman, A, Straus, S, eds., *Chronic fatigue syndrome,* Ciba Foundation Symposium 173. Chichester: John Wiley & Sons, 1993; 238–261.

Abbey, S, Garfinkel, P. Neurasthenia and chronic fatigue syndrome: The role of culture in the making of a diagnosis. *Am J Psychiatry* 1991; 148:1638–1646.

Abramson, L, Seligman, M, Teasdale, J. Learned helplessness in humans: A critique and reformulation. *Abnormal Psychol* 1978; 87:49–74.

Ames, M. Learning to live with incurable virus. *Chicago Tribune* 1985; June 9.

Anon. Nerves and nervousness. *The Spectator* 1894; 72:11–12.

Anon. Fatigue blamed on virus: Malingering disease proved genuine. *The Times* 1988; Jan 2.

Anon. The ME generation. *Sunday Telegraph Magazine,* 1989; Jan 22.

Anon. Mystery disease without a cure. *Daily Mail* 1990; Feb 8.

Anon. ME myths. *Sheffield Telegraph* 1990; Aug 7.

Anon. Justice for the neglected and maligned sufferers of ME. *Guardian* 1990; Aug 7.

Antoni, M, Brickman, A, Imia-Fins, A. Cognitive appraisals and coping strategies predict chronic fatigue syndrome disturbances (abstract). In *Proceedings of the International CFS/ME Research Conference.* Albany, New York, Oct 3/4, 1992.

Antoni, M, Brickman, A, Lutgendorf, S, Klimas, N, Imia-Fins, A, Ironson, G, Quillian, R, Miguez, M, van Riel, F, Morgan, R, Patarca, R, Fletcher, M. Psychosocial correlates of illness burden in chronic fatigue syndrome. *Clin Infect Dis* 1994; 18(Suppl 1):S73–S78.

Arnold, D, Bore, P, Radda, G, Styles, P, Taylor, D. Excessive intracellular acidosis of skeletal muscle on exercise in a patient with a post-viral exhaustion/fatigue syndrome. *Lancet* 1984; i:1367–1369.

Asher, R. The dangers of going to bed. *Br Med J* 1947; 4:976–968.

Astrom, A, Friman, G, Pilstrom, L. Effects of viral and mycoplasma infections on ultrastructure and enzyme activities in human skeletal muscle. *Acta Pathologica Microbiologica Scandinavica* 1976; (A)84:113–122.

Bandura, A. Self-efficacy: Toward a unifying theory of behavioral change. *Psychological Rev* 1977; 84:192–215.

Baszanger, I. Deciphering chronic pain. *Sociology of Health and Illness* 1992; 14:181–215.

Bearn, J, Wessely, S. Neurobiological aspects of the chronic fatigue syndrome. *Eur J Clin Investigation* 1994; 24:79–90.

Beevor, C. *Diseases of the nervous system: A handbook for students and practitioners.* London: H K Lewis, 1898.

Behan, P, Behan, W. The postviral fatigue syndrome. *CRC Critical Reviews in Neurobiology* 1988; 42:157–178.

Behan, W, More, I, Behan, P. Mitochondrial abnormalities in the postviral fatigue syndrome. *Acta Neuropathologica* 1991; 83:61–65.

Benjamin, J, Hoyt, R. Disability following post-vaccinal (yellow fever) hepatitis. A study of 200 patients manifesting delayed convalescence. *JAMA* 1945; 128:319–324.

Bennett, R, Clark, S, Campbell, S, Burckhardt, C. Low levels of somatomedin C in patients with the fibromyalgia syndrome. *Arthritis Rheum* 1992; 35:1113–1116.

Blakely, A, Howard, R, Sosich, R, Murdoch, J, Menkes, D, Spears, G. Psychological symptoms, personality and ways of coping in chronic fatigue syndrome. *Psychol Med* 1991; 21:347–362.

Blocq, P. Neurasthenia. *Brain* 1894; 14:306–334.

Booth, F. Physiologic and biochemical effects of immobilization on muscle. *Clinical Orthopaedics* 1987; 10:15–20.

Bragg, P. Kilroy was here. *Interaction 3* 1989; 503.

Brodsky, C. Depression and chronic fatigue in the workplace. *Primary Care* 1991; 18:381–396.

Bryan, J, Melville, J. The ME generation. *Observer Magazine,* 1989, Jan 22.

Buchwald, D, Garrity, D, Pascualy, R, Kith, P, Ashley, R, Wner, M, Kidd, P, Katon, W, Russo, J. Chronic fatigue syndrome. *Toxicol Ind Health* 1992; 8:157–173.

Butler, S, Chalder, T, Ron, M, Wessely, S. Cognitive behavior therapy in the chronic fatigue syndrome. *J Neurol Neurosurg Psychiatry* 1991; 54:153–158.

Cathebras, P, Robbins, J, Kirmayer, L, Hayton, B. Fatigue in primary care: Prevalence, psychiatric comorbidity, illness behavior and outcome. *J Gen Int Med* 1992; 7:276–286.

Charatan, F. Chronic fatigue in the US. *Br Med J* 1990; 301:1236.

Cheney, P. It's a dirty little war: proponents of a "psychoneurotic" cause of CIDS try again. *Christopher Street* 1989; 1:32–33.

Cherreson, A. Am I sick or just tired? *New Woman* Aug 1991.

Clark, A. Some observations concerning what is called neurasthenia. *Lancet* 1886; i:1–2.

Coats, A, Adamopoulos, S, Meyer, T, Conway, J, Sleight, P. Effects of physical training in chronic heart failure. *Lancet* 1990; 335:63–66.

Colby, J. *Guidelines for schools.* ME Support Centre, Harold Wood Hospital, 1992.

Collee, J. A Doctor writes. *Observer* 1991; Aug 25.

Crook, W. *Chronic fatigue syndrome and the yeast connection.* Jackson, TN: Professional Books, 1992.

Conant, S. Living with chronic fatigue. *Taylor* 1990.

Dainty, E. M.E. and I. *Nursing Standard* 1988; 84:49–50.

Dalrymple, T. Myalgic encephalomyelitis—my eye. *Medical Monitor* 1992; Feb 14.

David, A, McDonald, E, Mann, A, Pelosi, A, Stephens, D, Ledger, D, Rathbone, R. Tired, weak or in need of rest: Fatigue among general practice attenders. *Br Med J* 1990; 301:1199–1202.

David, A, Wessely, S, Pelosi, A. Post-viral fatigue: Time for a new approach. *Br Med J* 1988; 296:696–699.

Dawes, B, Downing, D. *Why M.E.? A guide to combatting post-viral illness.* London: Grafton, 1989.

DeLuca, J, Johnson, S, Natelson, B. Information processing efficiency in chronic fatigue syndrome and multiple sclerosis. *Arch Neurology* 1993; 50:301–304.

Denman, A. The chronic fatigue syndrome: A return to common sense. *Postgrad Med J* 1990; 66:499–501.

Dowsett, E, Welsby, P. Conversation piece. *Postgrad Med J* 1992; 68:63–65.

Editorial. Aching muscles after exercise. *Lancet* 1987; 2:1123–1125.

Edwards, R, Gibson, H, Clague, J, Halliwell, T. Muscle histopathology and physiology in chronic fatigue syndrome. In Kleinman, A, Straus, S, eds., *Chronic fatigue syndrome,* Ciba Foundation Symposium 173. Chichester: John Wiley & Sons, 1993; 102–131.

Eichner, E. Chronic fatigue syndrome: How vulnerable are athletes? *Physician and Sports Med* 1989; 16:157–160.

Eland, A. ME—not a middle class disease. *Social Work Today* 1988; Mar 24.

Fegan, K, Behan, P, Bell, E. Myalgic encephalomyelitis—report of an epidemic. *J Roy Coll Gen Pract* 1983; 33:335–337.

Feiden, K. *Hope and help for chronic fatigue syndrome.* New York: Prentice-Hall, 1990.

Finlay, S. Don't listen if your GP says it's "just nerves." *Scotsman* 1986; Aug 18.

Flett, K. Why ME? *Arena* 1990; Mar.

Folgering, H, Snik, A. Hyperventilation syndrome and muscle fatigue. *J Psychosom Res* 1988; 32:165–171.

Frank, A. Low back pain. *Br Med J* 1993; 306:901–909.

Frank, J. Emotional reactions of American soldiers to an unfamiliar disease. *Am J Psychiatry* 1946; 102:631–640.

Franklin, M, Sullivan, J. *The new mystery fatigue epidemic. M.E. What is it? Have you got it? How to get better.* London: Century, 1989.

Friman, G, Schiller, H, Schwartz, M. Disturbed neuromuscular transmission in viral infections. *Scand J Infect Dis* 1977; 9:99–103.

Friman, G, Wright, J, Ilback, N, Beisel, W, White, J, Sharp, D, Stephen, E, Daniels, W, Vogel, J. Does fever or myalgia indicate reduced physical performance capacity in viral infections? *Acta Medica Scandinavica* 1985; 217:353–361.

Gardner, K. *Interaction* 1988; 1:Winter.

Gibson, J, Halliday, D, Morrison, W, Stoward, P, Hornsby, G, Watt, P, Murdoch, G, Rennie, M. Decrease in human quadriceps muscle protein turnover consequent upon leg immobilization. *Clin Sci* 1987; 72:503–509.

Gibson, H, Carroll, N, Clague, J, Edwards, R. Exercise performance and fatiguability in patients with chronic fatigue syndrome. *J Neurol Neurosurg Psychiatry,* 1993; 156:993–995.

Gold, D, Bowden, R, Sixbey, J, Riggs, R, Katon, W, Ashley, R, Obrigewitch, R, Corey, L. Chronic fatigue: A prospective clinical and virologic study. *JAMA* 1990; 264:48–53.

Gow, J, Behan, W, Clements, G, Woodall, C, Riding, M, Behan, P. Enteroviral RNA sequences detected by polymerase chain reaction in muscle of patients with postviral fatigue syndrome. *Br Med J* 1991; 302:692–696.

Greenberg, D. Neurasthenia in the 1980s: Chronic mononucleosis, chronic fatigue syndrome and anxiety and depressive disorders. *Psychosomatics* 1990; 31:129–137.

Harding, T, De Arango, M, Baltazar, J, Climent, C, Abrahim, H, Ladrido-Ignacio, L, Srivinasa-Murthy, R, Wig, N. Mental disorders in primary health care: A study of their frequency and diagnosis in four developing countries. *Psychol Med* 1980; 10:231–241.

Hellinger, W, Smith, T, Van Scoy, R, Spitzer, P, Forgacs, P, Edson, R. Chronic fatigue syndrome and the diagnostic utility of Epstein–Barr virus early antigen. *JAMA* 1988; 260:971–973.

Helman, C. Feed a cold and starve a fever. *Cult Med Psychiatry* 1978; 7:107–137.

Hickie, I, Lloyd, A, Wakefield, D, Parker, G. The psychiatric status of patients with chronic fatigue syndrome. *Br J Psychiatry* 1990; 156:534–540.

Hinds, G, McCluskey, D. A retrospective study of the chronic fatigue syndrome. *Proc Roy Coll Physicians Edin* 1993; 23:10–14.

Hodgkinson, L., ME: The mystery disease. *Women's Journal* 1988; Nov.

Hodgkinson, N. Tired and alone, my mind reduced to porridge. *Sunday Times* 1987; Feb 21.

Hodgkinson, N. Virus research doctors prove shirkers really are sick. *Sunday Times* 1987; Jan 25.

Hoehn-Saric, R, McLeod, D. Locus of control in chronic anxiety disorders. *Acta Psychiatrica Scandinavic* 1985; 72:529–535.

Holford, N. ME. *Report on the Assistant Masters and Mistresses Association* 1989; Sept:12–13.

Hood, J. 10 minute rule bill on myaglic encephalomyelitis. *Hansard* 1988; Feb 23.

Ho-Yen, D. Patient management of the post-viral fatigue syndrome. *Br J Gen Pract* 1990; 40:37–39.

Ho-Yen, D. Post-viral fatigue does exist. *GP Magazine*. Sept 18 1987.

Hurry, J. The vicious circles of neurasthenia. *Br Med J* 1914; i:1404–1406.

Hurry, J. The vicious circles of neurasthenia and their treatment. London: Churchill, 1915.

Hyde, B, Bergmann, S. Akureyi disease (myalgic encephalomyelitis), forty years later. *Lancet* 1988; ii:1191–1192.

Imboden, J, Canter, A, Cluff, L. Brucellosis III. Psychologic aspects of delayed convalescence. *Arch Int Med* 1959; 103:406–414.

Jaffe, D, Terry, R, Spiro, A. Disuse atrophy of skeletal muscle. *Neurol Sci* 1978; 35:189–200.

Jamal, G, Hansen, S. Post-viral fatigue syndrome: Evidence for underlying organic disturbance in the muscle fibre. *Eur Neurology* 1989; 29:273–276.

Jelliffe, S. Dispensary work in nervous diseases. *J Nerv Ment Diseases* 1905; 32:449–453.

Johnson, J. Journey into fear. *Rolling Stone* 1987.

Jones, M, Mellersh, V. A comparison of the exercise response in anxiety states and normal controls. *Psychosom Med* 1946; 8:180–187.

Jones, M, Scarisbrick, R. Effect of exercise on soldiers with neurocirculatory asthenia. *Psychosom Med* 1946; 8:188–192.

Katon, W, Buchwald, D, Simon, G, Russo, J, Mease, P. Psychiatric illness in patients with chronic fatigue and rheumatoid arthritis. *J Gen Int Med* 1991; 6:277–285.

Katon, W, Russo, J. Chronic fatigue syndrome criteria: A critique of the requirement for multiple physical complaints. *Arch Intern Med* 1992; 152:1604–1609.

Katz, B, Andiman, W. Chronic fatigue syndrome. *J Pediatrics* 1988; 113:944–947.

Kent-Braun, J, Sharma, K, Chein, C, Weiner, M, Miller, R. Chronic fatigue syndrome: Pathophysiologic basis for muscular fatigue. *Neurology* 1993; 43:125–131.

Klug, G, McAuley, E, Clark, S. Factors influencing the development and maintenance of aerobic fitness; lessons applicable to the fibrositis syndrome. *J Rheumatol* 1989; (Suppl 19)16,S30–S39.

Kottke, F. The effect of limitation of activity upon the human body. *JAMA* 1966; 196:275–281.

Kroenke, K, Wood, D, Mangelsdorff, D, Meier, N, Powell, J. Chronic fatigue in primary care: Prevalence, patient characteristics and outcome. *JAMA* 1988; 260:929–934.

Lechky, O. Life insurance MDs sceptical when chronic fatigue syndrome diagnosed. *Can Med Assoc J* 1990; 143:413–415.

Lethem, J, Salde, P, Troup, J, Bentley, G. Outline of a fear-avoidance model of exaggerated pain perception—1. *Beh Res Ther* 1983; 21:401–408.

Lindstrom, I, Ohlund, C, Eek, C, Wallin, L, Peterson, L, Nachemson, A. Mobility, strength and fitness after a graded activity program for patients with subacute low back pain. A randomised prospective clinical study with a behavioral therapy approach. *Spine* 1992; 17:641–649.

Lloyd, A, Gandevia, S, Hales, J. Muscle performance, voluntary activation, twitch properties and perceived effort in normal subjects and patients with the chronic fatigue syndrome. *Brain* 1991; 114:85–98.

Lloyd, A, Hales, J, Gandevia, S. Muscle strength, endurance and recovery in the postinfection fatigue syndrome. *J Neurol Neurosurg Psychiatry* 1988; 51:1316–1322.

MacIntyre, A. ME: Post-viral fatigue syndrome: How to live with it. London: Unwin, 1989.

Mackenzie, J. Soldier's heart. *Br Med J* 1916; i:117–120.

Mantysaari, M, Antila, K, Peltonen, T. Blood pressure reactivity in patients with neurocirculatory asthenia. *Am J Hypertension* 1988; 1:132–139.

Manu, P, Matthews, D, Lane, T. Panic disorder among patients with chronic fatigue. *South Med J* 1991; 84:451–456.

Maros, K. Portrait of a plague. *Med J Australia* 1991; 155:132.

McCain, G, Bell, D, Mai, F, Holliday, P. A controlled study of the effects of a supervised cardiovascular fitness training program on the manifestations of primary fibromyalgia. *Arthritis Rheum* 1988; 31:1135–1141.

Merrigan, K. That old psychosomatic blues again. *Observer* 1991; Sept 8.

Merskey, H. Symptoms that depress the doctor: Too much pain. *Br J Hosp Med* 1984; 31:63–66.

Millenson, J. ME: An alternative view. *Interaction* 1992; 9:Spring.

Milner-Brown, H, Miller, R. Muscle strengthening through high-resistance weight training in patients with neuromuscular disorders. *Arch Phys Med Rehabil* 1988; 69:14–19.

Mitchell, J. Diagnosis and treatment of neurasthenia. *Johns Hopkins Hospital Bulletin* 1908; 19:41–43.

Monckton, C. The ME generation. *Evening Standard* 1988; July 25.

Montague, T, Marrie, T, Bewick, D, Spencer, A, Kornreich, F, Horacek, B. Cardiac effects of common viral illnesses. *Chest* 1988; 94:919–925.

Newham, D. The consequences of eccentric contractions and their relationship to delayed onset muscle pain. *Europ J App Physiology* 1988; 57:353–359.

Nooregaard, J, Bulow, P, Prescott, E, Jacobsen, S, Danneskiold-Samsoe, B. A four year follow-up study in fibromyalgia. Relationship to chronic fatigue syndrome. *Scand J Rheumatol* 1993; 22:35–38.

Paul, O. Da Costa's syndrome or neurocirculatory asthenia. *Br Heart J* 1987; 58:306–315.

Pawlikowska, T, Chandler, T, Hirsch, S, Wallace, P, Wright, D, Wessely, S. A population based study of fatigue and psychological distress. *Br Med J* 1994; 308:743–746.

Peel, M. Rehabilitation in postviral syndrome. *J Soc Occup Med* 1988; 38:44–45.

Pershing, H. The treatment of neurasthenia. *Med News* 1904; 84:637–640.

Philips, H. Avoidance behavior and its role in sustaining chronic pain. *Behav Res Therapy* 1987; 25:273–279.

Powell, R, Dolan, R, Wessely, S. Attributions and self esteem in depression and the chronic fatigue syndrome. *J Psychosom Res* 1990; 34:665–673.

Ramsay, M. *Introduction to Shepherd, C. Living with ME; A self help guide*. London: Heinemann, 1989.

Rankin, G. Neurasthenia: The wear and tear of life. *Br Med J* 1903; i:1017–1020.

Reeves, W, Pellett, P, Gary, H. The chronic fatigue syndrome controversy. *Ann Int Med* 1992; 117:343.

Reid, J, Ewan, C, Lowy, E. Pilgrimage of pain: The illness experiences of women with repetition strain injury and the search for credibility. *Soc Sci Med* 1991; 32:601–612.

Reilly, P. Fibromyalgia in the workplace: A "management" problem. *Ann Rheum Dis* 1993; 52:249–251.

Reilly, P, Littlejohn, G. Fibrositis/fibromyalgia syndrome; the key to the puzzle of chronic pain. *Med J Australia* 1990; 152:226–228.

Riley, M, O'Brien, C, McCluskey, D, Bell, N, Nicholls, D. Aerobic work capacity in patients with chronic fatigue syndrome. *Br Med J* 1990; 301:953–956.

Robbins, J, Kirmayer, L, Kapusta, M. Illness worry and disability in fibromyalgia. *Int J Psychiatry Med* 1990; 20:49–64.

Roeber, J. Industry of anxiety. *Vogue* 1989; Aug 178–179.

Rohling, M, Binder, L, Langhinrichsen-Rohling, J. Money matters: A meta-analytic review of the association between financial compensation and the experience and treatment of chronic pain. *Health Psychology* 1995; 14:537–547.

Rutherford, O, White, P. Human quadriceps strength and fatigability in patients with post-viral fatigue. *J Neurol Neurosurg Psychiatry* 1991; 54:961–964.

Seagrove, J. The ME generation. *Guardian* 1989; May 19.

Sensky, T. Patients' reactions to illness. *Br Med J* 1990; 300:622–623.

Sharpe, M, Hawton, K, Seagroatt, V, Pasvol, G. Follow up of patients with fatigue presenting to an infectious diseases clinic. *Br Med J* 1992; 305:347–352.

Shepherd, C. Fatigue that's viral, not hysterical. *MIMS Magazine* 1987; October 15.

Shepherd, C. Living with ME: A self-help guide. London: Heinemann, 1989.

Shorter, E. *From paralysis to fatigue: A history of psychosomatic illness in the modern era.* New York: Macmillan, 1992.

Smith, D. Myalgic encephalomyelitis. In *1989 Members Reference Book*. London: Royal College of General Practitioners: Sabre Crown Publishing, 1989; 247–250.

Stacey, S. Tired and tested. *Harpers & Queen* 1990; Oct.

Steincamp, J. *Overload: Beating M.E.* London: Fontana, 1989.

Stewart, D. The changing face of somatisation. *Psychosomatics* 1990a; 31:153–158.

Stewart, D. Emotional disorders misdiagnosed as physical illness: Environmental hypersensitivity, candiadisis hypersensitivity and chronic fatigue syndrome. *Int J Mental Health* 1990b; 19:56–68.

Stokes, M, Cooper, R, Edwards, R. Normal strength and fatigability in patients with effort syndrome. *Br Med J* 1988; 297:1014–1018.

Stone, R. Presentation, investigation and diagnosis of PVFS (ME) in general practice. In Jenkins, R, Mowbray, J, eds., *Post-viral fatigue syndrome*. Chichester: John Wiley & Sons, 1991; 221–226.

Undated fact sheet; ME Action Campaign 1989.

Urquhart, A. Austrian retrospect: Review of the writings of Professor Benedikt of Vienna. *J Mental Sci* 1889; 34:276–281.

Vignos, P. Physical models of rehabilitation in neuromuscular disease. *Muscle Nerve* 1981; 6:323–338.

Wagenmakers, A, Coakley, J, Edwards, R. Metabolic consequences of reduced habitual activities in patients with muscle pain and disease. *Ergonomics* 1988; 31:1519–1527.

Ware, N. Society, mind and body in chronic fatigue syndrome: an anthropological view. In Kleinman, A, Straus, S, eds., *Chronic fatigue syndrome,* Ciba Foundation Symposium 173. Chichester: John Wiley & Sons, 1993; 62–82.

Ware, N, Kleinman, A. Culture and somatic experience: The social course of illness in neurasthenia and chronic fatigue syndrome. *Psychosom Med* 1992; 54:546–560.

Watts, F. Attributional aspects of medicine. In Antaki, C, Brewin, C, eds., *Attributions and psychological change*. London: Academic Press, 1982; 135–155.

Webb, H, Parsons, L. Post viral fatigue syndrome, presentation and management in the neurology clinic. In Jenkins, R, Mowbray, J, eds., *The postviral fatigue syndrome (M.E.)*. Chichester: John Wiley & Sons, 1992.

Wessely, S. Myalgic encephalomyelitis—a warning. *J Roy Soc Med* 1989; 82:215–217.

Wessely, S. Old wine in new bottles: Neurasthenia and "ME." *Psychol Med* 1990; 20:35–53.

Wessely, S. The history of the postviral fatigue syndrome. *Br Med Bulletin* 1991; 47:919–941.

Wessely, S, Butler, S, Chalder, S, David, A. The cognitive behavioral management of the post-viral fatigue syndrome. In Jenkins, R, Mowbray, J, eds. *The postviral fatigue syndrome (M.E.)*. Chichester: John Wiley & Sons, 1991; 305–334.

Wessely, S, David, A, Butler, S, Chalder, T. The management of the chronic "postviral" fatigue syndrome. *J Roy Coll Gen Pract* 1989; 39:26–29.

Wessely, S, Powell, R. Fatigue syndromes: A comparison of chronic "postviral" fatigue with neuromuscular and affective disorders. *J Neurol Neurosurg Psychiatry* 1989; 42:940–948.

Wheeler, E, White, P, Reed, E, Cohen, M. Neurocirculatory asthenia (anxiety neurosis, effort syndrome, neurasthenia). *JAMA* 1950; 142:878–889.

White, P. Fatigue syndrome: Neurasthenia revived. *Br Med J* 1989; 298:1199–1200.

White, P, Thomas, J, Amess, J, Grover, S, Kangro, H, Clare, A. The existence of a fatigue syndrome after glandular fever. *Psychol Med* 1995; 25:907–916.

Willsher, K. I beat the disease of the 90s. *Daily Express* 1990; April 11.

Wilson, D, Widmer, R, Cadoret, R, Judiesch, K. Somatic symptoms: A major feature of depression in a family practice. *J Affect Dis* 1983; 5:199–207.

Wong, R, Lopaschuk, G, Zhu, G, Walker, D, Catellier, D, Burton, D, Teo, K, Collins-Nakai, R, Montague, T. Skeletal muscle metabolism in the chronic fatigue syndrome: In vivo assessment by 31P nuclear magnetic resonance spectroscopy. *Chest* 1992; 102:1716–1722.

Wood, G, Bentall, R, Gopfert, M, Edwards, R. A comparative psychiatric assessment of patients with chronic fatigue syndrome and muscle disease. *Psychol Med* 1991; 21:619–628.

Yunus, M. Diagnosis, etiology and management of fibromyalgia syndrome: An update. *Comprehensive Therapy* 1988; 14:8–20.

Zuber, J, Wilgosh, L. Prolonged immobilization of the body: Changes in performance and the electroencephalogram. *Science* 1963; 140:306–308.

10

Cognitive-Behavioral Therapy for Patients with Chronic Fatigue Syndrome: How?

Michael C. Sharpe, M.A., M.R.C.P., M.R.C.Psych.

*I*n Chapter 9, Wessely made the case for the application of cognitive-behavioral therapy (CBT) to the treatment of patients with chronic fatigue syndrome (CFS). In this chapter, I shall explain how CBT can be applied to the problem of CFS. The first step will be to describe the cognitive-behavioral approach and associated model of illness, and then to propose a cognitive-behavioral theory of CFS. The next step will be to outline the actual practice of therapy as employed in a recent treatment trial, and the final step will be to review the evidence for the efficacy of CBT in the treatment of CFS.

WHAT IS COGNITIVE-BEHAVIORAL THERAPY?

Description

CBT is an approach to the understanding and management of patients' problems. CBT is based on a model of human functioning that assumes: (1) cognitions (the way a person interprets events) are major determinants of behavior, emotion, and physiological state, and (2) these cognitions may be inaccurate and consequently lead to excessive emotional reactions and a failure to cope effectively. CBT helps patients to improve the accuracy of their appraisal of problems and thereby to reduce distress and improve coping behavior. The treatment interventions employed to do this include both cognitive and behavioral techniques. It is important to note that CBT is not a single specific treatment; rather, it is a category of therapies unified by the use of a cognitive-behavioral approach to guide treatment. For the interested reader, several useful accounts of the subject are available—for example, Hawton et al. (1989), Beck et al. (1979), and Persons (1989).

The Cognitive-Behavioral Model of Illness

According to the cognitive-behavioral model of illness, a patient's misinterpretation of symptoms may play an important role in the perpetuation of those symptoms. Perpetuation can occur in several ways: (1) "catastrophic" interpretations may lead to excessive emotional reactions, (2) the belief that the symptoms are beyond the person's control may lead to poor coping responses on behalf of the patient, and (3) both excessive emotional reactions and maladaptive coping may accentuate the physiological abnormalities giving rise to the symptoms. Thus, negative appraisal of the symptoms of cancer may lead to poor emotional adjustment and maladaptive coping behavior (Moorey & Greer, 1989). Catastrophic misinterpretation of the symptoms of anxiety may exacerbate physiological changes and give rise to panic (Clark, 1986).

The cognitive-behavioral model of illness differs from the conventional disease model in that clinically observable phenomena such as patients' beliefs and coping behavior are considered not only as manifestations of an underlying organic cause, but also as potentially important etiological factors in their own right. The cognitive-behavioral model also differs from an extreme psychological perspective such as that proposed for hysteria, which conceives of the illness as an exclusively mental phenomenon (Sharpe & Bass, 1992). These alternative conceptualizations of illness are schematically illustrated in Figure 10.1.

Cognitive-Behavioral Therapy

The practice of CBT is logically derived from the model. The therapy seeks to help the patient to achieve a more accurate understanding of the illness and, thereby, to cope more effectively. The therapist and patient work together in a collaborative fashion in order to clarify the patient's current understanding of their illness, to check this understanding against the best available evidence, and, where necessary, to replace the understanding with a more accurate appraisal of the situation. New ways of coping based on this improved understanding of the illness are then implemented and evaluated.

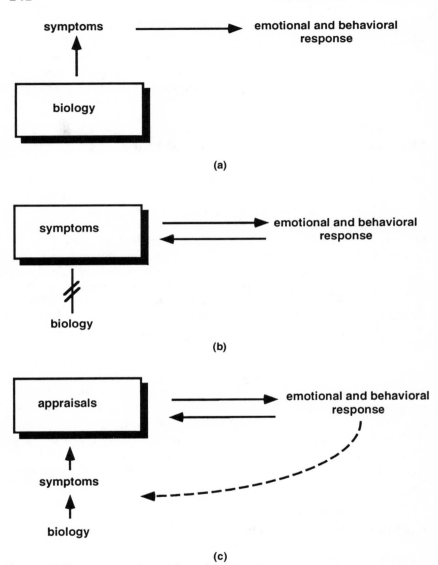

FIGURE 10.1. Illness conceptualizations: (a) simple disease model, (b) simple psychological model, and (c) cognitive behavioral model.

TABLE 10.1. Stages of a Course of Cognitive-Behavioral Therapy and the Structure of a Single Session

Stages of Therapy	Sessions
1. Assessment, formulation, and engagement	1 to 3
2. Reviewing thoughts and behavior	4 to 10
3. Reviewing unhelpful attitudes	8 to 12
4. Problem solving practical difficulties	10 to 14
5. Review and planning for the future	12 to 16

Structure of a Single Session
1. Review previous session and homework.
2. Review formulation of problem.
3. Reevaluate a specific thought, belief, or behavior.
4. Plan homework.

Through this evaluation of understanding, the patient is helped to overcome problems and attain desired goals. The patient is also encouraged to apply the approach that has been learned to other difficulties that are encountered.

Most courses of CBT are of relatively brief duration and consist of 10 to 20 one-hour treatment sessions. In addition, patients have homework assignments. The course of both the therapy and the individual session is structured. An outline of each is shown in Table 10.1.

Applications

The early applications of CBT focused on the treatment of patients attending psychological and psychiatric outpatient services. CBT has subsequently become a well-established treatment for depression, anxiety, phobias, panic disorder, obsessive–compulsive neurosis, and eating disorders (Beck, 1991). More recently, the range of application has widened to include patients attending general medical services (Emmelkamp & Van Oppen, 1993). Specific applications in this setting include the treatment of emotional disorders in patients with organic diseases such as cancer (Moorey & Greer, 1989), and the treatment of somatic complaints unexplained by organic disease (Sharpe et al., 1992). This latter application includes patients with medically unexplained pain syndromes (Klimes et al., 1990) and patients with poorly understood conditions such as irritable bowel syndrome (Greene & Blanchard, 1994).

WHAT IS CHRONIC FATIGUE SYNDROME?

Description

The term chronic fatigue syndrome is used to describe the clinical problem of the patient who presents with chronic disabling fatigue or exhaustion that is unexplained by organic disease. The most recent and widely agreed-on criteria are those published by the CDC (Fukuda et al., 1994; see also Chapter 1, this volume).

> *Case Vignette.* Ms. P was a 35-year-old teacher seen in the clinic. She presented to her physician with a history of 18 months' exhaustion. She was no longer able to work and had trouble walking more than half a mile. Other symptoms included poor concentration, interrupted sleep, headache, a sore throat, and tender neck glands. Her symptoms were made worse by activity. Physical examination was unremarkable. Basic laboratory investigations were all normal. Psychiatric assessment revealed a number of symptoms several of which suggested depression, but she did not meet diagnostic criteria for depressive disorder. A diagnosis of CFS was made.

Etiology and Treatment Options

A number of disease explanations have been suggested to explain the symptoms of CFS. These explanations include persistent virus infection, immune disturbance, metabolic abnormalities, and depression (Thomas, 1993; see also Chapters 3 and 4, this volume). Although there is considerable evidence supporting an etiological role for depressive disorder in CFS (Kendell, 1991) none of these disease theories has been generally accepted, and the cause of the syndrome remains controversial. Similarly, no specific biological treatment has been shown to be effective (Wilson et al., 1994; see Chapters 11 and 12, in volume).

A COGNITIVE-BEHAVIORAL MODEL OF CFS

The cognitive-behavioral approach to CFS has the potential to offer a novel basis for understanding an otherwise mysterious condition, as well as a logical approach to treatment (Surawy et al., 1995).

The Components of the Model

To construct a cognitive-behavioral model of CFS, we must consider not only the possible biological processes underlying fatigue, but also other

TABLE 10.2. Clinical Characteristics of Chronic Fatigue Syndrome

Cognitions	"I have a disease." "I can't do anything." "Symptoms indicate harm." "I'm not the sort of person who gets depressed."
Behavior	Avoidance of activity Oscillation in activity
Mood	Frustration Depression Anxiety
Physiology	Concomitants of emotion Physiological deconditioning Other factors
Environment	Relationship/occupational problems Unhelpful information and advice about the illness

aspects of the patient's clinical presentation, including illness beliefs, coping behaviors, emotional state, and social context. These characteristics of patients with CFS are listed in Table 10.2.

Case Vignette (continued). A more detailed assessment of Ms. P revealed that she believed her symptoms were caused by a persistent virus infection, and that activity worsened the illness. She had consequently coped by spending long periods in bed and by avoiding both physical and social activity as much as possible. She believed that there was nothing that she could do to influence the course of the illness, was preoccupied with the illness, and feared ending up in a wheelchair. She described being frustrated with the illness, and at times was tearful. Her doctor said that there was no treatment. Her partner encouraged her to rest and had bought her books about the illness. Prior to becoming ill, she had been under considerable work pressure, and had very high standards. She was now thinking of retiring on medical grounds. The following components of her presentation may be distinguished.

Cognitions

These may be divided into beliefs about the nature of the illness, the meaning attached to symptoms, and expressions of more general attitudes about achievement and social acceptability. Almost all patients with CFS attending hospital clinics believe that they are suffering from an organic disease (Powell et al., 1990; Sharpe et al., 1992). They tend to interpret exacerbations of symptoms occurring with activity either as a warning of impending "relapse," or as evidence of damage to the body (Petrie et al., 1995). In addition, their self-concept is commonly that of a strong, coping person. High

standards for performance and responsibility, and a tendency not to express
negative emotion are typical (Surawy et al., 1995).

Behavior

Most patients with CFS cope with the illness by avoiding activity or by actively pursuing rest (Sharpe et al., 1992). However, their strong desire to get
on with life and to do things often leads to oscillations between rest and
activity.

Emotion

Studies have demonstrated a high prevalence of emotional distress in patients
with CFS (Kendell, 1991). Although often described as depression, patients
commonly complain of frustration—an understandable reaction to their perception that their pursuit of activities is hindered by a disease process outside
their control. Emotional distress and frustration are associated with physiological changes (Sharpe & Bass, 1992; Surawy et al., 1995).

Physiology

The pathophysiology of CFS is poorly understood. Although it is possible
that there is an undiscovered, fixed disease process—perhaps a persistent
virus, or damage to the immune system—such a process has not been convincingly demonstrated. Research shows evidence for decreased physical
fitness (Riley et al., 1990), sleep disturbance (Morriss et al., 1993) and, in
some patients, hyperventilation (Saisch et al., 1994). Neuroendocrine abnormalities are also possible (Bakheit et al., 1992; Demitrack, 1994). All
these processes are potentially reversible and likely to be strongly influenced
by the emotional and coping responses described above. The patient's perception of physiological changes may be amplified by the focusing of attention on symptoms regarded as threatening (Salkovskis & Clark, 1990).

Social Context

The interpersonal and social environment may be particularly important in
chronic fatigue syndrome. Readily available information in magazines and
books may shape the person's interpretation of the symptoms (MacLean &

Wessely, 1994) and friends, family members, and physicians may further reinforce the patient's belief that he or she has a fixed disease process. Furthermore, occupational difficulties, loss of employment, and medical retirement are all likely to mitigate against a return to normal activity.

Interacting Processes

The processes outlined above may interact to perpetuate the symptoms and disabilities of CFS. This interaction is shown diagrammatically in Figure 10.2. An example of an interaction between the components would be as follows. If the disturbances in physiology are interpreted as evidence of a fixed disease process, several consequences may follow. First, the patient may become anxious, distressed, and frustrated by his or her plight. Second, the patient may resort to rest and avoidance of any activity that exacerbates symptoms. Third, both of these processes are likely to cause deconditioning and chronic autonomic arousal that, in turn, will give rise to further symptoms.

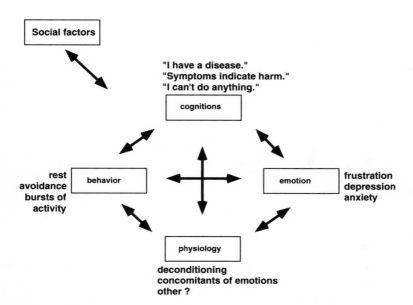

FIGURE 10.2. The cognitive-behavioral model of chronic fatigue syndrome.

The Cognitive-Behavioral Hypotheses

1. *The weak hypothesis.* This hypothesis assumes that the pathophysiology of CFS is largely irreversible, but considers that a fine-tuning of the patient's understanding and coping behavior may achieve some improvement in his or her quality of life.
2. *The strong hypothesis.* This model considers the pathophysiology of CFS to be entirely reversible and perpetuated *only* by the interaction of cognitions, behavior, and emotional processes. According to this model, CBT should not only improve the quality of the patient's life, but could be potentially curative.

The model that best describes CFS can only be determined by further research. However, whichever model turns out to be correct, the cognitive-behavioral approach offers a plausible, clinically based and potentially helpful form of treatment.

THE COGNITIVE-BEHAVIORAL TREATMENT OF CFS

This treatment will be described according to the five stages outlined in Table 10.1. Several general issues must be considered before starting (Wessely & Sharpe, 1995).

General Issues

Referral

Most patients will have presented initially to a physician. He or she has the important tasks of excluding organic disease and of preparing the patient for referral to the cognitive-behavioral therapist. The way in which the referral is made is important because it may determine whether the patient attends the initial interview (House, 1995).

Exclusion of Other Conditions

It is assumed that the patient has been adequately assessed for the presence of occult physical disease. The general assessment should include an examination of the patient's mental state, to assess for evidence of major psychiatric disorder and suicidal intent.

The Therapeutic Relationship

When using psychotherapeutic methods to treat patients with CFS, it may be particularly difficult to establish the positive therapeutic relationship essential for effective treatment. If the therapist is a psychiatrist or a psychologist, the patient is likely to be suspicious that his or her problems will be interpreted as "psychiatric," "all in the mind," or even malingered—explanations that are incompatible with the patient's self-image (Surawy et al., 1995).

This problem can usually be overcome by genuine and nonjudgmental interest in the patient's somatic symptoms and understanding of the illness. The role of the therapist is to help the patient to review his or her understanding of CFS by developing a shared sense of curiosity and by asking appropriate questions.

Stage 1. Assessment, Formulation, and Engagement

This first stage of therapy is crucial. It must provide information essential to the cognitive-behavioral formulation of the patient's problem and obtain the patient's active involvement in the process of treatment.

Assessment

The aim of the cognitive-behavioral assessment is to seek information about each of the facets of the patient's illness, as described above. The therapist should use all of the following sources to obtain the necessary information.

1. Interview of patient and informant
2. Patient-completed questionnaires
3. Patient diaries
4. Physiological measures

The patient's illness beliefs should be explored in detail and the "worst fears" should be examined. To investigate coping behavior, it is useful to obtain an account of the patient's current lifestyle. This account can then be inspected in more detail by asking the patient to go through a typical day, hour by hour. Patients are often reluctant to express emotions and may, in accordance with their attitudes about emotional expression, habitually present "a brave face" or cope with their feelings by ignoring them. Therefore, eliciting emotionally laden topics requires a trusting relationship and sensitivity. The context of the illness should also be considered, and it is important to interview and elicit beliefs about the illness from the patient's cohabitee or family. Obstacles to a return to work and the existence of financial benefits contingent on remaining ill should also be explored at an early stage.

Patient-completed questionnaires are useful supplements to the initial interview in the measurement of fatigue, disability, and emotional disorder (Fukuda et al., 1994), as well as illness beliefs (Schweitzer et al., 1994) and general attitudes such as perfectionism (Frost et al., 1994).

Although physiological changes are usually inferred from the patient's symptoms, specific provocation tests such as voluntary hyperventilation may reveal whether this process causes exacerbation of symptoms such as dizziness and paresthesia. Laboratory investigations of physiological abnormalities such as deconditioning, if available, may contribute to both the assessment and the education of the patient.

In the early stages of treatment, patients will be shown how to complete diaries. Initial diaries will record activity and may be used to provide information about the amount and patterns of activity and sleep. Once the patient understands the importance of becoming aware of the way he or she thinks about the situation, records of thoughts may be introduced.

Formulation

The next step is to construct a provisional cognitive-behavioral formulation of the illness. Although the general model as described above provides a guide, the heterogeneity of CFS makes an individualized formulation necessary. This formulation is not necessarily definitive, but may be modified or elaborated as therapy proceeds. The importance of the illness formulation is threefold:

1. It focuses attention on the factors that are perpetuating the illness as opposed to those (such as viral infection) that may have precipitated it.
2. It draws in psychological and social factors to complement a biological model of etiology.
3. It shows how the biological, psychological, and social components may interact in vicious circles.

Engagement

An important part of the collaborative approach is to share the formulation with the patient. Because the therapy requires the patient's active cooperation, it can proceed only when there is at least some willingness on the patient's behalf to consider this formulation. The way in which the formulation is introduced will depend on the degree of the patient's present willingness to consider a new interpretation of the difficulties. Patients who are mystified by their symptoms but are open to any positive explanation may be presented with the formulation in a fairly direct way. Patients who believe in a specific disease causation may need to have it presented more gradually. A patient may be asked to present his or her own explanation of the illness and then, in discussion with the therapist, to suggest modifications based on the assessment.

For patients who hold very strong beliefs about physical causation, the existing explanation and the new cognitive-behavioral formulation may be explicitly set up as competing alternatives. The therapist can explain that, at the moment, it is uncertain which explanation is best, and that the patients' disease explanation may be right. However, it would be unfortunate if they didn't consider the alternative, more optimistic view, because they would have missed an opportunity to improve their quality of life. The initial aims of therapy should be to set up predictions and to evaluate the usefulness of the cognitive-behavioral model.

An important early task is the setting of goals for therapy. A central part of reframing the patient's illness and its management is to move from a futile search for a specific cause of the disease to a pragmatic commitment to rehabilitation. The goals of this rehabilitation should be operationally defined, such as "being able to walk five miles twice a week." Setting realistic goals is also important. If someone has been severely disabled for several years, it is not realistic that he or she will be able to enjoy normal sporting activities within weeks; nor is it realistic to aim for a complete absence of symptoms. Indeed, one task of the therapy may be to reduce unrealistic expectations of health and ability.

Case Vignette (continued). After completing the assessment, a provisional cognitive-behavioral formulation was presented to Ms. P as an alternative to her simple disease model. [This formulation is illustrated in Figure 10.3.] She was skeptical of its validity but, because none of the previous physicians she had seen had been able to identify the cause or to offer treatment, she was interested in the idea of rehabilitation. She agreed to try CBT for 3 months. By that time, she wanted to be able to walk a mile, to go out socially twice each week, and to begin an art class.

Stage 2. Behavioral and Cognitive Interventions

This stage is concerned with teaching the patient to be aware of habitual ways of thinking about and responding to the illness, how to reevaluate these responses, and how to implement more accurate and helpful alternatives.

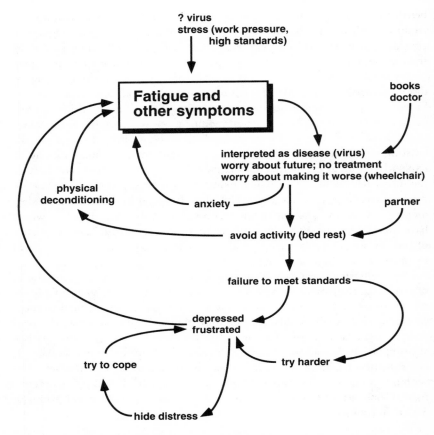

FIGURE 10.3. Provisional individual formulation for Ms. P.

Planning Therapy and Patients' Suitability

At this point, the clinician should consider how much treatment the patient will need. The formulation is a revelation for some patients. They may immediately start making suggestions about how they could change their behavior and lifestyle so as to unlock themselves from the vicious circles they now perceive. These patients may only need encouragement and follow-up to make sure that they remain on course.

For other patients, whose difficulties are long-standing and rooted in intractable social or personality difficulties, brief CBT is not appropriate. For these patients, one strategy is to manage them within a cognitive-behavioral framework, but to do it in a "slow motion" way, seeing them intermittently for months or even years.

The majority of patients are likely to fall into a middle group. They have had a fairly good premorbid functioning, but need help to reevaluate their understanding of their illness, to modify their coping behavior, and, perhaps, to make occupational, social, and lifestyle changes. These patients are the focus of the following account of therapy.

Assuming that a patient is willing to consider the cognitive-behavioral formulation, has identified realistic goals, and has agreed to attend a course of therapy, the work can begin. The aim of therapy is to change inaccurate cognitions and ineffective coping behavior. All therapeutic interventions are based on and guided by the formulation. Interventions may be divided into behavioral and cognitive, although, in practice, they are employed together. It is usual to begin with simple behavioral measures, move on to focus on thinking and illness beliefs, and then to focus on more general attitudes.

Reviewing Behavior

The first step in reviewing behavior is to find out what the patient's activity pattern is. One way to achieve this is for the patient to keep an hour-by-hour diary. The diary should include activities, rest, and sleep. Once the current pattern of activity is recorded, a behavioral experiment can be set up to test predictions about the effect of changes in activity. The majority of patients will have an overall reduced level of activity, and many may be resting and sleeping excessively. The aim of the experiment will be to evaluate the effect of increasing activity and planning rest and sleep. To have the best chance of producing sustainable improvements in functioning, the new activity level should be: (1) at a reasonable and tolerable level for the patient, (2) consistent day-to-day, (3) styled as a gradual increase aimed at the achievement of the realistic goals, and (4) rewarding for the patient.

Behavioral experiments should be set up as "no-lose" exercises. If the patient is able to increase activity, this is evidence of the benefit of this approach; if the patient cannot increase activity, the behavioral experiment will provide valuable information about the obstacles to be overcome.

Although some patients may improve with this simple approach, obstacles usually become apparent and indicate the need for a further consideration of psychological factors for the majority of patients.

Reviewing Thoughts

Cognitive factors are likely to emerge as important obstacles to increasing the level of activity and overcoming avoidance. These factors are best captured by having the patient record his or her thoughts, in writing, prior to and during activity so that they can be reviewed. One method for doing this is the "double-column technique," which requires writing thoughts in one column, considering the thoughts, and then listing alternatives in the second column. An example is shown in Table 10.3. Sometimes, as with the thought "It's hopeless, I will never get better," simple scrutiny may reveal to the patient that the original thought was negatively biased. In other cases, as with the thought "This treatment will make me worse," the inaccuracy may not be so obvious, and the patient should be encouraged to seek evidence—often by testing out the prediction. Some beliefs may prevent a patient from even beginning to make changes. These beliefs might include: "I've tried an increase in activity before and it didn't work" or "Activity is harmful for people with my disease." To address this block, the therapist should ask the patient how he or she knows that an activity is harmful, and whether a gradual, supervised activity program has previously been tried. Most often, patients will have tried sudden, large increases in activity, or increases in activity unaccompanied by a review of their understanding of the illness and symptoms. A collaborative review of the experience with a patient usually reveals why the attempt failed.

Problems may also occur when the patient starts to increase the level of activity but becomes increasingly concerned about the significance of worsening symptoms. If the patient interprets these symptoms as heralding a major relapse or even causing a deterioration in the disease, he or she will understandably back off from activity. To deal with this difficulty, it is important to review with the patient the evidence for and against a belief that the symptoms have sinister significance, and to encourage persistence with the behavioral experiment of a gradual, consistent increase in activity. Predicting an increase in symptoms with increase in activity is important, and the clinician should also help the patient to generate alternative, more benign explanations of this exacerbation. Alternative explanations include the effects of prolonged inactivity, anxiety, and oversensitivity to bodily sensations. The aim of the exercise is to help the patient to regard the symptoms as positive evidence of an effective challenge to the pathophysiology of the

TABLE 10.3. The Double-Column Technique

Column 1: Original Thought	Column 2: Alternative Thought
"It's hopeless, I will never get better."	"How do I know? I haven't given this new approach a try yet. I do know that some people do recover."
"This treatment will make me worse."	"It might, but I don't know that it will and if I don't try I won't find out. It has helped others."

illness. Persistent recording of thoughts, and challenging of these thoughts, may be required in some cases.

Case Vignette (continued). Ms. P agreed to try to adopt a gradual increase in activity, starting with a manageable level, as an experiment. She was initially dismayed at how little she was achieving. She was, however, able to institute daily walks and to adopt a more regular sleep pattern. When she found that she was able to do more, she became optimistic that she could recover.

Stage 3. Review of Unhelpful Attitudes

An attitude that frequently gets in the way of recovery is perfectionism accompanied by an all-or-nothing approach to activities. A related attitude is: "You should always do what other people ask of you." Both of these beliefs may lead to the patient's experiencing self-critical thoughts such as "I should try harder," and then to deviations from planned activity. If these attitudes are a major problem, the patient may be encouraged to review the advantages and disadvantages of keeping them. An example is shown in Table 10.4. A revised version of the attitude may then be discussed, and the patient can be encouraged to change his or her behavior accordingly.

Attitude change is a potentially difficult and long-term task. If time is short, a simpler method is to repeatedly encourage the patient (and a significant other) to make the rehabilitation program—rather than meeting external demands or unrealistic standards—the highest priority task in daily life.

Case Vignette (continued). Ms. P had difficulty sustaining her initial increase in activity. A review of her records indicated that she found it difficult to set time limits on tasks such as cleaning, and tended to continue much longer than planned in order to "do the job properly." She then felt tired, became worried that the illness was being exacerbated, and took to her bed.

TABLE 10.4. Reviewing Attitudes

Attitude:	"I must do everything perfectly."
Advantages:	Motivates me. I feel good if I think I've done something right.
Disadvantages:	I never get things finished. It makes me self-critical. My work always disappointments me. I never feel that I've finished. I find it difficult to plan gradually increasing activity.

This oscillation in activity prevented her from carrying out the experiment of a gradual and consistent increasing of activity.

After review, she agreed to focus all of her effort on her rehabilitation and to plan her activities by time rather than having to complete them perfectly. It became clear that unrealistic standards had been a cause of extreme overwork prior to her becoming ill. Several therapy sessions were, therefore, devoted to helping her adopt more realistic standards and to challenging the associated excessive self-criticism.

Stage 4. Problem Solving of Practical Difficulties

As the patient improves, external obstacles to recovery may become apparent. In particular, a patient who has been chronically disabled, off work, and perhaps receiving financial benefits, needs to make the financial and social transition from sickness to health. This may involve potential "loss of face" and may also mean loss of financial benefits without any certainty of an ability to return to remunerative employment. Issues present when the patient first became ill, such as difficulties at work, may also remain unresolved.

These problems are best dealt with by discussing them openly, helping the patient to make them more manageable by breaking them down into components, and then evaluating different solutions. This cognitive-behavioral technique is called problem solving (Hawton et al., 1989).

> *Case Vignette (continued).* As Ms. P improved, the issue of her return to work became more urgent. When asked how she felt about this, she admitted that she had become disillusioned with teaching and wanted to work as an interior designer—an occupation for which she had previously trained. Her career transition was examined as a problem to be solved. She decided to return to teaching part-time while she built up a clientele for her design work.

Stage 5. Consolidating Gains and Planning for the Future

By the end of therapy, the therapist and patient should have a final collaboratively generated formulation of the illness. It is very useful, at this point, for the patient to produce a written document that includes the formulation and a list of the things learned from the therapy. This document can also include practical guidelines for how the patient can continue rehabilitation and cope with relapse. My experience has shown that patients often refer to these documents subsequently.

Case Vignette (continued). By the end of therapy, Ms. P had achieved her goals of walking a mile each day and going out socially twice weekly, and she was planning to return to her job on a part-time basis. She was very pleased with her progress, although she still believed that her original illness had been viral. She regarded her rigid perfectionism as a problem and was actively working on being more flexible in her work standards. Her summary of therapy included instructions on "what to do if she relapsed" and a "guide to staying healthy."

Problems and Additional Interventions

One of the factors driving patients' continuing distress is a combination of worry about their symptoms and concern at their inability to function. Therefore, a more benign understanding of the illness and evidence of improvement usually results in a resolution of distress. However, other issues such as unresolved grief and chronic relationship difficulties often emerge during therapy. If these issues are important, they may have to be dealt with. However, in many cases, the issues can be deferred and the patient may go on to deal with them after an adequate level of rehabilitation has been reached.

Severe Depression

Antidepressant medication may have a role in therapy when the patient suffers a high level of distress. Antidepressant drugs and CBT have been used in combination in patients with depression, although it is not always clear that the combination is significantly better than either method used alone (Beck et al., 1985).

Persistent Sleep Problems

Sleep problems will usually respond to the simple intervention of helping the patient to adopt a regular sleep pattern and minimizing daytime sleep. If this intervention is ineffective and poor sleep remains a problem, sleep hygiene techniques such as a relaxing bedtime routine may be useful. Sedative antidepressant drugs taken at bedtime may also help to regularize sleep.

Interference by Family

The therapist should interview a member of the patient's family as part of the assessment. This meeting is particularly important in the case of children and adolescents. Some family members may hold strong views about the nature of the illness, and may tell the patient to persist with rest. In these cases, the use of cognitive techniques to persuade the family of the potential benefits of the cognitive-behavioral approach is desirable. In a small number of cases, the patient's family may strongly resist rehabilitation efforts. It may then appear that the patient's sick role is necessary for the stability of the family. Such cases can be very difficult to manage but may benefit from family therapy.

Administration of Therapy

Individual or Group

The advantage of individual cognitive-behavioral therapy is that it can be closely tailored to each patient. Cognitive-behavioral groups require careful patient selection and are demanding on the group leaders. However, group CBT has been used in related conditions (Stern & Fernandez, 1991) and has the potential benefit that patients often give greater credence to the challenging of their beliefs and behavior by other patients than by a therapist. However, groups can also be problematic and can degenerate into patients' discussing symptoms and swapping alternative remedies. At present, an individual approach is preferred.

How Many Sessions?

Some patients can benefit greatly from simple assessment and advice; others might require 20 or more sessions and a minority require long-term therapy and follow-up. An average number would be 10 to 20 individual sessions over a 4- to 6-month period, perhaps with 1 or 2 follow-up or "booster" sessions.

Informational Aids

Patients can be helped to get the most out of their therapy sessions in a variety of ways. One way is for all the therapy sessions to be tape-recorded and for the patient to be given the "homework" of listening to the tape at home. Written summaries outlining certain components of the therapy can also be useful to the patient. Topics might include an outline of CBT, the cognitive-behavioral approach to chronic fatigue syndrome, and detailed sheets explaining how to record and evaluate unhelpful thoughts and beliefs. Other written material, including excerpts from books and articles, may occasionally be useful. Self-help books on the cognitive-behavioral approach, especially those that deal with issues such as perfectionism, also have a place.

Who Should Give the Therapy?

Although the general principles of treatment can be applied by any clinician, complex or difficult cases require the skills of a trained cognitive-behavioral therapist who is used to working with patients who present with somatic, rather than psychological symptoms. Unfortunately, such therapists are rare, and this problem may be a major impediment to developing effective services. Experience has shown that therapists accustomed to working with psychiatric populations often have difficulty engaging and working with patients suffering from chronic fatigue syndrome, without additional training and supervision.

Evidence for the Effectiveness of CBT in CFS

Until recently, studies evaluating the effectiveness of CBT in patients with CFS had been inconclusive, largely because the available studies had employed a variety of research designs and had evaluated different forms of CBT.

Early Studies

The first attempt to apply CBT to patients suffering from CFS was an uncontrolled evaluation of a rehabilitation-oriented therapy with a behavioral emphasis. Many patients refused to participate, but a substantial proportion of those who did take part attained a sustained improvement in functioning that was maintained at long-term follow-up (Bonner et al., 1994; Butler et al., 1991).

The second study was a randomized, controlled trial that compared standard medical care with a brief rehabilitative type of CBT that had a behavioral emphasis, and did not challenge the patients' illness beliefs. The investigators found no difference between these treatments in terms of functional impairment at the final 3-month follow-up evaluation (Lloyd et al., 1993).

The therapy evaluated in both these trials had a rehabilitative orientation but paid relatively little attention to patients' beliefs. A later study used a nonrandomized design to evaluate the effectiveness of CBT with a cognitive emphasis aimed at improving adjustment to illness rather than rehabilitation, compared with a waiting list condition (Friedberg & Krupp, 1994). Compliance was good, and the patients who received CBT reported some reduction in depression, but no reduction in disability.

These early studies suggested that (1) to achieve patient compliance, treatment should address illness beliefs, and (2) that if a reduction in disability is to be obtained, therapy should aim for rehabilitation rather than accommodation to illness.

Recent Studies

Two trials of a rehabilitative form of CBT that paid attention to patients' illness beliefs have been recently completed. One was performed by our group in Oxford and the other by Dr. Wessely and his colleagues at King's College in London.

In Oxford, we randomized patients to receive either 16 sessions of individual CBT or standard medical care (Sharpe et al., 1996). The therapy had a strong cognitive emphasis. Patients experimented with graded increases in activity, attribution of symptoms to physical disease was questioned, and unrealistic personal expectations were reviewed. Outcome was evaluated at 12 months after randomization.

At King's College Hospital in London, patients were randomized to either a similar form of CBT or to relaxation therapy (Deale & Wessley, submitted). In both of these studies, the patients who received CBT achieved a significant reduction in disability at the final follow-up. These new findings suggest that intensive CBT that combines both cognitive and behavioral components can be an effective therapy for many patients with CFS.

CONCLUSION

The cognitive-behavioral model offers a plausible and constructive understanding of what is otherwise a mysterious illness. CBT leads to a flexible, individualized approach to treatment that is well-suited to a heterogeneous condition. Although the initial evidence for the efficacy of this approach was mixed, the most recent studies suggest that it can produce not only better illness adjustment but also a significant reduction in disability for the majority of patients. Given the financial impact of chronic fatigue syndrome, this type of treatment is likely to be cost-effective. The growing evidence that CBT is an effective treatment for patients with chronic fatigue syndrome has major implications for medical services and for how patients with this chronically disabling condition are managed.

REFERENCES

Bakheit, AMO, Behan, PO, Dinan, TG, O'Keane, VO. Possible upregulation of hypothalamic 5-hydroxytraptamine receptors in patients with postviral fatigue syndrome. *Br Med J* 1992; 304:1010–1012.

Beck, AT. Cognitive therapy. A 30-year retrospective. *Am Psychol* 1991; 46:368–375.

Beck, AT, Hollon, SD, Young, JE, Bedrosian, RC, Budenz, D. Treatment of depression with cognitive therapy and amitriptyline. *Arch Gen Psychiatry* 1985; 42:142–148.

Beck, AT, Rush, AJ, Shaw, BF, Emery, G. *Cognitive therapy of depression.* New York: Guilford Press, 1979.

Bonner, D, Ron, M, Chalder, T, Wessely, S. Chronic fatigue syndrome: A follow up study. *J Neurol Neurosurg Psychiatry* 1994; 57:617–621.

Butler, S, Chalder, T, Ron, M, Wessely, S. Cognitive behavior therapy in chronic fatigue syndrome. *J Neurol Neurosurg Psychiatry* 1991; 54:153–158.

Clark, DM. A cognitive approach to panic. *Behav Res Ther* 1986; 24:461–470.

Demitrack, MA. Chronic fatigue syndrome: A disease of the hypothalamic–pituitary–adrenal axis? *Ann Med* 1994; 26:1–5.

Emmelkamp, PMG, Van Oppen, P. Cognitive interventions in behavioral medicine. *Psychother Psychosom* 1993; 59:116–130.

Friedberg, F, Krupp, LB. A comparison of cognitive-behavioral treatment for chronic fatigue syndrome and primary depression. *Clin Infec Dis* 1994; 18(suppl 1):S105–S109.

Frost, RO, Marten, P, Lahart, C, Rosenblate, R. The dimensions of perfectionism. *Cogn Ther Res* 1994; 14:449–468.

Fukuda, K, Straus, SE, Hickie, I, Sharpe, MC, Dobbins, JG, Komaroff, AL. Chronic fatigue syndrome: A comprehensive approach to its definition and management. *Ann Int Med* 1994; 121:953–959.

Greene, B, Blanchard, EB. Cognitive therapy for irritable bowel syndrome. *J Consul Clin Psychol* 1994; 62:576–582.

Hawton, K, Salkovskis, P, Kirk, J Clark, D. *Cognitive behavior therapy for psychiatric problems.* Oxford: Oxford University Press, 1989.

House, A. The patient with medically unexplained symptoms: Making the initial psychiatric contact. In Mayou, R, Bass, C, Sharpe, M, eds., *Treatment of functional somatic symptoms.* Oxford: Oxford University Press, 1995; 89–102.

Kendell, RE. Chronic fatigue, viruses and depression. *Lancet* 1991; 337:160–162.

Klimes, I, Mayou, RA, Pearce, MJ, Coles, L, Fagg, JR. Psychological treatment for atypical non-cardiac chest pain: A controlled evaluation. *Psychol Med* 1990; 20:605–611.

Lloyd, AR, Hickie, I, Brockman, A, Hickie, C, Wilson, A, Dwyer, J, Wakefield, D. Immunologic and psychologic therapy for patients with chronic fatigue syndrome: A double-blind, placebo-controlled trial. *Am J Med* 1993; 94:197–203.

MacLean, G, Wessely, S. Professional and popular views of chronic fatigue syndrome. *Br Med J* 1994; 308:776–777.

Moorey, S, Greer, S. *Psychological therapy for patients with cancer: A new approach.* Oxford: Heinemann Medical Books, 1989.

Morriss, R, Sharpe, MC, Sharpley, A, Cowen, P, Hawton, KE, Morris, J. Abnormalities of sleep in patients with chronic fatigue syndrome. *Br Med J* 1993; 306:1161–1164.

Persons, JB. *Cognitive therapy in practice: A case formulation approach.* New York: W. W. Norton, 1989.

Petrie, K, Moss-Morris, R, Weinman, J. The impact of catastrophic beliefs on functioning in chronic fatigue syndrome. *J Psychosom Res* 1995; 39:31–38.

Powell, R, Dolan, R, Wessely, S. Attributions and self-esteem in depression and chronic fatigue syndromes. *J Psychosom Res* 1990; 34:665–673.

Riley, MS, O'Brien, CJ, McCluskey, DR, Bell, NP, Nicholls, DP. Aerobic work capacity in patients with chronic fatigue syndrome. *Br Med J* 1990; 301:953–956.

Saisch, SG, Deale, A, Gardner, WN, Wessely, S. Hyperventilation and chronic fatigue syndrome. *Q J Med* 1994; 87:63–67.

Salkovskis, PM, Clark, DM. Affective responses to hyperventilation: A test of the cognitive model of panic. *Behav Res Ther* 1990; 28:51–61.

Schweitzer, R, Robertson, DL, Kelly, B, Whiting, J. Illness behavior of patients with chronic fatigue syndrome. *J Psychosom Res* 1994; 38:41–49.

Sharpe, MC, Bass, C. Pathophysiological mechanisms in somatization. *Int Rev Psychiatry* 1992; 4:81–97.

Sharpe, MC, Hawton, KE, Seagraott, V, Pasvol, G. Patients who present with fatigue: A follow up of referrals to an infectious diseases clinic. *Br Med J* 1992; 305:147–152.

Sharpe, MC, Hawton, KE, Simkin, S, Surawy, C, Klimes, I, Peto, TEA, Warrell, D Seagroatt, V. Cognitive therapy for chronic fatigue syndrome: A randomized controlled clinical trial. *Br Med J* 1996; 312:22–26.

Sharpe, MC, Peveler, R, Mayou, R. The psychological treatment of patients with functional somatic symptoms: A practical guide. *J Psychosom Res* 1992; 36:515–529.

Stern, R, Fernandez, M. Group cognitive and behavioral treatment for hypochondriasis. *Br Med J* 1991; 303:1229–1231.

Surawy, C, Hackmann, A, Hawton, K, Sharpe, M. Chronic fatigue syndrome: A cognitive approach. *Behav Res Ther* 1995; 33:535–544.

Thomas, PK. The chronic fatigue syndrome: What do we know? *Br Med J* 1993; 306:1557–1558.

Vercoulen, JH, Swanink, CM, Fennis, JF, Galama, JM, Van der Meer, JW, Bleijenberg, G. Dimensional assessment of chronic fatigue syndrome. *J Psychosom Res* 1994; 38:383–392.

Wessely, S, Sharpe, MC. Chronic fatigue, chronic fatigue syndrome and fibromyalgia. In Mayou, R, Bass, C, Sharpe, M. ed., *Treatment of functional somatic symptoms.* Oxford: Oxford University Press, 1995; 285–312.

Wilson, A, Hickie, I, Lloyd, A, Wakefield, D. The treatment of chronic fatigue syndrome: Science and speculation. *Am J Med* 1994; 96:544–550.

11

Psychopharmacological Principles in the Treatment of Chronic Fatigue Syndrome

Mark A. Demitrack, M.D.

> . . . the man who can insure belief in his opinions and obedience to his decrees secures very often most brilliant and sometimes easy success. . . .
>
> —S. WEIR MITCHELL (1904)

The idea that the central nervous system plays a principal role in the clinical expression of chronic fatigue syndrome, as has been discussed elsewhere in this volume, was a theoretical position that dates at least to Beard's writings, if not earlier. Neurasthenia was felt to arise fundamentally as a result of a disruption in the integrity of nervous tissue, a "dephosphorization," in susceptible individuals, with ensuing subtle changes in brain neurochemistry. Beard (1880) opined that "the one principle on which neurasthenia is to be treated is by the concentration of all possible tonic influence on the nervous system—air, sunlight, water, food, rest, diversion, muscular exercise, and the internal administration of those remedies . . . which directly affect the central nervous system. . . ."

Treatment approaches, not surprisingly, have focused considerable attention on various preparations whose primary mode of action was felt to be on the nervous system itself. For example, general electrization, principally applied to the spinal cord and brain, was proposed as a specific therapy. The majority of the recommended prescription medications appear to have exerted their clinical effects principally due to their psychoactive properties, whether sedating or stimulating. Stea and Fried (1993) have pointed out that the emergence of neurasthenia as a popular clinical diagnosis occurred during a period of time marked also by the easy availability of patent medications—therapeutic preparations that were registered under commercial trademark and sold direct to the general public. As with the prescription medications given by physicians, these medications were often composed of substances whose principal (and sometimes sole) mechanism of action was a psychoactive compound contained in the recipe.

Considered in this historical context, parallels with the present-day therapeutics for chronic fatigue syndrome are striking. For instance, it is becoming increasingly apparent that, as with the putative historical antecedent of neurasthenia, many of the clinical symptoms of chronic fatigue syndrome suggest a prominent role for the central nervous system, whether as a secondary response to a primary alteration in physiological function, or as the principal locus of pathophysiological disturbance. On this basis alone, it may not be surprising that, among the conventional medications that have been proposed to have therapeutic merit in the clinical management of chronic fatigue syndrome, psychopharmacological agents (e.g., antidepressants and sedative-hypnotics) are key resources for the clinician. As did their historical counterparts, patients with chronic fatigue syndrome nowadays make use of a wide array of modern-day patent medications in the form of nutritional supplements, vitamins, minerals, and herbal preparations. Because the interaction of these preparations with conventional medications is not always known, it is important for the clinician to specifically inquire whether the patient is actively using any of these preparations, and, if so, to review the chemical composition. Many of these compounds are directly marketed to patients through local distributors or national buyers' clubs; unfortunately, few have been subjected to rigorous clinical trial, relying more on anecdote and testimonial for their usefulness.

This chapter focuses on the rationale and use of psychopharmacological agents as adjunctive therapies in the clinical approach to patients with chronic fatigue syndrome. Because of the symptom similarity among chronic fatigue syndrome and several other illnesses, most notably fibromyalgia (see Chapter 1, this volume), a selective review of the use of these medications in this latter condition will also be given. Several important conceptual issues are raised by these studies, and they merit comment regarding the use of psychopharmacological agents in the management of chronic fatigue syndrome. An overview of the current peer-reviewed, published literature describing the use of these agents in patients with chronic fatigue syndrome will be presented, and the chapter concludes by providing a framework for a logical approach to treatment.

PSYCHOPHARMACOLOGY OF CHRONIC FATIGUE: A RATIONALE

As this chapter is being written, there are no well-conducted, blinded, placebo-controlled treatment trials establishing the efficacy of psychopharmacological agents in the treatment of chronic fatigue syndrome. Nevertheless, these medications remain among the most commonly prescribed empiric approaches to the pharmacotherapy of this condition, for several important clinical and theoretical reasons. These reasons are summarized in Table 11.1 and are discussed in this section.

Probably the most mundane reason for using psychopharmacological agents is that psychiatric symptoms are intrinsic to the experience of chronic fatigue syndrome for the vast majority of patients. Indeed, these symptoms often account for a substantial portion of the morbidity and decline in quality of life associated with this illness. An extensive series of studies performed to date, using well-designed, structured psychiatric interview techniques and rigorously applied psychiatric diagnostic criteria, have affirmed the reality of this observation (Gold et al., 1990; Hickie et al., 1990; Katon et al., 1991; Kruesi et al., 1989; Manu et al., 1988, 1989; Taerk et al., 1987; Wessely & Powell, 1989). In the majority of these studies, the prevalence of formally diagnosable psychiatric illness was higher in patients with chronic fatigue syndrome than in the general population or among other comparable somatically ill patients. More often than not, the psychiatric illness preceded the onset of the fatigue syndrome. In only one study was the prevalence of psychiatric illness reported to be similar in magnitude to that of the general population, and to follow, rather than precede, the development of the chronic fatigue (Hickie et al., 1990). Regardless of their source, the emergence of psychiatric symptoms in patients with chronic fatigue syndrome places patients at morbid risk for serious clinical complications such as suicide, and hence cannot

TABLE 11.1. Clinical and Theoretical Reasons for the Use of Psychopharmacological Agents in the Management of Chronic Fatigue Syndrome

- Psychiatric symptoms and syndromes are ubiquitous in the clinical presentation of chronic fatigue syndrome (chronic fatigue syndrome as a phenotypic variation of a primary psychiatric illness).

- Chronic fatigue syndrome may emerge as a interactive consequence of disruptions in the integrity of the nervous and immune systems (chronic fatigue syndrome as a novel neuroendocrine/neuroimmune disease process).

- Psychotropic medications may have benefits in the treatment of a variety of undifferentiated somatic symptoms (e.g., headache, arthralgias, myalgias, gastrointestinal discomfort, and sleep disturbances).

be ignored. For this reason, the use of psychopharmacological agents may be indicated.

However, it is often difficult, if not impossible, to determine whether the psychiatric symptoms represent a primary disease process, a secondary clinical condition, or a cormorbid illness modifying the primary disease state. The reasons for the presence of psychiatric symptoms in patients with chronic fatigue syndrome remain a topic of profound controversy. Katon and Russo (1992) have argued that a possible explanation may be a definitional one. They have demonstrated that the stipulation within the original Centers for Disease Control and Prevention (CDC) case definition for chronic fatigue syndrome, which requires patients to manifest multiple, unexplained physical symptoms, merely seems to select individuals who have an increased burden of both current and lifetime psychiatric illness. The result is an obscuring, rather than a clarifying, of the delineation of what is already probably a heterogeneous population of individuals. In other words, their work would suggest that the reason for the high prevalence of psychiatric symptoms in individuals with CDC-defined chronic fatigue syndrome is that the vast majority of these individuals do indeed have a primary psychiatric diagnosis that is a sufficient explanation for their illness. From this perspective, referring to a separate "chronic fatigue syndrome," merely reflects an attributional bias on the part of the patient and clinician by ascribing the illness to an external, most often viral, cause. This view is, therefore, compatible with the idea that chronic fatigue syndrome represents an idiosyncratic phenotypic variation of a primary psychiatric illness. In this model, the substantial clinical response to psychopharmacological treatment in essence reflects the response of the underlying primary psychiatric syndrome.

The previous argument has been vigorously countered by the assertion that the primary pathophysiological disturbance in patients with chronic fatigue syndrome is fundamentally immunological, not psychiatric. In other words, the psychiatric syndromes, when present, are secondary to a primary, persistent immune dysfunction. This view arose, in part, as the result of initial reports of abnormal patterns of antibody responses to certain viral antigens, along with nonspecific elevations in antinuclear antibodies and immune complexes in patients with persistent, unexplained fatigue (Jones et al., 1985; Straus et al., 1985; Tobi et al., 1982). Subsequent observations of disturbances in humoral and cellular immune mechanisms, such as immunoglobulin subclass deficiencies, defects in natural killer cell or other T-cell subset number and function, and abnormal levels of serum cytokines, have further increased interest in this view (Calgiuri et al., 1987; Chao et al., 1990, 1991; Cheney et al., 1989; Kibler et al., 1985; Klimas et al., 1990; Landay et al., 1991; Lloyd et al., 1989; Straus et al., 1989, 1993; Tosato et al., 1985). This model is attractive because it is known that many of the biochemical components of the immune response (e.g., the interleukins and other cytokines) have important neuroactive properties, producing symptoms that are important elements of the clinical expression of chronic fatigue syndrome (e.g., feverishness, myalgias, arthralgias, and disturbances in sleep and activity).

However, a discrete separation between chronic fatigue syndrome as a purely "psychological" or "physiological" condition is probably not feasible, nor may such an approach be desirable. For example, a more complete understanding of the immunological findings reported in patients with chronic fatigue syndrome must be integrated with the emerging body of literature studying such biological aberrations in patients with primary psychiatric illness, or during periods of profound psychological stress (Kronfol, 1994; O'Leary, 1990). This work clearly suggests that immunological disturbances, some of which are remarkably similar to those described in patients with chronic fatigue syndrome, may be observed in various psychologically challenged populations. Examples of these observations include alterations in both cellular immunity (e.g., reductions in natural killer-cell activity, and variations in lymphocyte subset number) and humoral immunity (e.g., elevations in cytokine levels and alterations in immunoglobulin production). More complex issues are raised by the observation that susceptibility to infectious illnesses and the pattern of recuperation from those illnesses may be affected by antecedent psychological state (see Chapters 1 and 4, this volume). Furthermore, certain viral illnesses may be associated with a wide range of psychiatric symptoms during the recuperative phase, long after evidence of clinical infection has subsided. It has long been known that infectious mononucleosis provides provocative examples of such persistent clinical syndromes. Isaacs (1948) described a series of 53 patients with clinically substantiated infectious mononucleosis whose illness subsequently evolved into a clinical condition characterized by profound fatigue, "out of proportion to the physical data . . . ," along with exhaustion, aching of legs, weakness, depression, mild feverishness, and low blood pressure. In 1976, Cadie and colleagues reported on a series of 36 patients with serologically proven infectious mononucleosis. Patients were evaluated by personal interview, and completed a questionnaire assessing psychiatric symptoms during the 3 months before and the 12 months after the onset of the infectious episode. Cadie et al. observed a significant increase in the prevalence of depression and anxiety states, and more evident somatic complaints in women, but not in men. Hendler and Leahy (1978) described 2 patients with serologically proven infectious mononucleosis, in whom psychiatric and neurological symptoms developed in the recuperative phase of the illness. Interestingly, in one patient they described, the symptoms responded to treatment with tranylcypromine. In these latter two reports, the clear delineation between cause and effect was obscure, and a more interactive model of illness development seemed appropriate.

An intimate connection exists between the immune and nervous systems; for example, receptors for immune substances and the immune substances themselves exist in the central nervous system, while receptors for classical central nervous system neurotransmitters exist on the surfaces of immune cells, and immune cells manufacture neuropeptide species active in the central nervous system (Figure 4.1). Hence, a variety of apparently disparate clinical syndromes may actually arise from disturbances of this neuroendocrine/neuroimmune network. Placing the development of an illness such as chronic fatigue syndrome in such a framework fosters a less parochial view of disease pathogenesis, and enables one to see the possible consequence of commonality in clinical symptomatology, despite subtle differences in disease pathogenesis. The bidirectionality implied by such an illness model also poses questions about the true mechanism of action of psychotropic agents in the treatment of chronic fatigue syndrome. In other words, is the clinical effect due solely to an influence of the medications on the nervous system directly, or should more subtle, indirect actions of the drug be considered, taking into account the potential nervous system/immune system interactions? What might these alternate mechanisms of action tell us about the nature of the disease itself?

A final reason that may also assist in explaining the rationale and empiric usefulness of psychopharmacological agents in the treatment of chronic fatigue syndrome is the pragmatic observation that psychotropic agents may have multiple symptomatic uses. For example, these medications are commonly used in the management of such undifferentiated symptoms as generalized pain, sleep disturbances, allergic phenomena, gastrointestinal discomfort, or headaches. From this clinical vantage point, it can also readily be appreciated that chronic fatigue syndrome shares symptom similarity not only with major psychiatric illnesses, but also with several other poorly understood clinical conditions, most notably fibromyalgia, a clinical condition for which several psychopharmacological agents appear to have demonstrated efficacy. Given that the symptoms shared by these two conditions are clinically redundant and do not, in and of themselves, confer diagnostic specificity on the clinical syndrome in which they occur, the precise reason why a particular neuroactive active agent is helpful may be due to any one of its multiple clinical effects. This latter point is an important one to keep in mind when ascribing a unitary etiological mechanism to clinically diverse syndromes that, nevertheless, may share a common pharmacotherapy.

THE USE OF PSYCHOPHARMACOLOGICAL AGENTS IN RELATED CLINICAL SYNDROMES: WHAT CAN BE LEARNED?

As noted in the preceding section and elsewhere in this volume, chronic fatigue syndrome shares many clinical similarities with fibromyalgia (Buchwald et al., 1987; Goldenberg et al., 1990). Because of the clinical and pathophysiological resemblance between these two conditions, an examination of the existing literature on the use of psychopharmacological agents in the treatment of fibromyalgia may be particularly instructive, at the very least because it may serve to highlight some important conceptual pitfalls with regard to the use of these medications. Early attempts at medication therapy of fibromyalgia led to the observation that the tricyclic compound, cyclobenzaprine, showed substantial promise in relieving many of the symptoms of this illness (Campbell et al., 1982). This initial finding has led to a series of studies of the tricyclic antidepressants themselves, and, more recently, of several other neuroactive agents. The results of this work are summarized in Table 11.2, and several points relevant to the discussion of chronic fatigue syndrome treatment are addressed in the paragraphs that follow.

Initial results were not encouraging. Wysenbeek and colleagues (1985) reported an open treatment trial using imipramine in doses ranging from 50 to 75 milligrams per day, in a series of 20 patients with primary fibrositis, as defined by the criteria of Smythe (1981). Only two favorable responses to treatment were reported; in one of these, treatment was ultimately limited by adverse effects of the medication. Overall, 19 patients stopped therapy during the 3-month period of observation, 14 because of a specific lack of response. The specific rationale for the dosage chosen arose from the existing clinical practice of the treatment of this illness, but the modest dosage and the absence of serum drug levels are obvious confounds in understanding the meaning of these results. More importantly, though, it was clear to these investigators that the complexity of the behavioral accompaniments of the condition were profound. This complexity made a more definitive interpretation of the meaning of an open treatment trial particularly problematic. However, no objective measures of behaviors or their potential relation to treatment response were provided.

At this point, two important pathophysiological observations about fibromyalgia had entered the literature. The first was the finding by Moldofsky and colleagues of a high prevalence of a characteristic arousal pattern occurring during non-REM sleep in patients with fibromyalgia (Moldofsky et al., 1975). This polysomnographic abnormality was comprised of a significant intrusion of alpha rhythms into the normally slow-wave delta sleep typical of the deeper stages of sleep. This was an extremely intriguing finding, given the common clinical observation that patients with fibromyalgia described their sleep as "nonrefreshing," and, conversely, improvement in clinical symptoms was often heralded by a return to restful nocturnal sleep. It was also well-known that the indoleamine neurotransmitter serotonin played an important role in the regulation of slow-wave sleep. Hence, it was of additional interest when the same investigators subsequently reported an inverse relationship between plasma-free tryptophan (a serotonin precursor) and pain severity in patients with fibromyalgia (Moldofsky et al., 1978). Such findings

TABLE 11.2. Studies Reporting the Use of Psychopharmacological Agents for the Treatment of Fibromyalgia

Study	Design	Medication	Patient Group	Results
Wysenbeek et al. (1985)	Open trial; 3 months	Imipramine	19 females, 1 male; mean age: 46.9 years	1 patient reported sustained improvement, 19 discontinued treatment (14 due to nonresponse)
Carette et al. (1986)	Double-blind, placebo-controlled, 9 weeks	Amitriptyline	54 females, 5 males; mean age: 41.0 years	Significant improvement in morning stiffness and pain, sleep quality, and global improvement; no change in tender points
Goldenberg et al. (1986)	Double-blind, placebo-controlled, 6 weeks	Amitriptyline, naproxen, or combination therapy	59 females, 3 males; mean age: 43.8 years	Amitriptyline showed superiority over placebo or naproxen alone on all outcome measures, including tender points
Caruso et al. (1987)	Double-blind, placebo-controlled, 8 weeks	Dothiepin	52 females, 8 males; mean age: 46.0 years	Dothiepin significantly better than placebo on all outcome measures, including tender points
Tavoni et al. (1987)	Double-blind, placebo-controlled, 21 days	S–Adenosylmethionine IM injection	17 patients (gender not specified)	S–AMe improved depressive symptoms and pain scores; a significant correlation was seen between mood and pain symptoms

Bennett et al. (1988)	Double-blind, placebo-controlled, 12 weeks	Cyclobenzaprine	126 females, 4 males; mean age: 49.4 years	Significant improvement in pain (including tender points) and sleep quality with active drug treatment; 52% placebo dropout rate compared to 16% for active drug
Hamaty et al. (1989)	Double-blind, placebo-controlled, crossover, 5 months	Cyclobenzaprine	6 females, 1 male; mean age: 48.6 years	No significant drug effect on pain, but a significant improvement in sleep quality
Scudds et al. (1989)	Double-blind, placebo-controlled, crossover, 10 weeks	Amitriptyline	32 females, 4 males; mean age: 39.9 years	Significant improvement in pain, tender-point severity, and well-being on active drug
Quimby et al. (1989)	Double-blind, placebo-controlled, 6 weeks	Cyclobenzaprine	40 females; mean age: 45 years	Significant improvement in stiffness and aching, sleep quality, and overall function; 67% of patients could distinguish drug from placebo
Caruso et al. (1990)	Double-blind, placebo-controlled, 30 days	5-Hydroxytryptophan	7 females, 43 males; mean age: 47.4 years	All clinical measures improved with active drug treatment; placebo resulted in significant and sustained improvement in sleep and pain severity

(continued)

271

TABLE 11.2 (Continued)

Study	Design	Medication	Patient Group	Results
Russell et al. (1991)	Double-blind, placebo-controlled, 6 weeks	Alprazolam, ibuprofen, or both	69 females, 9 males; mean age: 47.3 years	Improvement in patient self-assessment and tender points (by palpation but not by dolorimeter) in combined therapy group
Drewes et al. (1991)	Double-blind, placebo-controlled, 12 weeks	Zopiclone	41 females; mean age: 50 years	Significant improvement of sleep quality and a reduction in daytime tiredness; no effect on pain or other constitutional symptoms
Jaeschske et al. (1991)	n-of-1 trial design, 2–4 weeks per trial	Amitriptyline	22 females, 1 male; mean age: 55.2 years	A significant symptom reduction in favor of drug occurred in 30% of trials, and a significant reduction in tender-point score was evident in 17% of trials; onset of action was rapid
Geller et al. (1989)	Case report	Fluoxetine	Female, age 29	Complete remission of symptoms
Finestone & Ober (1990)	Case report	Fluoxetine	2 females, ages 41 and 49	Complete remission of symptoms
Tyber (1990)	Case report	Lithium augmentation	3 females, ages 48, 49, and 56	Complete remission of symptoms

were compelling justification for the further investigation of centrally neuroactive substances in the treatment of fibromyalgia, despite the apparently discouraging results of Wysenbeek and coworkers. These results further increased interest in the use of lower treatment doses of these agents, due to the prominence of hypnotic qualities of these agents at those dosages.

The first literature report of a controlled treatment trial of a tricyclic antidepressant was reported by Carette and colleagues in 1986. In this work, they performed a 9-week double-blind, placebo-controlled trial comparing 50 milligrams of amitriptyline with placebo in patients meeting criteria for primary fibromyalgia as defined by Smythe. Again, no specific behavioral descriptors were included in the subject characterization. Clinical endpoints included the patients' report of morning stiffness, pain, sleep quality, and global symptom change, and the physician's measurement of tender-point severity and global improvement. Overall, amitriptyline appeared effective in improving sleep quality and in the sense of global symptom change, by patient self-report and physician assessment. However, no other clinical parameter was significantly different when comparing placebo to active drug. It is of note that no specific comment was provided regarding the potential for a dose-dependent drug effect. Would the use of higher doses of medication, or a specific threshold blood level have been associated with a more obvious clinical benefit? Despite this omission, several important comments provided by the investigators are worth emphasizing. Most important, the majority of the patients taking an active drug were able to correctly determine whether they were taking an active drug or not, because the anticholinergic effects of the medication were prominent. Moreover, the placebo response rate of the overall group was notable, with 50% of patients reporting symptom relief on placebo. In 31% of subjects, this response was "meaningful" in the definition of the investigators. In other words, in patients with fibromyalgia, as in chronic fatigue syndrome, the patients' expectancy of treatment effect is high. Much of the source for the substantial placebo response has been ascribed to the dramatic contrast between the lack of seriousness or even outright disdain with which the patients' symptoms are often greeted by many physicians, in comparison to the participation as a subject in a scientific study. A scientifically rigorous and compassionate treatment approach may present itself as an attractive clinical setting, and, hence, may be of therapeutic benefit in and of itself. Among the most important conclusions of this study, then, may have been the extent to which it laid the groundwork pointing to the need for a more multidimensional approach to clinical management. Medications play an important adjunctive role in clinical care, but may be most effective when coupled with the poorly understood contextual factors that may be responsible for the "nonspecific treatment" effects of the study.

The results apparent in the study by Carette and colleagues have been echoed in subsequent work. For example, Goldenberg and coworkers (1986), in a 6-week, double-blind, placebo-controlled comparison of 25 milligrams of amitriptyline at bedtime, and 500 milligrams of naproxen twice daily, or both, found that either of the amitriptyline-containing arms of the study performed significantly better than placebo or naproxen alone on several representative clinical measures. Similarly, Caruso and colleagues (1987) documented the benefit of dothiepin, a tricyclic antidepressant, in an 8-week, double-blind, placebo-controlled study at a dose of 75 milligrams at bedtime. A pronounced placebo response was evident in this study also. The report was additionally noteworthy for its consideration of the potential role of depressive or other behavioral symptoms in the production or perpetuation of the fibromyalgia syndrome. Unlike the earlier reports, these authors noted a clear effect of the medication as distinguished from placebo at the 8-week endpoint of the study, an onset of effect more compatible with the typical latency of clinical effect for antidepressant medications. The absence of specific behavioral descriptors, though, leaves much of the interpretation of the results to hypothetical discussion.

The study by Tavoni and colleagues (1987) was the first to employ specific self- and observer-rated instruments for the assessment of depressive symptoms. These symptoms were examined in relation to the subjective physical symptoms of the disease, and its response to treatment—in this case, the intramuscular administration of S-adenosylmethionine, a methyl donor with putative antidepressant effect. Tavoni et al. conducted a 21-day, double-blind, placebo-controlled crossover design. At baseline, a clear positive association was noted between depression scores and pain severity. In response to active treatment, both pain measures and depressive symptoms significantly improved. The investigators argued that the response to clinical treatment with antidepressant medications in patients with primary fibromyalgia is inextricably linked to the mood state of the individual; however, a clear cause-and-effect relationship is not readily apparent. In another study, Quimby and coworkers (1989) noted that pretreatment Beck Depression Inventory scores were positively associated with the magnitude of improvement in sleep quality in response to treatment with cyclobenzaprine. In their report, they also underscored the ability of subjects to accurately identify active drug, and the role that such expectancy may play in the overall response to treatment. In the study by Caruso and colleagues (1990), psychiatric status was assessed by unstructured interview and by the Hamilton rating scale for depression. Individuals diagnosed with major depression using these instruments were excluded from study. All others participated in a double-blind, placebo-controlled trial of 100 milligrams of 5-hydroxytryptophan for a 30-day trial. Active treatment in this study resulted in an improvement in measures of tender-point severity, pain intensity, amount of sleep, level of anxiety, fatigue, and morning stiffness, along with significant improvement in global disease severity. However, placebo-treated patients also reported a significant improvement in sleep and pain intensity, along with a transient improvement in stiffness and number of tender points.

The complexity of the clinical presentation of patients suffering from a multidetermined condition such as fibromyalgia is well-noted in the report by Bennett and colleagues (1988). They examined the specific efficacy of up to 40 milligrams of cyclobenzaprine versus placebo in a 12-week, double-blind trial in patients with primary or secondary fibromyalgia. Psychiatric exclusions in that study consisted only of those patients with psychosis or significant manipulative behavior, or individuals who were unable to discontinue psychiatric medications for the duration of the study. Overall, the cyclobenzaprine-treated group showed superiority of clinical response on self-reported outcome measures of pain severity and sleep disturbance. Nevertheless, interpretation of the results was confounded by several factors. First, response to treatment was variable and by no means universal. The medication was clearly not effective as monotherapy for this condition. Second, the rate of placebo response, as in the other cited studies, was high, as was the difficulty in ensuring proper blinding of the study, due to the prominence of anticholinergic side effect in the actively treated group. In acknowledging these issues, Bennett emphasized the need for a more comprehensive appreciation of the causative and perpetuating factors in this clinical condition by pointing out: "It is evident that fibrositis affects the quality of life by reducing patients' vigor and making them tentative about exercise because of postexertional pain and stiffness. In this sense, fibrositis is a disease of *dysfunction.* . . ."

Taken in aggregate, the results of these studies suggest that psychopharmacotherapy is a useful adjunctive tool for the treatment of pain, fatigue, sleep difficulty, and affective symptoms in patients with fibromyalgia. Despite this fact, a specific and readily apparent unitary mechanism of action that could account for this efficacy has remained elusive. Although beyond the scope of this chapter, it is useful to note that similar observations on the use of these medications as part of a comprehensive treatment approach have been made in other complex, multidetermined clinical conditions, such as chronic pain, headache, and the irritable bowel syndrome (Egbunike & Chaffee, 1990; Greenbaum et al., 1987; Max, 1990; Max et al., 1992; Sindrup et al., 1990).

What can be learned from this work with respect to studies in chronic fatigue syndrome? An answer to this question can be found, in part, from several methodological points that have emerged over time from the studies discussed in this section. A first point that should be made is that many psychotropic medications are biochemically broad in action, and the relative importance of specific effects may vary with the dose employed. Few studies to date have examined a truly broad range of doses, or have related these doses and their clinical effect to blood levels of the particular medication. Indeed, the initial rationale for the use of antidepressants in the treatment of fibromyalgia was based on a rather narrowly focused view of disease pathogenesis—namely, serotonin dysfunction. Accumulated data would suggest that, on the contrary, rather than emerging from a single pathophysiological defect, fibromyalgia, like chronic fatigue syndrome, arises as a clinically evident condition as a result of the complex interplay of a variety of factors that may be dispersed across the lifetime of the individual. Among these factors are the current, predominant symptom profile of the patient. However, rarely considered factors, which should be studied in future work on treatment response, include the detailed personal and family medical and psychiatric history of the individual, coping strategies and resulting attitudes toward disease attribution, and gender. Consideration of such factors and others in the subsequent generation of treatment studies may help in providing more precise answers regarding:

- How do these medications work?
- What is the relationship between the effect of the drug and the psychological state of the individual?
- How long should these medications be administered?
- Should the administration of medication be sequenced in any particular way with regard to other therapeutic modalities?
- What is the proper dosing scheme?
- Can the response to medication provide any additional information about the underlying disease biology?

Despite the questions that remain, much can be learned, from the existing literature about the use of these medications in fibromyalgia, that may be of immense use in the development of treatment strategies in patients with chronic fatigue syndrome. The following section presents a brief survey of published studies that report the use of these medications in chronic fatigue syndrome.

CHRONIC FATIGUE SYNDROME: EMPIRICAL TREATMENT TRIALS

As noted earlier, at the time this chapter is being written, there are no randomized, double-blind, placebo-controlled treatment trials of psychotropic medication in patients with chronic fatigue syndrome. However, several reports of open-treatment trials of single- or multiple-case series have been published. In addition, there is one report of a double-blind, placebo-controlled, single-case study. The studies reviewed in this section are summarized in Table 11.3. The reader is also referred to a recent publication by Goodnick and colleagues (1993) for additional discussions of this topic.

In part due to the similarity in clinical presentation to fibromyalgia, and because of the diffuse range of symptoms reported in patients with chronic fatigue syndrome, antidepressants were very early recommended as symptomatically useful. For instance, in 1987, Jones noted in his uncontrolled case series that, "approximately 70% [of patients] reported clinical improvement with low doses of doxepin. . . ." In two case reports, Goodnick (1990) described the successful resolution of chronic fatigue syndrome with the use of bupropion. In both instances, symptom resolution was substantial by subjective symptom report, and in one case was achieved at a rather low dose of bupropion (100 milligrams twice daily). Although in both cases the clinical effect was accompanied by a substantial reduction in mood, as reflected in Beck Depression Inventory scores, the degree of change in physical symptoms, such as recurrent upper respiratory tract infections and feverishness, was equally profound.

Gracious and Wisner (1991) subsequently provided a more detailed report of psychotropic medication response in a patient with chronic fatigue syndrome. Their report is of particular interest because it provides a detailed, categorical diagnostic assessment of the patient's current and past psychiatric status and her presenting symptom pattern with respect to the 1988 CDC case definition of chronic fatigue syndrome. Furthermore, dosage and serum level of the antidepressant, nortriptyline, are reported. The patient was studied in a double-blind, placebo-controlled case design, with an A-B-A-B pattern of alternating active drug placebo administration over an interval of 15 weeks, during which time serial mood and chronic fatigue symptoms were assessed. Periods of drug administration were clearly associated with a subjective and measurable amelioration of affective and physical symptoms, although resolution of illness was incomplete.

In a larger series than his initial case report, Goodnick and colleagues (1992) reported on the clinical response to bupropion of 9 patients with CDC-defined chronic fatigue syndrome who had failed a previous 12-week trial of fluoxetine. Five of the subjects met criteria for a mood disorder concurrent with the diagnosis of chronic fatigue syndrome. A maximal dose of 300 milligrams per day of bupropion was used in this study. After 8 weeks, there was a significant fall in Beck Depression Inventory and Hamilton Depression Scale ratings. In 6 subjects, the depressive symptom reduction was at least 40%, considered a "response" to treatment. In this latter subgroup, the trough plasma bupropion level was more often $\geq$ 30 nanograms/milliliter.

Two recent uncontrolled, open-treatment studies have documented a symptomatic benefit of the serotonin-reuptake inhibitors, fluoxetine and sertraline. Klimas and colleagues (1993) have reported on two separate patient

TABLE 11.3. Psychopharmacological Agents in the Treatment of Chronic Fatigue Syndrome: Published Reports

Study	Design	Medication	Patient Group	Results
Goodnick et al. (1990)	Case report	Bupropion	2 female, ages 61 and 48	Improvement in self-reported mood and physical complaints
Gracious et al. (1991)	Double-blind, placebo-controlled, single-case study; 15 weeks	Nortriptyline	Female, age 35	Improvement of self-rated depression and physical complaints during active treatment phases
Berlin et al. (1992)	Case report; 4 weeks	Fluoxetine	Female, age 41; male, age 46	Improvement of chronic fatigue, "energizing effect," decreased sleep; syndrome precipitated by poison with ciguatera toxin
Goodnick et al. (1992)	Open-treatment trial; 8 weeks	Bupropion	7 females, 2 males; mean age: 43.4 years	Improvement of self- and observer-rated depressive symptoms
Klimas et al. (1993)	Open-treatment trial; 3 months (Cohort 1), 8 weeks (Cohort 2)	Fluoxetine	Cohort 1 (n = 25) Cohort 2 (28 females, 7 males; mean age: 42 years)	Cohort 1: 87% "clinical improvement" with treatment Cohort 2: Significant improvement in Karnofsky score with treatment
Behan et al. (1994)	Open-treatment trial; 6 months	Sertraline	39 females, 40 males; mean age: 35.4 years	"Substantial abatement of symptoms," with a 72% reduction in self-reported fatigue

278

cohorts, 25 and 35 patients each. In the first cohort, a response rate of a "moderate to marked" degree was reported in 46% of the subjects by 8 weeks, at a dose of 20 milligrams per day. The total response rate increased to 87% at 3 months' follow-up. In the second cohort under study, a significant increase in Karnofsky score (a global measure of functional status) was seen in all subjects, compared with their pretreatment score, regardless of the presence or absence of depressive symptoms. The daily dose of fluoxetine in this latter cohort was again 20 milligrams daily. In the largest case series to date, Behan and coworkers (1994) reported on the use of sertraline, 50 milligrams daily, in 79 patients with chronic fatigue arising in the aftermath of an apparent viral infection. A strict case definition was not employed, nor was there specific quantitation of comorbid psychiatric symptoms. However, they noted "a substantial abatement of symptoms," with a 72% reduction of fatigue in the overall sample.

It is of interest that, in many instances in these reports, medication benefit was evident on the affective as well as the physical symptoms of the disease. The meaning of this observation is, however, unknown in the absence of more detailed clinical subgrouping, in particular the use of a nonpsychiatrically ill chronic fatigue sample. Equally noteworthy is that, with the exception of the report by Gracious and Wisner, these are uncontrolled, open-treatment trials. Given the substantial nonspecific treatment effect evident in the studies of fibromyalgia, and also in the available controlled studies of nonpsychotropic medications in patients with chronic fatigue syndrome (Chapter 12, this volume), caution must be exercised in the interpretation of the results. On the other hand, it becomes important to ask what these nonspecific factors are and whether they can be quantified. For instance, do they represent psychological interventions inherent in the patient/clinician interactions? Are they variations in the attributional bias of the patient or physician regarding the nature of the illness? Or do they relate to confounding illness-associated behaviors (e.g., changes in activity, sleep habits, or dietary practice)? Clarification of these issues will be essential in future work in this area.

A LOGICAL APPROACH TO THE PSYCHOPHARMACOLOGY OF CHRONIC FATIGUE

A complete understanding of the pathophysiology of chronic fatigue syndrome is not available. Unfortunately, in the absence of reliable information, speculative hypotheses may develop the compelling force of established fact. These principles then foster treatment proposals that may have heuristic merit for future research, but may, in their present form, be detrimental to the well-being of the patient. Therefore, education of both the patient and

the treating physician is essential. This education may, at times, involve utilizing appointment times to discuss articles appearing in the medical and lay
media, differentiating research hypotheses from clinically useful treatments,
and differentiating both of the latter from irrational pseudoscience. The
treatment context must establish a common ground for discussion of such
issues.

As discussed elsewhere in this volume, an emerging explanatory model
for the development of chronic fatigue syndrome emphasizes the heterogeneous nature of this illness. The specific antecedent factors that place an individual at risk for this illness may vary widely from person to person. As a
result, a clinical management plan that is multidimensional in character is
suggested as an essential starting point for treatment. Given that psychopharmacological medications as a class may be broad in clinical effect, it is
reasonable to presume that they may play a significant role in such a multidimensional treatment model. The material reviewed in this chapter would
support that view. This section will summarize the elements of a logical approach to the pharmacotherapy of chronic fatigue syndrome (Table 11.4),
keeping such a treatment framework in mind.

Many patients may be reluctant to entertain psychotropic medications as
part of their treatment, despite their evident usefulness. The stigma associated with the use of the medications is immense, and, for some patients, may
be an insurmountable obstacle to their use. To provide a context to address
this issue and others like it, a collaborative approach to treatment is essential.
Such collaboration should ideally foster exchange of clinical information and
development of a treatment consensus between patient and clinician. This
framework should also underscore the lack of current definitive diagnostic
testing, and the view that chronic fatigue syndrome is, at the present time, a
diagnosis of exclusion that does not fall neatly into any discrete clinical domain. Therefore, if novel symptoms emerge during the course of treatment,
careful ongoing psychiatric and medical evaluation, or specialty consultation,
and collaborative discussion are necessary to avoid premature diagnostic closure. This format also establishes a neutral ground to discuss behavioral
symptoms, their meaning for the patient, and any possible pharmacothera-
peutic or other treatment interventions.

If pharmacotherapy is chosen as a treatment option by the patient, it is
often best employed as a targeted intervention designed to provide specific
symptomatic relief. Such interventions should be directed at specific functional symptom domains (e.g., musculoskeletal pain, sleep quality, fatigue, or
subjective cognitive changes), specific psychiatric symptoms (e.g., anxiety or
depression), or formally evident psychiatric syndromes. In our experience
and from the evidence reviewed above, there is no compelling argument to
pursue any one particular psychopharmacological agent in the treatment of
chronic fatigue syndrome. Therefore, the selection of a specific drug should

TABLE 11.4. Recommendations for a Logical Pharmacotherapy of Chronic Fatigue

- Establish a collaborative patient/physician treatment framework.
- Avoid premature diagnostic closure.
- Determine what self-administered, over-the-counter medications the patient is already taking and assess closely for interaction with the proposed medication.
- Discuss the role of medication and identify clear treatment goals:

    Psychiatric syndromes

    Domains of symptomatic distress (e.g., musculoskeletal pain, poor sleep quality, fatigue, subjective cognitive changes, and mood or anxiety symptoms)
- Choice of agent should be based on:

    The predicted side-effect profile

    The patient's preference

    Medical contraindications to the use of a particular medication
- Begin therapy at the lowest possible dose, and increase the dose gradually; observe and discuss side effects during treatment, clarifying issues of significant medical concern.
- Attempt thorough trial to known optimal target dose of drug or until maximum clinical effect is evident.
- Ongoing discussion of the patient's specific response pattern should occur, clarifying the patient's expectations about the treatment.
- Do not continue treatment indefinitely without evidence of clear clinical response; if necessary, discontinue treatment and reassess during medication-free state.
- Avoid polypharmacy, assess treatment response to one agent at a time.
- Frame pharmacotherapy with respect to other aspects of the treatment plan; use medication as setting a context for a multidimensional treatment framework.

be based on the symptomatic or syndrome targets agreed on by the patient and clinician prior to initiating therapy, and by the acceptability or desirability of the medication's side-effect profile (e.g., sedating agents taken at bedtime may be preferable when insomnia is a problem). On the other hand, it should be noted that patients with chronic fatigue syndrome may be extremely sensitive to, or apprehensive about, the side effects of medications; hence, small initial dosages may be desired, and gradual increases in dose may then follow. Distinction between sensitivity to the predictable side effects of medications (e.g., anticholinergic effects of tricyclic antidepressants or the activating effects of the selective serotonin reuptake inhibitors) and true allergic reactions should be attended to and clarified for the patient. However, there is no reason to believe that modified doses are routinely necessary for patients with chronic fatigue syndrome. Indeed, a patient's report of a previous treatment failure may reflect inadequate dosing or duration of treatment.

At the present time, it is unrealistic to present medication as a sole treatment for this illness. Indeed, properly framing the illness and its treatment in a multidisciplinary perspective is a crucial step in the initial stages of treatment. Eliciting the patient's active participation in his or her own recovery is essential; recuperation is not something that is done "to" a patient, but rather "with" a patient. In this regard, Goldenberg's caution is worth noting: although antidepressant medications have clear-cut short-term benefits in the treatment of fibromyalgia, evidence for specific long-term usefulness is lacking (Goldenberg, 1989). This caveat is equally relevant for the use of these compounds in patients with chronic fatigue syndrome. Medications may function largely in a short-term time frame, providing sufficient symptomatic relief to allow other, more enduring nonpharmacological therapeutic interventions to take hold. Future work may be usefully directed at understanding how pharmacotherapy may blend with these nonpharmacological strategies in the development of a comprehensive, multidimensional treatment approach.

REFERENCES

Beard, GM. *A practical treatise on nervous exhaustion (neurathenia). Its symptoms, nature, sequences, treatment.* New York: William Wood, 1880.

Behan, PO, Haniffah, BAG, Doogan, DP, Loudon, M. A pilot study of sertraline for the treatment of chronic fatigue syndrome. *Clin Inf Dis* 1994; 18(Suppl 1):S111.

Bennett, RM, Gatter, RA, Campbell, SM, Andrews, RP, Clark, SR, Scarola, JA. A comparison of cylcobenzaprine and placebo in the management of fibrositis. *Arthritis Rheum* 1988; 31(12):1535–1542.

Berlin, RM, King, SL, Blythe, DG. Symptomatic improvement of chronic fatigue with fluoxetine in ciguatera fish poisoning [letter]. *Med J Australia* 1992; 157:567.

Buchwald, D, Goldenberg, DL, Sullivan, JL, Komaroff, AL. The "chronic active Epstein–Barr virus infection" syndrome and primary fibromyalgia. *Arthritis Rheum* 1987; 30(10):1132–1136.

Cadie, M, Nye, FJ, Storey, P. Anxiety and depression after infectious mononucleosis. *Brit J Psychiatry* 1976; 128:559–561.

Calgiuri, M, Murray, C, Buchwald, D, Levine, H, Cheney, P, Peterson, D, Komaroff, AL, Ritz, J. Phenotypic and functional deficiency of natural killer cells in patients with chronic fatigue syndrome. *J Immunol* 1987; 139:3306–3313.

Campbell, SM, Gatter, RA, Clark, S, Bennett, RM. A double-blind study of cyclobenzaprine versus placebo in patients with fibrositis (abstract). *Arthritis Rheum* 1982; 27:S76.

Carette, S, McCain, GA, Bell, DA, Fam, AG. Evaluation of amitriptyline in primary fibrositis. *Arthritis Rheum* 1986; 29(5):655–659.

Caruso, I, Sarzi Puttini, PC, Boccassini, L, Santandrea, S, Locati, M, Volpato, R, Montrone, F, Benvenuti, C, Beretta, A. Double-blind study of dothiepin versus placebo in the treatment of primary fibromyalgia syndrome. *J Int Med Res* 1987; 15:154–159.

Caruso, I, Sarzi Puttini, P, Cazzola, M, Azzolini, V. Double-blind study of 5-hydroxytryptophan versus placebo in the treatment of primary fibromyalgia syndrome. *J Int Med Res* 1990; 18:201–209.

Chao, CC, Gallagher, M, Phair, J, Peterson, PK. Serum neopterin and interleukin-6 levels in chronic fatigue syndrome. *J Inf Dis* 1990; 162:1412–1413.

Chao, CC, Janoff, EN, Hu, S, Thomas, K, Gallagher, M, Tsang, M, Peterson, PK. Altered cytokine release in peripheral blood mononuclear cell cultures from patients with the chronic fatigue syndrome. *Cytokine* 1991; 3:292–298.

Cheney, PR, Dorman, SE, Bell, DS. Interleukin-2 and the chronic fatigue syndrome. *Ann Int Med* 1989; 110:321.

Drewes, AM, Andreasen, A, Jennum, P, Nielsen, KD. Zopiclone in the treatment of sleep abnormalities in fibromyalgia. *Scand J Rheumatol* 1991; 20:288–293.

Egbunike, IG, Chaffee, BJ. Antidepressants in the management of chronic pain syndromes. *Pharmacotherapy* 1990; 10(4):262–270.

Finestone, DH, Ober, SK. Fluoxetine and fibromyalgia. *JAMA* 1990; 264(22): 2869–2870.

Geller, SA. Treatment of fibrositis with fluoxetine hydrochloride (Prozac). *Am J Med* 1989; 87:594–595.

Gold, D, Bowden, R, Sixbey, J, Riggs, R, Katon, WJ, Ashley, R, Obrigewitch, RM, Corey, L. Chronic fatigue: A prospective clinical and virologic study. *JAMA* 1990; 264(1):48–53.

Goldenberg, DL. A review of the role of tricyclic medications in the treatment of fibromyalgia syndrome. *J Rheumatol* 1989; 16(suppl 19):S137–S139.

Goldenberg, DL, Felson, DT, Dinerman, H. A randomized, controlled trial of amitriptyline and naproxen in the treatment of patients with fibromyalgia. *Arthritis Rheum* 1986; 29(11):1371–1377.

Goldenberg, DL, Simms, RW, Geiger, A, Komaroff, AL. High frequency of fibromyalgia in patients with chronic fatigue seen in a primary care practice. *Arthritis Rheum* 1990; 33(3):381–387.

Goodnick, PJ. Bupropion in chronic fatigue syndrome [letter]. *Am J Psychiatry* 1990; 147:1091.

Goodnick, PJ, Sandoval, R. Psychotropic drug treatment of chronic fatigue syndrome and related disorders. *J Clin Psychiatry* 1993; 54(1):13–20.

Goodnick, PJ, Sandoval, R, Brickman, A, Klimas, NG. Bupropion treatment of fluoxetine-resistant chronic fatigue syndrome. *Biol Psychiatry* 1992; 32(9):834–838.

Gracious, B, Wisner, KL. Nortriptyline in chronic fatigue syndrome: A double-blind, placebo-controlled single case study. *Biol Psychiatry* 1991; 30:405–408.

Greenbaum, DS, Mayle, JE, Vanegeran, LE, Jerome, JA, Mayor, JW, Greenbaum, RB, Matson, RW, Stein, GE, Dean, HA, Halvorsen, NA. Effects of desipramine on irritable bowel syndrome compared with atropine and placebo. *Dig Dis Sci* 1987; 32:257–266.

Hamaty, D, Valentine, JL, Howard, R, Howard, CW, Wakefield, V, Patten, MS. The plasma endorphin, prostaglandin and catecholamine profile of patients with fibrositis treated with cyclobenzaprine and placebo: A 5-month study. *J Rheumatol* 1989; 16(suppl 19):S164–S168.

Hendler, N, Leahy, W. Psychiatric and neurologic sequelae of infectious mononucleosis. *Am J Psychiatry* 1978; 135(7):842–844.

Hickie, I, Lloyd, A, Wakefield, D, Parker, G. The psychiatric status of patients with chronic fatigue. *Br J Psychiatry* 1990; 156:534–540.

Isaacs, R. Chronic infectious mononucleosis. *Blood* 1948; 3:858–861.

Jaeschske, R, Adachi, J, Guyatt, G, Keller, J, Wong, B. Clinical usefulness of amitriptyline in fibromyalgia: The results of 23 N-of-1 randomized controlled trials. *J Rheumatol* 1991; 18:447–451.

Jones, JF, Ray, G, Minnich, LL, Hicks, MJ, Kibler, R, Lucas, DO. Evidence for active Epstein–Barr virus infection in patients with persistent, unexplained illnesses: Elevated anti-early antigen antibodies. *Ann Int Med* 1985; 102(1):1–7.

Jones, JF, Straus, SE. Chronic Epstein-Barr virus infection. *Ann Rev Med* 1987; 38:195–209.

Katon, WJ, Buchwald, DS, Simon, GE, Russo, JE, Mease, PJ. Psychiatric illness in patients with chronic fatigue and those with rheumatoid arthritis. *J Gen Int Med* 1991; 6:277–285.

Katon, WJ, Russo, J. Chronic fatigue syndrome: A critique of the requirement for multiple physical complaints. *Arch Int Med* 1992; 152:1604–1609.

Kibler, R, Lucas, DO, Hicks, MJ, Poulos, BT, Jones, JF. Immune function in chronic active Epstein–Barr virus infection. *J Clin Immunol* 1985; 5:46–54.

Klimas, NG, Morgan, R, Van Riel, F, Fletcher, MA. Observations regarding the use of an antidepressant, fluoxetine, in chronic fatigue syndrome. In Goodnick, PJ, Klimas, NG, eds., *Chronic fatigue and related immune deficiency syndromes.* Washington, DC: American Psychiatric Press, Inc., 1993; 95–108.

Klimas, NG, Salvato, FR, Morgan, R, Fletcher, MA. Immunological abnormalities in chronic fatigue syndrome. *J Clin Microbiol* 1990; 28:1403–1410.

Kronfol, Z. Immune function in depression and anxiety. In den Boer, J, Sitsen, JM, eds., *Handbook of depression and anxiety: A biological approach.* New York: Marcel Dekker, 1994; 515–527.

Kruesi, MJP, Dale, JK, Straus, SE. Psychiatric diagnoses in patients with the chronic fatigue syndrome. *J Clin Psychiatry* 1989; 50:53–56.

Landay, AL, Jessop, C, Lennette, ET, Levy, JA. Chronic fatigue syndrome: Clinical condition associated with immune activation. *Lancet* 1991; 338(8769): 707–712.

Lloyd, AR, Wakefield, D, Boughton, CR, Dwyer, JM. Immunological abnormalities in the chronic fatigue syndrome. *Med J Austral* 1989; 151:122–124.

Manu, P, Lane, TJ, Matthews, DA. The frequency of the chronic fatigue syndrome in patients with symptoms of persistent fatigue. *Ann Int Med* 1988; 109:554–556.

Manu, P, Matthews, DA, Lane, TJ, Tennen, H, Hesselbrock, V, Mendola, R, Affleck, G. Depression among patients with a chief complaint of chronic fatigue. *J Aff Dis* 1989; 17:165–172.

Max, MB. Towards physiologically based treatment of patients with neuropathic pain. *Pain* 1990; 42:131–133.

Max, MB, Lynch, SA, Muir, J, Shoaf, SE, Smoller, B, Dubner, R. Effects of desipramine, amitriptyline, and fluoxetine on pain in diabetic neuropathy. *N Engl J Med* 1992; 326:1250–1256.

Moldofsky, H, Scarisbrick, P, England, R, Smythe, HA. Musculoskeletal symptoms and non-REM sleep disturbance in patients with "fibrositis syndrome" and healthy subjects. *Psychosom Med* 1975; 37:341–351.

Moldokfsky, H, Warsh, JJ. Plasma tryptophan and musculoskeletal pain in nonarticular rheumatism (fibrositis syndrome). *Pain* 1978; 5:65–71.

O'Leary, A. Stress, emotion, and human immune function. *Psychol Bull* 1990; 108(3):363–382.

Quimby, LG, Gratwock, GM, Whitney, CD, Block, SR. A randomized trial of cyclobenzaprine for the treatment of fibromyalgia. *J Rheumatol* 1989; 16(suppl 19):S140–S143.

Russell, IJ, Fletcher, EM, Michalek, JE, McBroom, PC, Hester, GG. Treatment of primary fibrositis/fibromyalgia syndrome with ibuprofen and alprazolam. *Arthritis Rheum* 1991; 34(5):552–560.

Scudds, RA, McCain, GA, Rollman, GB, Harth, M. Improvements in pain responsiveness in patients with fibrositis after successful treatment with amitriptyline. *J Rheumatol* 1989; 16(Suppl 19):S98–S103.

Sindrup, SH, Gram, LF, Brosen, K, Eshoj, O, Mogensen, EF. The selective serotonin reuptake inhibitor paroxetine is effective in the treatment of diabetic neuropathy symptoms. *Pain* 1990; 42:135–144.

Smythe, HA. Fibrositis and other diffuse musculoskeletal syndromes. In Kelley, WN, Harris, ED, Jr, Ruddy, S, Sledge, CB, eds., *Textbook of rheumatology*, first edition. Philadelphia: W. B. Saunders Co., 1981; 485–493.

Stea, J, Fried, W. Remedies for a society's debilities. Medicines for neurasthenia in Victorian America. *NY State J Med* 1993; 93(2):120–127.

Straus, SE, Dale, JK, Peter, JB, Dinarello, CA. Circulating lymphokine levels in the chronic fatigue syndrome. *J Infect Dis* 1989; 160:1085–1086.

Straus, SE, Fritz, S, Dale, J, Gould, B, Strober, W. Lymphocyte phenotype analysis suggests chronic immune stimulation in patients with chronic fatigue syndrome. *J Clin Immunol* 1993; 13(1):30–40.

Straus, SE, Tosato, G, Armstrong, G, Lawley, T, Preble, OT, Henle, W, Davey, R, Pearson, G, Epstein, J, Brus, I. Persisting illness and fatigue in adults with evidence of Epstein–Barr virus infection. *Ann Int Med* 1985; 102(1):7–16.

Taerk, GS, Toner, BB, Salit, IE, Garfinkel, PE, Ozersky, S. Depression in patients with neuromyasthenia (benign myalgic encephalomyelitis). *Int J Psychiatry Med* 1987; 17(1):49–56.

Tavoni, A, Vitali, C, Bombardieri, S, Pasero, G. Evaluation of S-adenosylmethionine in primary fibromyalgia: A double-blind crossover study. *Am J Med* 1987; 83(suppl 5A):S107–S110.

Tobi, M, Morag, A, Ravid, Z, Showers, I, Feldman-Weiss, V, Michaeli, Y, Ben-Chetrit, E, Shalit, M, Knobler, H. Prolonged atypical illness associated with serological evidence of persistent Epstein–Barr virus infection. *Lancet* 1982; 9:61–64.

Tosato, G, Straus, SE, Henle, W, Pike, SE, Blaese, RM. Characteristic T-cell dysfunction in patients with chronic active Epstein–Barr virus infection (chronic infectious mononucleosis). *J Immunol* 1985; 134:3082–3088.

Tyber, MA. Lithium carbonate augmentation therapy in fibromyalgia. *Can Med Assoc J* 1990; 143(9):902–904.

Weir-Mitchell, S. The evolution of the rest treatment. *J Nerv Ment Dis* 1904; 31:368–373.

Wessely, S, Powell, R. Fatigue syndromes: A comparison of chronic "postviral" fatigue with neuromuscular and affective disorders. *J Neurol Neurosurg Psychiatry* 1989; 52:940–948.

Wysenbeek, AJ, Mor, F, Lurie, Y, Weinberger, A. Imipramine for the treatment of fibrositis. *Ann Rheum Dis* 1985; 44:752–753.

12

Medically Oriented Therapy for Chronic Fatigue Syndrome and Related Conditions

N. Cary Engleberg, M.D.

S ince the recent resurgence of interest in chronic, idiopathic fatigue states began, numerous reports of treatment efforts have appeared in the medical literature. These reports range from double-blind, placebo-controlled trials in large research institutes to anecdotal reports from individual physicians. Yet, as this chapter is being written, there is still no clearly efficacious or generally accepted drug therapy for these patients. This is not a surprising state of affairs when one considers how little we actually understand about the biological factors that contribute to these perplexing chronic fatigue states.

Because we understand so little about the pathophysiology of chronic fatigue, many thoughtful physicians have opted to focus therapy on specific symptoms *per se*. Accordingly, they have tried medications that relieve symptoms of fatigue, pain, sleep, and mood disorders associated with other medical or psychiatric disorders. Several medications that have established records of efficacy and safety in treating symptoms of depression, fibromyalgia, and multiple sclerosis have been recommended for treatment of patients with chronic fatigue syndrome (CFS), often without the benefit of controlled studies in these patients. For example, it is a common experience that antidepressants often ameliorate certain symptoms in CFS patients, even in those who do not have a prominent mood disorder. In the absence of a clear understanding of the biology of chronic fatigue states, an individualized, symptom-directed approach to therapy would seem to be safe and potentially effective. Some of the nonpsychotropic medications used in this way will be reviewed below. The use of antidepressants and other psychotropic agents in CFS was reviewed in Chapter 11 of this volume.

Alternatively, certain drugs have been selected for trial in CFS patients for more specific reasons. In several formal studies, specific drugs are tested in order to validate or to refute a particular concept of the pathophysiology of the syndrome. Hence, antiviral agents have been used to examine the hypothesis that specific viruses are involved in the pathogenesis, various immunomodulators have been used because of the popular notion that an immune dysfunction is driving the pathological process, and various nutritional supplements have been given with the intent of correcting a specific deficiency. None of these approaches has yielded convincingly positive results to date, and the pathophysiological mechanism of most chronic fatigue cases remains obscure.

A prevailing problem with the published experience on drug therapy is the notable paucity of carefully controlled trials. There is instead a preponderance of uncontrolled trials, case reports, and anecdotes in the literature. Another serious concern is the question of case definition (Fukuda et al., 1994; Holmes et al., 1988; Katon & Russo, 1992; Schluederberg et al., 1992; Straus, 1992b). The Centers for Disease Control and Prevention (CDC) has published, and revised, a case definition for chronic fatigue syndrome (see Chapter 1, this volume) that has been adopted by several major research centers. Unfortunately, therapeutic trials have not always adhered to this definition. Even when the definition is used, the criteria may be interpreted and weighted differently by different investigators in assembling patient groups. Patient groups used at different institutions may not be comparable; hence, a drug that seems to be efficacious in one selected population may not be useful in populations selected elsewhere.

Finally, a variety of medicinal and herbal products have been recommended as "general tonics." Some of these medications are formulated pharmaceutical agents; others are undefined mixtures of substances that are more properly considered "alternative medicines." Without editorializing about the value of such remedies, they will not be discussed here unless they have been the subject of a peer-reviewed report in the medical literature.

SYMPTOM-DIRECTED THERAPY

Analgesic and Anti-Inflammatory Agents

Pain is often a particularly troublesome symptom in CFS patients. Although there is no clinical or histological evidence of an inflammatory basis for this pain, anti-inflammatory agents are occasionally used for their analgesic effects. Unfortunately, there is no published literature to support the notion that these agents work better than placebo in CFS. However, there have been a few double-blinded, placebo-controlled trials of nonsteroidal anti-inflammatory agents (NSAIDs) in the fibromyalgia syndrome. In these studies, NSAIDs used alone appear to have only marginal (if any) efficacy (Goldenberg, 1989). In a 6-week study of 62 fibromyalgia patients, Goldenberg et al. (1986) concluded that naproxen, 500 mg twice daily, did not significantly improve pain, although there was a trend toward pain reduction when this drug was combined with nightly amytriptyline (25 mg). Likewise, Russell et al. (1991) found minor improvement in tender points and in patient-reported pain, using a combination of ibuprofen and alprazolam, but no significant benefit with either agent alone.

S-Adenosylmethionine is a basic molecule that can donate methyl groups and affect a variety of biological processes. The drug produces anti-inflammatory, analgesic, and antidepressant effects. For pain due to osteoarthritis, S-adenosylmethionine is felt to be an equivalent of NSAIDs. In a short-term, crossover study of 17 patients with fibromyalgia by Tavoni et al. (1987), therapy with this agent produced significant reduction in the number of tender points as well as significant improvements in depression rating scales, when compared with placebo. Thus, it was difficult to assess whether the primary effect of the drug was analgesic or psychotropic. A subsequent study by Jacobsen et al. (1991) evaluated a 6-week course of therapy in 44 patients. Again, symptoms of pain, fatigue, and stiffness were improved, but so was mood as evaluated by the Face scale. Tender-point score, muscle strength, and depression (as measured by the Beck Depression Inventory) were similar for drug and placebo in this study.

Corticosteroids have also been used in cases of fibromyalgia syndrome, primarily for their anti-inflammatory effects. This treatment approach has significance for CFS, in light of the recent observations linking impaired activation of the hypothalamic–pituitary–adrenal (HPA) axis with this syndrome (Demitrack et al., 1991), and with fibromyalgia (Crofford et al., 1994; Griep et al., 1993). A double-blind, placebo-controlled trial to assess the effects of "replacement" doses of hydrocortisone of the symptoms of CFS is currently in progress, but the results are not available at the time this chapter is being assembled. However, there has been a report of a double-blind, crossover trial of prednisone in 20 patients with fibromyalgia (Clark et al., 1985). In this study, patients took placebo or prednisone for 14 days each, and they were assessed functionally and symptomatically at 2 and 4 weeks. Rather than improvement, there was a trend toward deterioration during prednisone therapy.

There are no published data on the efficacy of anti-inflammatory agents in CFS on which to base a therapeutic recommendation. By extrapolation from patients with the overlapping syndrome of fibromyalgia, one might expect little consistent efficacy from NSAIDs and potential deterioration with corticosteroids. NSAIDs may offer some benefit as adjunctive therapy with some psychotropic agents, and it may be reasonable to continue to use them in individual patients who experience a favorable analgesic response. In contrast, corticosteroids should be avoided until the effects of these agents on the symptoms of CFS and the HPA axis are better understood. S-Adenosylmethionine may be a useful agent, but it is not clear whether the favorable responses with this agent are due to its anti-inflammatory or psychotropic effects.

Muscle Relaxants

As for anti-inflammatory agents, there are no controlled trials of muscle relaxants in CFS. However, there are two published studies showing that the tricyclic, cyclobenzaprine (Flexeril), is more effective than placebo in improving some of the symptoms of fibromyalgia (Bennett et al., 1988; Quimby et al., 1989). In the first of these studies by Bennett et al., 120 patients (116 women) were given either cyclobenzaprine 40 mg per day (divided doses) or placebo for a 12-week course. Fifty-two percent of the patients in the placebo group, but only 16% of the patients in the treatment group, dropped out of the study because of lack of efficacy. There were significant improvements in self-evaluation of pain and sleep quality, and a trend toward improvement of fatigue. A smaller, 6-week controlled study of 40 female patients with fibromyalgia by Quimby et al. revealed a similar improvement in sleep and general well-being, but little effect on patient-evaluated pain or fatigue. Unfortunately, many of the patients in the study were aware of the drug's effects and were able to identify the test drug. How this awareness might have skewed the patients' self-evaluation is unknown. A third group studying plasma levels of neurotransmitters in 7 fibromyalgia patients compared cyclobenzaprine with placebo in a double-blind, crossover trial lasting 9 weeks in each phase of the study (Hamaty et al., 1989). Again, there was improvement in sleep quality but not in reported pain. Subsequently, Reynolds et al. (1991) confirmed the beneficial effect of cyclobenzaprine in a formal sleep study, using a double-blind, crossover design. Nine patients who completed the study showed prolonged sleep time and improvement in evening fatigue. Their analysis showed no effect of the drug on pain, tender points, dolorimetry, mood, or sleep EEG patterns.

Finally, there is one reported trial comparing carisoprodol (Soma) in a fixed combination with acetaminophen and caffeine (Somadril) with placebo in 43 patients treated for 8 weeks (Vaeroy et al., 1989). In this double-blind trial, active treatment improved pain, sleep quality, and general well-being. In addition, a higher tolerance to pressure pain at tender points was noted. Some improvement in these parameters was also noted in the placebo group during the trial; however, all patients in this study were permitted access to other medications as needed for symptom relief. It was noted that patients taking placebo were more likely than active treatment patients to require analgesics or NSAIDs (56.5% vs. 20%; $p = .015$) or psychotropic agents (43% vs. 0%; $p = .0008$). The lesser requirement for additional drug therapy again supports the efficacy of this drug combination. These studies generally support the use of tricyclic muscle relaxants as adjuncts in fibromyalgia. They may also be useful in some patients with CFS. The findings with the carisoprodol-containing combination are encouraging, but they have not been reproduced.

Fatigue

A significant degree of drug experimentation has been directed at the problem of fatigue in patients with multiple sclerosis (MS). Mild central nervous system stimulants (e.g., methylphenidate), anti-cholinesterase agents (e.g., pyridostigmine), and muscle relaxants (e.g., baclofen) have been tried to alleviate this symptom without success. Fortuitously, T. J. Murray (1985) discovered that some MS patients experienced remarkable improvement in their fatigue while taking the antiviral drug, amantadine, for prevention of type A influenza. In fact, apart from its antiviral activity, amantadine is known to have neurotropic effects, including increased release of norepinephrine from terminal nerve fibers and an increase in dopaminergic activity (making the drug a potential adjunct in Parkinson's disease).

In a double-blind, crossover study of 32 evaluable, fatigued MS patients, amantadine, 100 mg twice daily, produced a prompt improvement in fatigue in 66% versus 22% improvement in response to placebo (Murray, 1985). Improvement was judged to be "marked" in 31% and "moderate" in an additional 16% of patients while taking amantadine. In contrast, no patient reported marked improvement while taking placebo, and only one patient reported moderate improvement. At the end of the trial, 23 of the 32 patients selected amantadine for long-term therapy, no patient selected placebo, and 9 preferred no further drug therapy. Improvement in some responders was sustained for up to 2 years.

An attempt to reproduce these findings in a 10-week, crossover study of 115 MS patients showed less impressive, but nonetheless significant effects of the drug (Canadian MS Research Group, 1987). Notably, an important placebo effect was also observed. Moreover, although amantadine appeared to reduce the fatigue rating, this improvement was not associated with reduced disability in terms of daily living activities. In addition, insomnia occurred more frequently with amantadine therapy than with placebo. To objectify further the response to amantadine, Cohen and Fisher (1989) conducted a double-blind, controlled study employing daily patient diary ratings of seven parameters and patient performance on seven neuropsychological tests. Amantadine therapy produced small improvements in overall energy level, concentration, problem solving, and sense of well-being. In addition, patients taking amantadine performed slightly better on the Stroop Interference test, a measure of attentional focus in the presence of distracting information. Rosenberg and Appenzeller (1988) compared six MS patients who responded to amantadine with four MS patients who did not respond in a blinded, controlled trial. The responders had significantly higher levels of β-endorphin/β-lipotropin than nonresponders. The nonresponders had higher lactate and lower pyruvate levels than the responders. Rosenberg and Appenzeller suggested that the drug might be exerting its effect by a central release of catecholamines, similar to that induced by the antihypertensive drug, clonidine.

In more recent reports, amantadine has been used with success in open studies to ameliorate the fatigue of the postpolio syndrome (Dunn, 1991) and the symptom of refractory pain in MS patients (Chiba et al., 1992). The drug has not been formally tested in CFS patients; however, there is a published anecdotal report of improvement in a single patient with postinfectious fatigue and myalgia following an Epstein–Barr virus (EBV) infection (Wiggs, 1991). A more formal evaluation of the drug in CFS patients will be needed before it can be recommended for this indication.

SPECIFIC THERAPEUTIC AGENTS
(EXCLUDING PSYCHOTROPICS)

Anti-Infective Agents

There is lengthy literature implicating various infective agents in CFS (see Chapters 4 and 7, this volume). For potential pathogens that are amenable to therapy, the hypothesis that these agents are actively involved in producing symptoms is testable in a therapeutic trial. Two proposed etiological agents, EBV and *Candida* sp., are treatable entities. Controlled studies evaluating acyclovir and nystatin, respectively, have been conducted to test whether active therapy for these agents would influence the clinical course of CFS patients.

Acyclovir

In 1988, Straus et al. published the results of a blinded, placebo-controlled trial of intravenous and oral acyclovir in 27 patients with CFS. The 8 men and 19 women who participated were selected if they met the CDC criteria for CFS for 1 year or more, and if they had either high titer antibodies against EBV early antigens or undetectable antibody to EBV nuclear antigen

(EBNA). The serological criteria were applied in order to select a subgroup of CFS patients who were most likely to have active EBV infection as a factor in their illness. Thirteen of the patients had a mononucleosis-like illness at the onset of their CFS, and 6 of these were heterophile-positive cases of acute infectious mononucleosis.

The patients were randomized and hospitalized to receive intravenous acyclovir (500 mg per m²) or placebo every 8 hours for 7 days. After discharge, the patients continued to take acyclovir (800 mg) or placebo orally 4 times a day for 30 days. After a 6-week medication washout period, the patients were readmitted and crossed-over to the opposite arm of the study for an identical course of medication. At various intervals, the patients were examined by physicians and tested for EBV antibodies and certain immunological parameters. To assess clinical improvement, the patients completed self-evaluations each evening of the study. Twenty-four patients completed the trial (three had reversible renal failure with acyclovir and were dropped from further analysis).

Twenty-one scored themselves improved during one phase of treatment: eleven during the acyclovir phase, and ten during the placebo phase. Four patients had sustained improvement that lasted for one or more years; three of these patients perceived that their improvement began during the placebo phase. There were no significant changes in EBV serology or various immunological parameters during either treatment phase. In addition, patients whose fatigue syndrome began with infectious mononucleosis did not respond differently to acyclovir than did other patients in the study.

The antiviral therapy used in this study should have been adequate to inhibit active replication of EBV. Although the study was small, the sample size was large enough to have detected a three-fold difference in improvement between drug and placebo with a power of .80. The failure of the drug to influence the symptoms or the serological or immunological features of CFS, therefore, supports the conclusion that active EBV infection is not responsible for the syndrome, although the authors acknowledge that the study does not rule out a role for EBV in the immunopathology of CFS (Pagano, 1989; Straus, 1989). From a more practical perspective, the study offers little support for the empiric use of acyclovir in CFS patients. Instead, acyclovir and other antivirals should be reserved for the extremely rare and severe disorders in which EBV causes a documented progressive infection (Straus, 1992a).

Nystatin

In 1978, Truss theorized that some patients might develop chronic fatigue as a consequence of hypersensitivity to endogenous *Candida* sp. This notion was popularized in the lay press, and countless patients were subsequently diagnosed with this hypersensitivity syndrome (a.k.a. "the yeast connection") by their health care providers or by themselves. The relationship between candidal colonization and the putative syndromes has never been confirmed in the scientific or medical literature. Moreover, a study by Renfro et al. (1989) suggests that 8 patients carrying this diagnosis were indistinguishable from 92 CFS patients with respect to history, symptoms, physical findings, and laboratory measurements. Therefore, in the absence of clear scientific data implicating candidal colonization as the unique cause of the syndrome, most of these cases are properly absorbed into the working definition of CFS.

If intestinal colonization with *Candida* is critical to the expression of this syndrome, then antifungal therapy should ameliorate symptoms. A controlled study by Dismukes et al. in 1990 addressed this question. Forty women with a history of vaginal candidiasis and three of five symptoms associated with the hypersensitivity syndrome (i.e., gastrointestinal complaints, allergic respiratory symptoms, premenstrual distress, depression, and cognitive difficulties) were randomized in a crossover study. The four 8-week treatment blocks used combinations of oral nystatin (or oral placebo) *plus* vaginal nystatin (or vaginal placebo). All four combinations (including oral placebo plus vaginal placebo) had positive effects overall. With respect to the vaginal symptoms of candidiasis, there were significant differences between the nystatin-containing regimens and the double placebo regimen. In contrast, there was no difference in the improvement of systemic symptoms among any of the regimens. This study casts additional doubt on the notion that candidal colonization produces symptoms in these patients, and strongly challenges the value of systemic antifungal therapy for such patients.

Supplemental Nutrients

Magnesium

In 1991, Cox et al. compared red cell (RBC) magnesium levels from 20 CFS patients with those of 20 healthy controls and found a small but significant mean difference between the two groups (0.1 mmol/liter). Based on this finding, they conducted a randomized, controlled trial to assess the effects of magnesium supplementation (Cox et al., 1991). Thirty-two patients satisfying the "Australian criteria" for CFS (see Chapter 1, this volume) were recruited; 15 were randomized to receive $MgSO_4$ (1 g) every week for 6 weeks, and 17 received placebo injections on the same schedule. At the end of treatment, the patients completed a health assessment profile that contained questions in six categories. In general, patients in both study arms experienced improvement in most categories. However, the active treatment group reported significantly more improvement than the placebo group in energy level, pain, and emotional reactions. The active treatment and placebo groups did not differ with respect to sleep, social isolation, or physical mobility. Pre- and posttreatment RBC magnesium measurements demonstrated that both groups had initially low levels, but the levels in the treatment group rose sharply during the trial. Plasma magnesium levels were normal in both groups, before and after the trial.

The Cox study stimulated a flurry of letters to the *Lancet*. In an attempt to reproduce the laboratory findings, two investigators reported no differences in RBC magnesium levels comparing their CFS patients and controls (Deulofeu et al., 1991; Gantz, 1991). A third letter questioned the competence of the commercial laboratory employed by the Cox study in measuring levels (Richmond, 1991). Young and Trimble (1991) pointed out that the RBC magnesium level provides a poor indication of total body magnesium stores or magnesium concentrations in other cells, and they suggested that a symptomatic syndrome of magnesium deficiency should be expected to manifest other clinical features (e.g., hypokalemia, hypocalcemia, and cardiac arrhythmias) that are not features of CFS. These authors also questioned the therapeutic significance of the administered dose of less than 1 mmol per day. The recommended daily dietary intake is 12 mmol per day (Young & Trimble, 1991).

If there is no true magnesium deficiency state in CFS, then the positive effects of treatment in the Cox study are not easily explained. Parenteral magnesium has been advocated as treatment for other medical conditions in the past, and the possibility that it increases the perception of "energy" in some nonspecific way must be ruled out (Shepherd, 1991). Because the findings of Cox et al. have not yet been replicated, it is premature to recommend the use of intramuscular magnesium sulfate in CFS patients.

Essential Fatty Acids

The human requirement for the essential fatty acids, linoleic and α-linolenic acids (EFAs), is not completely understood. It is known that these long-chain, unsaturated lipids are sequentially desaturated and lengthened in cells to form arachidonic, dihomo-γ-linolenic, and eicosapentaenoic acids. These latter three acids are the sole precursors for the synthesis of several important second-messenger molecules (i.e., prostaglandins, thromboxanes, and leukotrienes). A few medical conditions (e.g., atopic dermatitis) have been associated with a defect in the desaturation of the EFAs and the formation of these three important precursors (Horrobin & Manku, 1990). With respect to chronic infections, it is known that the second-messenger molecules derived from the EFA pathway are required for the antiviral effects of γ-interferon.

In 1988, Williams et al. reported diminished EFA desaturating activity in sera taken from patients several months after acute infectious mononucleosis. More importantly, these changes were prolonged in the minority of patients who reported persistent fatigue and malaise 7 months after the acute infection. It is not known whether these subtle changes are causally related to the fatigue or are simply a molecular marker of prolonged symptoms. Taking a theoretical view of the findings, Horrobin (1990) hypothesized that some viral infections (e.g., EBV) may actively block EFA metabolism at the first desaturating step in order to prevent antiviral immunity mediated through γ-interferon and to prolong infection. This hypothesis has not been tested directly. If correct, Horrobin suggests that supplementation with fatty acids from the EFA metabolic pathway, downstream of the putative enzymatic defect, might reverse this abnormality.

Accordingly, Behan et al. (1990) conducted a double-blind, placebo-controlled treatment trial with a mixture of primrose and fish oils (Efamol Marine) that is rich in EFA pathway fatty acids distal to the putative desaturation blockade. Sixty-three patients (36 females, 27 males) with chronic fatigue, myalgia, and psychiatric symptoms for 1 to 3 years following a definite viral infection were randomized to active treatment or placebo, and evaluated at 1 and 3 months. Assessment by both patients and physicians at 1 month favored the active treatment. In addition, although much of the improvement in the placebo group regressed at 3 months, the active treatment group showed sustained improvement. By end of the trial, the physicians reported improvement in 85% of the active treatment group, but in only 17% of the placebo group ($p < .0001$).

To date, these encouraging results have not been reproduced (mentioned in McCluskey, 1993). In addition, the findings apply to a group of patients that may not be typical of CFS patients, because the CDC definition was not used. For now, it is reasonable to remain circumspect about the utility of Efamol Marine, given the lack of published experiences and the nontrivial cost of treatment.

Selenium

Selenium is an essential trace element. Selenocysteine is a component of the enzyme glutathione peroxidase, a critical defense against oxidant damage of biological systems. Patients receiving prolonged intravenous fluid therapy may experience muscle pain and weakness associated with low selenium levels. These clinical symptoms are relieved by administering selenomethionine. Low selenium blood levels are also typically found in geographical regions where the soil content of this trace element is low. In China, a selenium-responsive cardiomyopathy has been described (Tasman-Jones, 1992).

Because of the low soil selenium levels in New Zealand, patients complaining of chronic fatigue in that country have been treated with selenium supplementation with alleged efficacy. Robinson et al. (1981) explored the efficacy of this therapy in a double-blind trial comparing either sodium selenite or selenomethionine with placebo in patients complaining of fatigue, headache, paresthesia, palpitation, muscle aches, and tender points. Although blood selenium and glutathione peroxidase levels rose only in the active treatment groups, symptomatic improvement was equivalent among the groups. Approximately 50% of patients in all groups improved. Thus, the authors were unable to show any relationship between relative selenium deficiency and the patients' fibromuscular rheumatism.

LEFAC and Kutapressin

Injectable bovine liver extract–folic acid–cyanocobalamin (LEFAC) has been widely used for the treatment of CFS in some communities. Similarly, Kutapressin, a porcine liver extract developed as a by-product of vitamin B-12 production, has also been widely prescribed. Human liver extract (Chisari, 1978), Kutapressin (Tewksbury & Stahmann, 1965), and methyl-B12 (Sakane et al., 1982) are all reputed to have immunomodulatory effects *in vitro,* but the specific effects of these preparations *in vivo* have never been studied in humans or animals.

Kaslow et al. (1989) used LEFAC in a double-blind, placebo-controlled trial of patients meeting CDC criteria for CFS. Preparations of LEFAC or placebo were self-administered intramuscularly daily for 1 week, and were followed with the alternate preparation for a second week. At the end of this blinded period, the patients were offered a 2-week open-label course of LEFAC. A functional status questionnaire was administered at 0, 1, 2, and 4 weeks. Significant but equivalent improvements were seen after both placebo and LEFAC, when compared to the entry evaluations; however, there was no difference when postplacebo and post-LEFAC questionnaires were compared. The authors concluded that 1 week of LEFAC was not superior to placebo for treatment of CFS. A comparable trial with Kutapressin has not been reported.

Coenzyme Q_{10} (CoQ_{10})

This enzyme is normally synthesized in a variety of tissues where it complexes with mitochondrial cytochromes and serves as an electron carrier in cellular respiration. Relative deficiencies of the enzyme, often along with other enzymes or cofactors, have been found in some of the rare mitochondrial encephalomyopathic disorders. Most of these disorders feature elevated blood or cerebrospinal fluid lactate and pyruvate levels as a consequence of impaired cellular oxidative respiration. For example, the Kearn–Sayre syndrome (KSS) is a diagnostic triad consisting of ophthalmoplegia, retinal degeneration, and cardiac conduction abnormalities. Patients with this condition have muscle weakness, abnormal muscle biopsy findings, and levels of CoQ_{10} in their muscles that are typically 20% to 30% of normal. Treatment of five adult KSS patients with 150 mg per day of CoQ_{10} resulted in objective improvement in all cases (Ogasahara et al., 1986). There are also reports of patients with a similar condition (i.e., mitochondrial myopathy, encephalopathy, lactic acidosis, and strokelike episodes [MELAS]), who showed marked improvement on CoQ_{10} at doses of 150–300 mg per day (Abe et al., 1991; Goda, et al., 1987). In one study, a reduction of cerebrospinal fluid (CSF) lactate was demonstrated along with resolution of a high-intensity MRI signal in the occipital lobe of the brain and resolution of an intractable seizure disorder. In a more recent study, a severe hereditary and tissue-specific deficiency in the synthesis of CoQ_{10} was documented in two adolescent sisters (Ogasahara et al., 1989). Both children had experienced progressive muscle weakness, abnormal fatigability, and impaired central nervous system function since early childhood. In a direct assay of mitochondrial CoQ_{10}, these children were found to have only 3.7% of the normal level observed in 10 controls. Both adolescents improved clinically on the drug. In all of these experiences, the response to the coenzyme can be objectified by monitoring blood lactate or pyruvate levels.

CoQ_{10} appears to be beneficial for patients who have certain mitochondrial encephalomyopathies. Although these conditions are quite rare and severe, comparisons with CFS are inevitable, given the shared, prominent symptoms. MELAS is associated with fatigue, muscle weakness, and headaches that are often exacerbated by exercise, as well as by central nervous system dysfunction (in addition to other, more severe symptoms). Popular publications, advertisements in support group literature, and uncontrolled treatment experiences argue that there is a role for CoQ_{10} in the treatment of CFS, and testimonials of miraculous responses to this drug are occasionally reported. However, the evidence that CFS represents a limited mitochondrial myopathy is weak (see Chapter 9, this volume). In addition, there are no formal trials using CoQ_{10} for CFS that would allow one to determine whether the drug has any beneficial effect at all. Finally, because myopathic disorders are not easily recognized or diagnosed, one must consider the possibility that a miraculous response to CoQ_{10} might have occurred because a patient with metabolic myopathy was incorrectly diagnosed as having CFS.

Immunotherapy

Intravenous Immunoglobulin

In addition to other evidence of immune dysregulation in CFS patients, immunoglobulin class and subclass deficiencies have frequently been reported (see Chapters 4 and 7, this volume). Treatment of CFS with intravenous immunoglobulin (IV-Ig) has been suggested with the thought that some of the symptoms of the syndrome might be attributable to a deficit of some antigen-specific antibody, or that IV-Ig might have some other beneficial immunomodulatory effect. Two studies have assessed the role of this treatment modality.

Peterson and his colleagues (1990), in Minneapolis, randomized 30 patients meeting CDC criteria for CFS to receive either IV-Ig (1 g/kg) or IV-placebo monthly for 6 months in a double-blind manner. They observed improvements in some symptoms in about 20% of patients in both groups. There were no observable differences in symptoms, functional status, or sense of well-being between the two groups. Interestingly, levels of IgG1, which were subnormal in 7 of the 14 patients in the active treatment group, increased to normal after the third dose of IV-Ig. In contrast, levels of IgG3, which were low in 9 of these patients, also increased overall, but 6 patients still had subnormal levels at 6 months. There was no measurable change in these subclasses in patients who received placebo. Peterson et al. found no therapeutic benefit of IV-Ig in spite of the significant changes in immunoglobulin subclass levels. The study was small and may not have detected a slight improvement with treatment; however, there was no striking trend in the data to suggest this possibility.

In the same journal issue, Lloyd and his colleagues (1990) from Sydney reported the results of their double-blind, placebo-controlled trial. Their subjects were 49 adults (25 males and 24 females) with a diagnosis of CFS based on the so-called Australian criteria, which differ somewhat from the CDC criteria used in the Minnesota study (see Chapter 1, this volume). Also, in contrast to the Minnesota trial, the patients were given 2 g/kg IV-Ig or IV-placebo at monthly intervals for 3 months. Based on a physician's blinded assessment, 43% of patients in the active treatment group, but only 12% in the placebo group were improved ($p = .03$) at the completion of the trial. A psychiatrist's assessment failed to show significant differences between the two groups. There were also no overall differences observed in the group scores on the Quality of Life, Hamilton Depression, and Zung scales. There were differences in the mean scores on these scales when the 10 patients from the IV-Ig treatment group identified as "responders" were compared with "nonresponders." The authors suggested that the favorable clinical responses in "responders" represented a dichotomous ("all-or-none") phenomenon. Therefore, the improvement was not reflected in the mean scores for the whole group, including the "nonresponders." Lloyd et al. also observed that a therapeutic response among those receiving IV-Ig was predicted by certain immunological parameters (e.g., CD4 lymphocyte count) at entry into the study, and that "a substantial return of symptoms and disability" occurred in most of the responders after cessation of IV-Ig therapy.

In summary, the Australian study demonstrated a significant difference between IV-Ig treatment and placebo only in a physician's judgment of improvement. Psychiatric evaluation and other standardized assessment instruments failed to show differences between the groups. However, in a 3-year follow-up study that reexamined the status of patients who had received IV-Ig during the trial, there was no sustained difference in global outcome, Karnovsky score, or delayed-type hypersensitivity between the responders and nonresponders (Wilson et al., 1994). Six of eight nonresponders and five of twelve responders had improved, but nearly all were still symptomatic. The analysis of these patients, and of others who had participated in CFS treatment trials, showed that the age of onset, duration of illness, "neuroticism," premorbid psychiatric diagnoses, and cell-mediated immune function were not predictors of outcome at 3 years. In contrast, the assignment of a psychiatric diagnosis during the follow-up period or the patient's belief that the symptoms were exclusively attributable to a physical cause were factors that predicted a poor outcome. Lloyd et al. concluded that illness attitudes and coping skills were more critical elements of recovery than were immunological factors.

In spite of the possible efficacy demonstrated in the Australian study, Straus suggested, in an accompanying editorial (Straus, 1990), three reasons why the use of IV-Ig should not be recommended for CFS: (1) the expense is prohibitive; (2) there is no evidence that any benefit would extend for more than 3 months after the cessation of therapy; and (3) there were considerable adverse reactions in both studies. A fourth reason would be that the only two studies to evaluate IV-Ig therapy arrived at conflicting conclusions about its possible efficacy.

Dialyzable Leukocyte Extract (DLE)

DLE has been shown to transfer delayed-type hypersensitivity in patients with disorders of cell-mediated immunity. Because this preparation is less expensive than IV-Ig, Lloyd and coworkers (1993) compared the efficacy of DLE treatment versus placebo with or without intensive cognitive-behavioral therapy for patients with CFS. Again, these investigators used their own diagnostic criteria to recruit and to randomize 90 patients (68 females, 22 males). DLE was prepared from sonicates of 5×10^8 leukocytes from healthy, single donors and administered intramuscularly as a course of

8 biweekly injections. The patients were reevaluated at the end of treatment and 3 months later, to assess their physical state (Visual analog and Karnovsky performance scales), psychologic states (Profile of Mood States subscales), and immunological status (T-cell subsets, DTH skin testing). The only significant difference found was a small improvement in the Visual analog scale in patients who received both DLE and cognitive-behavioral therapy. There was a strong correlation between symptomatic improvement and the patients' belief that they have received DLE ($p < .001$), but no significant correlation with actual therapy, suggesting a potent placebo effect. In summary, this study demonstrates no benefit of leukocyte extract therapy in CFS patients.

Ampligen

Ampligen is mismatched, double-stranded RNA in the form poly(I):poly (C12,U) that induces interferon and possesses some intrinsic antitumor activity (Carter et al., 1985). In tissue culture, Ampligen acts synergistically with zidovudine to inhibit human immunodeficiency virus (Mitchell et al., 1987). Subsequently, the drug was administered in phase I trials to HIV-positive patients, and some potentially beneficial effects were noted (Armstrong et al., 1992; Carter et al., 1987).

Because of the demonstrated immunomodulatory effects of this drug, a double-blind, placebo-controlled study of Ampligen therapy in 92 severely ill patients with CFS was reported in 1991. The results have been reported publicly, but the details of the study have not been published (Cotton, 1991). In this study, twice-weekly injections of 400 mg of Ampligen produced an 8-point increase in Karnovsky score, but there was no improvement among controls receiving placebo injections. In addition, treadmill testing showed physiological deterioration in control patients but not in those receiving Ampligen. The authors of the study interpreted these findings as proof of a beneficial effect of Ampligen on CFS. Nevertheless, in spite of this optimistic conclusion, an Investigational New Drug application to the Food and Drug Administration was put on hold, pending more data on the incidence of hepatic toxicity, abdominal pain, and arrhythmia that may be associated with the drug's use. Less severe but more common adverse effects of fever and rash were also observed in the trial.

The potential use of Ampligen in CFS patients is not an issue at present because the drug is not available, even for investigational use. However, several aspects of the controlled trial deserve comment. First, the measurable improvement was small relative to the unknown risk associated with the drug. Second, the occurrence of adverse effects associated with Ampligen administration may have unwittingly unblinded the study. Third, the failure to show any improvement in the placebo group (which is so typical of CFS treatment trials) and the demonstration of actual deterioration in this group again suggest the possibility that the study was not truly blinded. Given these experimental concerns and the FDA's concern about the toxicity of Ampligen, the drug should not be accepted as a therapeutic alternative for CFS patients until the safety concerns are clarified, the initial study is peer-reviewed and published, and the favorable results are reproduced independently.

The same authors have recently reported a small, uncontrolled experience with prolonged intravenous Ampligen therapy (12 to 48 weeks) in 15 patients (Strayer et al., 1995). They report gradual improvement in Karnovsky score, from a mean of 47 at entry, to 85 at 60 weeks. In addition, several other objective criteria (e.g., exercise testing, blood HHV-6 assay, neuropsychological testing, and SCL-90-R scores) showed improvement over time. Compared to historical placebo-treated CFS patients, these patients had remarkable and sustained response, although there have been no previous groups treated with placebo of a quality and duration comparable to Ampligen. In addition, it is not clear how patients were selected for this extended treatment trial, and the study suffers from an unexplained loss of patient data points during the latter phases of follow-up.

Lentinus Edodes (Shiitake Mushrooms)

Shiitake mushrooms have been prized in traditional Chinese medicine for their potential medical benefits. Recent studies in Japanese journals suggest putative immunomodulating, antitumor, and antiviral activities, as well as a potential effect on urinary sodium excretion that may result in lower blood pressure (Kabir et al., 1987; Takehara et al., 1979). They are often recommended in lay publications for use in CFS, although there are no published scientific studies to support their value in treatment of this diagnosis. In addition, there is a small body of literature documenting hypersensitivity alveolitis and dermatitis among mushroom pickers who are continuously exposed to these fungi (Matsui et al., 1992). Although these mushrooms may well provide a source of useful pharmaceuticals, more study of the active agents is needed before they can be recommended as rational therapy for CFS.

Vasoactive Agents

Mineralocorticoids and Beta-Blockers

In a small preliminary study, cardiologists from the Johns Hopkins University reported on the response of seven persistently fatigued adolescents to a 3-stage tilt-table protocol that included stimulation with intravenous isoproterenol during the later stages. All seven patients developed significant hypotension or syncope, and all reported the reproduction of symptoms of light-headedness or fatigue during the test (Rowe et al., 1995). Speculating that neurally-mediated hypotension might be a feature of the chronic fatigue syndrome, these investigators repeated similar studies in a group of adolescent and adult patients (median age: 34 years) who met the 1988 diagnostic criteria (Bou-Holaigah et al., 1995). Syncope or presyncope plus a 25mmHg decline in blood pressure, with no associated increase in heart rate, was observed in 22 of 23 chronic fatigue patients but in only 4 of 14 healthy controls. Reasoning that this response was similar to that observed among previously described patients with neurally-mediated hypotension (also known as "vasodepressor syncope"), the investigators treated fatigued patients for this syncopal disorder. Their open-labeled treatment consisted of a mineralocorticoid (fludrocortisone) plus dietary salt, atenolol, disopyramide, or some combination of these agents. Nine of the 22 tilt-positive patients responded to this therapy.

A preliminary report by a separate group of investigators corroborates the presence of autonomic dysfunction in 16 patients with fibromyalgia who also met the 1994 criteria for chronic fatigue syndrome (Clauw et al., 1995). After documenting comparable blood pressures in the supine position, tilting to 60° resulted in significantly lower pulse pressures in these patients than in age- and gender-matched, healthy controls (36.8 ± 8.2 vs. 50.0 ± 9.1; $p = .01$ at 15 minutes). Other controlled studies by these authors, using ambulatory Holter monitoring and measurement of serum neuropeptides, support their interpretation that a mild reduction of sympathetic activity accounts for these vasomotor phenomena. This interpretation is also supported by an independent study that documented reduced serum levels of the norepinephrine metabolite, 3-methoxy, 4-hydroxyphenylglycol, in chronic fatigue patients (Demitrack et al., 1992), and it is also consistent with the expected reduction in sympathetic tone associated with the hypocortisolism that has been repeatedly observed in patients with both chronic fatigue syndrome and fibromyalgia (Crofford et al., 1994; Demitrack et al., 1991; Griep et al., 1993).

Together, these findings fit with the conceptualization of the chronic fatigue syndrome as a heterogeneous disorder that may include autonomic dysfunction as a factor in some cases. However, our physiologic understanding of these phenomena is currently incomplete. We do not know whether the response of chronic fatigue patients to the tilt protocol involves the same dysfunctional reflex that occurs in vasodepressor syncope or whether it represents a more generalized dysautonomia. In addition, the respective contributions of mild hypocortisolism, prolonged physical inactivity, and anxiety provoked by the tilting or the infusion of a beta-adrenergic agent are unknown. The treatment offered by the Johns Hopkins group is rational only if one assumes one particular physiologic explanation for the positive tilt-table tests. In addition, the efficacy of their treatment (41% response) is not remarkably greater than the placebo effect reported in other, controlled treatment studies. Until the physiology is better understood and the claim of treatment efficacy is confirmed by a placebo-controlled, double-blinded study, this approach to diagnosis and treatment for chronic fatigue syndrome should be regarded with caution.

Nifedipine

Numerous other medications have been tried in CFS patients, and anecdotal reports of efficacy have been published. One example of these is the instructive and remarkable report by Adolphe (1988), which suggested a role for nifedipine in an individual patient's recovery (Adolphe, 1988). The patient was a 20-year-old male with symptoms lasting for 4 years. His case met both major criteria, 10 of 11 minor criteria, and all 3 physical criteria for CFS (Holmes et al., 1988). In January 1988, the patient was treated for a presumed urinary tract infection with Bactrim. Simultaneously, he was started on nifedipine (10 mg three times a day) for his headache, which was judged to be migraine-like, and because he complained of numbness of his hands and purplish discoloration of his right arm (which were interpreted as circulatory phenomena). A marked improvement in all of his symptoms, including the chronic fatigue, occurred within 5 days of treatment. After an unintentional 3-day lapse in his nifedipine treatment, his symptoms recurred. The symptoms once again disappeared within 72 hours of reinstituting nifedipine therapy. Subsequent attempts to discontinue nifedipine also resulted in a relapse of symptoms within 72 hours. The reason for the efficacy of this drug in this particular case is unknown; however, it seems to have been remarkably efficacious for this patient either because of its calcium channel blocking activity or because it was an unusually effective placebo. This author has treated many CFS patients who were taking or had taken calcium channel blockers for headache relief or hypertension, but who did not experience such a dramatic treatment effect. What this case illustrates is the notion that CFS signs and symptoms may have diverse physiological origins in different individuals. It also demonstrates that individual assessment and treatment of this disorder are essential until its pathophysiology is better understood.

CONCLUSIONS

Taken together, the body of information reviewed in this chapter can be summarized in a few simple statements:

- Some drugs have been useful for relief of symptoms in individual patients.

- The lack of a clear understanding of the pathophysiology of CFS means that etiologically based drug therapy is not currently possible.
- No drug trial to date has provided convincing and reproducible proof of substantial efficacy in CFS patients or evidence for a particular pathophysiological model of the disorder.
- Some of the still unproven drug therapies can be harmful or prohibitively expensive and should be avoided until more data support their use.

REFERENCES

Abe, K, Fujimura, H, Nishikawa, Y, Yorifuji, S, Mezaki, T, Hirono, N, Nishitani, N, Kameyama, M. Marked reduction in CSF lactate and pyruvate levels after CoQ therapy in a patient with mitochondrial myopathy, encephalopathy, lactic acidosis and stroke-like episodes (MELAS). *Acta Neurol Scand* 1991; 83:356–359.

Adolphe, AB. Chronic fatigue syndrome: Possible effective treatment with nifedipine. *Am J Med* 1988; 85:892.

Armstrong, JA, McMahon, D, Huang, XL, Pazin, GJ, Gupta, P, Rinaldo, CR, Jr, Schoenfeld, DA, Gaccione, P, Tripoli, CA, Bensasi, S. A phase I study of ampligen in human immunodeficiency virus-infected subjects. *J Infect Dis* 1992; 166:717–722.

Behan, PO, Behan, WMH, Horrobin, D. Effect of high doses of essential fatty acids on the postviral fatigue syndrome. *Acta Neurol Scand* 1990; 82:209–216.

Bennett, RM, Gatter, RA, Campbell, SM, Andrews, RP, Clark, SR, Scarola, JA. A comparison of cylcobenzaprine and placebo in the management of fibrositis. *Arthritis Rheum* 1988; 31(12):1535–1542.

Bou-Holaigah, I, Rowe, PC, Kan, J, Calkins, H. The relationship between neurally mediated hypotension and the chronic fatigue syndrome. *JAMA* 1995; 274:961–967.

Canadian MS Research Group. A randomized controlled trial of amantadine in fatigue associated with multiple sclerosis. *Can J Neurol Sci* 1987; 14:273–278.

Carter, WA, Hubbell, HR, Krueger, LJ, Strayer, DR. Comparative studies of ampligen (Mismatched Double-Stranded RNA) and interferons. *J Biol Response Mod* 1985; 4(6):613–620.

Carter, WA, Strayer, DR, Brodsky, I, Lewin, M, Pellegrino, MG, Einck, L, Henriques, HF, Simon, GL, Parenti, DM, Scheib, RG. Clinical, immunological, and virological effects of ampligen, a mismatched double-stranded RNA, in patients with AIDS or AIDS-related complex. *Lancet* 1987; 1:1286–1292.

Chiba, S, Ito, M, Matsumoto, H. Amantadine treatment for refractory pain and fatigue in patients with multiple sclerosis [letter]. *Can J Neurol Sci* 1992; 19:309.

Chisari, FV. Regulation of human lymphocyte function by a soluble extract from normal human liver. *J Immunol* 1978; 121:1279–1286.

Clark, S, Tindall, E, Bennett, RM. A double blind crossover trial of prednisone versus placebo in the treatment of fibrositis. *J Rheumatol* 1985; 12(5):980–983.

Clauw, DJ, Radulovic, D, Katz, P, Baraniuk, J, Barbey, JT. Tilt table testing as a measure of dysautonomia in fibromyalgia. *J Musculoskeletal Pain* 1995; 3(Suppl 1):10.

Cohen, RA, Fisher, M. Amantadine treatment of fatigue associated with multiple sclerosis. *Arch Neurol* 1989; 46:676–680.

Cotton, P. Treatment proposed for chronic fatigue syndrome; research continues to compile data on disorder [news]. *JAMA* 1991; 266:2667–2668.

Cox, IM, Campbell, MJ, Dowson, D. Red blood cell magnesium and chronic fatigue syndrome. *Lancet* 1991; 337:757–760.

Crofford, LJ, Pillemer, SR, Kalogeras, KT, Cash, JM, Michelson, D, Kling, MA, Sternberg, EM, Gold, PW, Chrousos, GP, Wilder RL. Hypothalamic–pituitary–adrenal axis perturbations in patients with fibromyalgia. *Arthritis Rheum* 1994; 37(11):1583–92.

Demitrack, MA, Dale, JK, Straus, SE, Laue, L, Listwak, SJ, Kruesi, MJP, Chrousos, GP, Gold PW. Evidence for impaired activation of the hypothalamic–pituitary–adrenal axis in patients with chronic fatigue syndrome. *J Clin Endo Metab* 1991; 73(6):1224–1234.

Demitrack, MA, Gold, PW, Dale, JK, Krahn, DD, Kling, MA, Straus, SE. Plasma and cerebrospinal fluid monoamine metabolism in patients with chronic fatigue syndrome: Preliminary findings. *Biol Psychiatry* 1992; 32:1065–1077.

Deulofeu, R, Gascon, J, Gimenez, N, Corachan, M. Magnesium and chronic fatigue syndrome [letter]. *Lancet* 1991; 338:641–640.

Dismukes, WE, Wade, JS, Lee, JY, Dockery, BK, Hain, JD. A randomized, double-blind trial of nystatin therapy for the candidiasis hypersensitivity syndrome. *N Engl J Med* 1990; 323:1717–1723.

Dunn, MG. Post-polio fatigue treated with amantadine [letter]. *Arch Neurol* 1991; 48:570.

Fukuda, K, Straus, SE, Hickie, I, Sharpe, MC, Dobbins, JG, Komaroff, A, and the International Chronic Fatigue Syndrome Study Group. The chronic fatigue syndrome: A comprehensive approach to its definition and study. *Ann Intern Med* 1994; 121(12):953–959.

Gantz, NM. Magnesium and chronic fatigue syndrome [letter]. *Lancet* 1991; 338:66–60.

Goda, S, Hamada, T, Ishimoto, S, Kobayashi, T, Goto, I, Kuroiwa, Y. Clinical improvement after administration of coenzyme Q10 in a patient with mitochondrial encephalomyopathy. *J Neurol* 1987; 234:62–63.

Goldenberg, DL. Treatment of fibromyalgia syndrome. *Rheum Dis Clin North Am* 1989; 15:61–71.

Goldenberg, DL, Felson, DT, Dinerman, H. A randomized, controlled trial of amitriptyline and naproxen in the treatment of patients with fibromyalgia. *Arthritis Rheum* 1986; 29(11):1371–1377.

Griep, EN, Boersma, JW, deKloet, ER. Altered reactivity of the hypothalamic–pituitary–adrenal axis in the primary fibromyalgia syndrome. *J Rheumatol* 1993; 20(3):469–474.

Hamaty, D, Valentine, JL, Howard, R, Howard, CW, Wakefield, V, Patten, MS. The plasma endorphin, prostaglandin and catecholamine profile of patients with fibrositis treated with cyclobenzaprine and placebo: A 5-month study. *J Rheumatol* 1989; 16(suppl 19):S164–S168.

Holmes, GP, Kaplan, JE, Gantz, NM, Komaroff, AL, Schonberger, LB, Straus, SE, Jones, JF, Dubois, RE, Cunningham-Rundlls, C, Pahwa, S, Tosato, G, Zegans, LS, Purtilo, DT, Brown, N, Schooley, RT, Brus, I. Chronic fatigue syndrome: A working case definition. *Ann Int Med* 1988; 108:387–389.

Horrobin, DF. Post-viral fatigue syndrome, viral infections in atopic eczema, and essential fatty acids. *Med Hypotheses* 1990; 32:211–217.

Horrobin, DF, Manku, MS. Clinical biochemistry of essential fatty acids. In Horrobin, DF, ed., *Omega-6 essential fatty acids; pathophysiology and roles in clinical medicine,* 21–53. New York: Allen R. Liss, Inc., 1990.

Jacobsen S, Danneskiold-Samsoe, B, Andersen, RB. Oral S-adenosylmethionine in primary fibromyalgia. Double-blind clinical evaluation. *Scand J Rheumatol* 1991; 20:294–302.

Kabir, Y, Yamaguchi, M, Kimuri, S. Effect of shiitake (lentinus edodes) and maitake (grifola frondosa) mushrooms on blood pressure and plasma lipids of spontaneously hypertensive rats. *J Nutr Sci Vitaminol* 1987; 33:341–346.

Kaslow, JE, Rucker, L, Onishi, R. Liver extract–folic acid–cyanocobalamin vs placebo for chronic fatigue syndrome. *Arch Intern Med* 1989; 149: 2501–2503.

Katon, W, Russo, J. Chronic fatigue syndrome criteria. A critique of the requirement for multiple physical complaints. *Arch Int Med* 1992; 152:1604–1616.

Lloyd, AR, Hickie, I, Brockman, A, Hickie, C, Wilson, A, Dwyer, J, Wakefield, D. Immunologic and psychologic therapy for patients with chronic fatigue syndrome: A double-blind, placebo-controlled trial. *Am J Med* 1993; 94(2): 197–203.

Lloyd, A, Hickie, I, Wakefield, D, Boughton, C, Dwyer, J. A double-blind, placebo-controlled trial of intravenous immunoglobulin therapy in patients with chronic fatigue syndrome. *Am J Med* 1990; 89:561–568.

Matsui, S, Nakazawa, T, Umegae, Y, Mori, M. Hypersensitivity pneumonitis induced by shiitake mushroom spores. *Intern Med* 1992; 31:1204–1206.

McCluskey, DR. *Pharmacological approaches to the therapy of chronic fatigue syndrome,* Ciba Foundation Symposium. 1993; 173:280–297.

Mitchell, WM, Montefiori, DC, Robinson, WE, Jr, Strayer, DR, Carter, WA. Mismatched double-stranded RNA (ampligen) reduces concentration of zidovudine (azidothymidine) required for in-vitro inhibition of human immunodeficiency virus. *Lancet* 1987; 1:890–892.

Murray, TJ. Amantadine therapy for fatigue in multiple sclerosis. *Can J Neurol Sci* 1985; 12:251–254.

Ogasahara, S, Engel, AG, Frens, D, Mack, D. Muscle coenzyme Q deficiency in familial mitochondrial encephalomyopathy. *Proc Natl Acad Sci USA* 1989; 86:2379–2382.

Ogasahara, S, Nishikawa, Y, Yorifuji, S, Soga, F, Nakamura, Y, Takahashi, M, Hashimoto, S, Kono, N, Tarui, S. Treatment of the Kearns-Sayre syndrome with coenzyme Q10. *Neurology* 1986; 36:45–53.

Pagano, JS. Acyclovir treatment of the chronic fatigue syndrome [letter]. *N Engl J Med* 1989; 321:188.

Peterson, PK, Shepard, J, Macres, M, Schenk, C, Crosson, J, Rechtman, D, Lurie, N. A controlled trial of intravenous immunoglobulin G in chronic fatigue syndrome. *Am J Med* 1990; 89:554–560.

Quimby, LG, Gratwock, GM, Whitney, CD, Block, SR. A randomized trial of cyclobenzaprine for the treatment of fibromyalgia. *J Rheumatol* 1989; 16(suppl 19):140–143.

Renfro, L, Feder, HM, Lane, TJ, Manu, P, Matthews, DA. Yeast connection among 100 patients with chronic fatigue. *Am J Med* 1989; 86:165–168.

Reynolds, WJ, Moldofsky, H, Saskin, P, Lue, FA. The effects of cyclobenzaprine on sleep physiology and symptoms in patients with fibromyalgia. *J Rheumatol* 1991; 18:452–454.

Richmond, C. Magnesium and chronic fatigue syndrome [letter]. *Lancet* 1991; 337:1095.

Robinson, MF, Campbell, DR, Stewart, RD, Rea, HM, Thomson, CD, Snow, PG, Squires, IH. Effect of daily supplements of selenium on patients with muscular complaints in Otago and Canterbury. *N Zealand Med J* 1981; 93:289–292.

Rosenberg, GA, Appenzeller, O. Amantadine, fatigue, and multiple sclerosis. *Arch Neurol* 1988; 45:1104–1106.

Rowe, PC, Bou-Holaigah, I, Kan, JS, Calkins, H. Is neurally mediated hypotension an unrecognised cause of chronic fatigue? *Lancet* 1995; 345:623–634.

R ssell, IJ, Fletcher, EM, Michalek, JE, McBroom, PC, Hester, GG. Treatment of primary fibrositis/fibromyalgia syndrome with ibuprofen and alprazolam. A double-blind, placebo-controlled study. *Arthritis Rheum* 1991; 34:552–560.

Sakane, T, Takada, S, Kotani, H, Tsunematsu, T. Effects of methyl-B12 on the in vitro immune functions of human T-lymphocytes. *J Clin Immunol* 1982; 2:101–109.

Schluederberg, A, Straus, SE, Peterson, P, Blumenthal, S, Komaroff, AL, Spring, SB, Landay, A, Buchwald, D. Chronic fatigue syndrome research. Definition and medical outcome assessment. *Ann Int Med* 1992; 117(4):325–331.

Shepherd, C. Magnesium and chronic fatigue syndrome [letter]. *Lancet* 1991; 337:1095.

Straus, SE. Acute progressive Epstein–Barr virus infections. *Ann Rev Med* 1992a; 43:437–449.

Straus, SE. Acyclovir treatment of the chronic fatigue syndrome [reply to Pagano, JS]. *N Engl J Med* 1989; 321:188.

Straus, SE. Defining the chronic fatigue syndrome. *Arch Int Med* 1992b; 152:1569–1570.

Straus, SE. Intravenous immunoglobulin treatment for the chronic fatigue syndrome. *Am J Med* 1990; 89:551–553.

Straus, SE, Dale, JK, Tobi, M, Lawley, T, Preble, O, Blaese, RM, Hallahan, C, Henle, W. Acyclovir treatment of the chronic fatigue syndrome: Lack of efficacy in a placebo-controlled trial. *N Engl J Med* 1988; 319(26):1692–1698.

Strayer, DR, Carter, W, Strauss, KI, Brodsky, I, Suhadolnik, RJ, Ablashi, D, Henry, B, Mitchell, WM, Bastien, S, Peterson, D. Long term improvement in patients with chronic fatigue syndrome treated with ampligen. *J Chr Fatigue Syndr* 1995; 1:35–53.

Takehara, M, Kuida, K, Mori, K. Antiviral activity of virus-like particles from lentinus edodes (shiitake). Brief report. *Arch Virol* 1979; 59:269–274.

Tasman-Jones, C. Disturbances of trace mineral metabolism. In Wyngaarden, JB, Smith, LH, Jr, Bennett, JC, eds., *Cecil textbook of medicine,* 18th edition. Philadelphia: W. B. Saunders Co., 1992; 1183–1185.

Tavoni, A, Vitali, C, Bombardieri, S, Pasero, G. Evaluation of S-adenosylmethionine in primary fibromyalgia. A double-blind crossover study. *Am J Med* 1987; 83:107–110.

Tewksbury, DA, Stahmann, MA. Potentiation of bradykinin by a liver extract. *Arch Biochem Biophys* 1965; 112:453–458.

Truss, CO. Tissue injury induced by *Candida* alliance: Mental and neurological manifestations. *Orthomol Psychiatry* 1978; 7:17–37.

Vaeroy, H, Abrahamsen, A, Forre, O, Kass, E. Treatment of fibromyalgia (fibrositis syndrome): A parallel double blind trial with carisoprodol, paracetamol and caffeine (somadril comp) versus placebo. *Clin Rheumatol* 1989; 8:245–250.

Wiggs, JW. Amantidine, the old anti-Parkinson medication, being useful in the fatigue syndrome that often accompanies multiple sclerosis [letter]. *S D J Med* 1991; 44:279.

Williams, LL, Doody, DM, Horrocks, LA. Serum fatty acid proportions are altered during the year following acute Epstein–Barr virus infection. *Lipids* 1988; 23:981–988.

Wilson, A, Hickie, I, Lloyd, A, Hadzi-Pavlovic, D, Boughton, C, Dwyer, J, Wakefield, D. Longitudinal study of chronic fatigue syndrome. *Br Med J* 1994; 308:756–759.

Young, IS, Trimble, ER. Magnesium and chronic fatigue syndrome [letter]. *Lancet* 1991; 337:1094–1095.

Index